MW01074619

PDR®
GUIDE TO TERRORISM RESPONSE

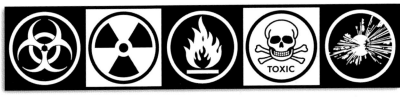

Biological   Nuclear   Incendiary   Chemical   Explosive

Contributing Editors:
John G. Bartlett, MD • Michael I. Greenberg, MD, MPH

A resource for
• Physicians • Nurses
• Emergency Medical Services
• Law Enforcement • Firefighters

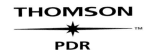

THOMSON
PDR

Director, Editorial Services: Bette LaGow
Chief Project Editor: Neil Chesanow
Project Editor: Harris Fleming
Senior Editor: Lori Murray
Senior Production Editor: Gwynned Kelly

Director, Clinical Content: Thomas Fleming, PharmD
Drug Information Specialists: Michael DeLuca, PharmD, MBA; Kajal Solanki, PharmD; Greg Tallis, RPh; Catherine H. Chyu, PharmD

Director of Operations: Robert Klein
Project Managers: John Castro, Noel Deloughery
Production Design Supervisor: Adeline Rich
Senior Electronic Publishing Designer: Livio Udina
Electronic Publishing Designers: Bryan C. Dix, Carrie Faeth, Monika Popowitz
Production Associates: Joan K. Akerlind, Shannon Reilly

Research Manager and Corporate Librarian: Kate Mason-Page
Research Analysts: Tim Gardiner, Melissa Herb
Editorial Manager, Toxicology: Joanne B. Brownhill, DVM
Senior Clinical Writer: Laurel H. Pye, MA
Consultant: Richard G. Kuiters

Contributing Editors
John G. Bartlett, MD
Chief, Division of Infectious Diseases
Johns Hopkins University School of Medicine
Baltimore, MD
Founding Co-Director
Center for Civilian Biodefense Strategies
Pittsburgh, PA

Michael I. Greenberg, MD, MPH
Professor of Emergency Medicine
Drexel University College of Medicine
Professor of Public Health
Drexel University School of Public Health
Philadelphia, PA

With contributions from: Matthew Salzman, MD; John Curtis, MD; Kimber Bogush, MD; and Sobia Ansari, MD of the Department of Emergency Medicine, Drexel University College of Medicine, Philadelphia, PA

THOMSON PDR
Senior Vice President, PDR Sales and Marketing: Dikran N. Barsamian
Vice President, PDR Services: Brian Holland
Vice President, Product Management: William T. Hicks
Senior Director, Brand and Product Management: Valerie E. Berger
Associate Product Manager: Andrea Colavecchio

Senior Director, Publishing Sales and Marketing: Michael Bennett
Director, Trade Sales: Bill Gaffney
Associate Director, Marketing: Jennifer M. Fronzaglia
Senior Marketing Manager: Kim Marich
Direct Mail Manager: Lorraine M. Loening
Manager, Marketing Analysis: Dina A. Maeder
Promotion Manager: Linda Levine

Director, Client Services: Stephanie Struble
Director of Finance: Mark S. Ritchin

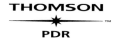

Officers of Thomson Healthcare, Inc.: *President and Chief Executive Officer:* Kevin King; *Chief Financial Officer:* Paul Hilger; *Chief Medical Officer:* Rich Klasco, MD, FACEP; *Chief Technology Officer:* Frank Licata; *Executive Vice President, Medstat:* Carol Diephuis; *Executive Vice President, Micromedex:* Jeff Reihl; *Senior Vice President, Marketing:* Timothy Murray; *Vice President, Finance:* Joseph Scarfone; *Vice President, Human Resources:* Pamela M. Bilash

ISBN: 1-56363-550-X

TABLE OF CONTENTS

PART SIX: MEDICAL MANAGEMENT IN AN INCENDIARY ATTACK

PART SEVEN: MEDICAL MANAGEMENT IN AN EXPLOSIVE ATTACK

PART EIGHT: MEDICAL MANAGEMENT IN A NUCLEAR/RADIATION ATTACK

PART NINE: DRUGS FOR TERRORISM RESPONSE

HOW TO USE THIS BOOK

The *PDR® Guide to Terrorism Response* is designed to quickly provide different professionals the information they need in just the right amount of detail to do their jobs decisively and effectively in the event of a terrorism attack. Here's how the guide is organized:

Part One: Terrorism Incident Management

Law enforcement, firefighting, emergency medical services, and hazmat personnel are responsible for managing the scene of a terrorism incident, including helping victims, identifying the terrorism agent used, ensuring that secondary devices or armed assailants are not present, managing the flow of traffic as emergency vehicles arrive on the scene, and more. This series of quick checklists for which tasks to perform when every second counts will serve as useful reminders.

Part Two: Signs & Symptoms

In a terrorism incident, it is crucial to know whether the agent used was biological or chemical, and if so, which one. This series of concise charts quickly takes you from body system to body system listing the most obvious signs and symptoms of illness or injury that you are seeing in victims and suggesting which terrorism agent or agent type may be the cause. Possible agents are cross-referenced to Part Three: Terrorism Agents in Brief or Part Four/Five, where applicable.

Part Three: Terrorism Agents in Brief

Once you have an idea of which terrorism agent produced the most obvious signs and symptoms you are seeing in victims, this series of concise charts briefs you on key details about the agent, further information on signs and symptoms, self-protection measures so you can keep helping others and avoid becoming a casualty, and administering first aid to victims. These charts cover the most likely biological and chemical terrorism agents, as well as how to treat victims of an incendiary, explosive, or nuclear/radiation incident. For more detailed information, each chart is cross-referenced to a monograph or article on medical management in subsequent sections of the book.

Part Four: Biological Terrorism Agents in Depth

For hospital emergency department and laboratory personnel, physicians and nurses in the field who are among the first responders, and clinicians in private practice to whom victims may turn for help, these clinical monographs quickly brief you on all Category A (most likely) and most Category B (less likely but still possible) biological terrorism agents identified by the federal Centers for Disease Control and Prevention (CDC). Background details, hospital preparation, personal protection, decontamination, quarantine procedures, clinical presentation, disease features, diagnosis, treatment (including drugs, dosages, and regimens), and prevention are covered for each agent.

Part Five: Chemical Terrorism Agents in Depth

For medical and laboratory personnel, these concise clinical monographs brief you on the most likely chemical agents to be used in a terrorism incident as identified by the CDC. For each agent, background details, routine use, potential terrorist use, mechanism of action, potential routes of exposure, target organs/systems, clinical features, diagnosis, laboratory testing and imaging, and treatment and disposition are discussed.

Part Six: Medical Management in an Incendiary Attack

For emergency department physicians and nurses, these four clinical articles comprehensively discuss medical management of a major burn injury—including assessment, resuscitation, intensive care management, and control of infection—as well as the assessment and management of smoke inhalation injury. Tables, figures, and clinical pathways present crucial information at a glance.

Part Seven: Medical Management in an Explosive attack

Here is a primer for clinicians on explosions and blast injuries; details on blast lung injury, which presents unique triage, diagnostic, and management challenges; and an authoritative article on the medical management of suicide bombing victims.

Part Eight: Medical Management in a Nuclear/Radiation Attack

These three documents from the CDC cover what a hospital emergency department must do to prepare for mass casualties from a radiological incident, as well as how to treat acute radiation syndrome and cutaneous radiation injury. Included are FDA recommendations for the administration of potassium iodide and the radiation detection and measurement instruments every hospital should now consider standard equipment.

Part Nine: Drugs for Terrorism Response

In concise monographs for quick reference, here you'll find antidotes to biological and chemical terrorism agents—from antibiotics to combat anthrax and plague to drug treatment for nerve agent victims—recommended by experts. Each monograph includes brand name, how the drug is supplied, therapeutic class, indication, dosage, contraindications, warnings/precautions, pregnancy considerations, interactions, and adverse reactions.

PART ONE

TERRORISM INCIDENT MANAGEMENT

CHECKLISTS FOR FIRST RESPONDERS IN THE FIELD

Sources: Department of Homeland Security, Federal Emergency Management Agency, United States Fire Administration, Department of Homeland Security Office for Domestic Preparedness, United States Department of Justice Office of Justice Programs, and Richard G. Kuiters, consultant to the Department of Homeland Security.

TERRORISM INCIDENT
MANAGEMENT

TERRORISM INCIDENT MANAGEMENT

CHECKLISTS FOR FIRST RESPONDERS IN THE FIELD

Terrorists strike when they believe the timing is advantageous and potential victims are unprepared for an attack. As such, first responders must react swiftly, knowledgeably, and decisively to save lives, protect themselves, and effectively manage the incident, whether it is a biological, chemical, incendiary, explosive, or nuclear/radiation attack.

Law enforcement, firefighting, emergency medical services, and hazmat personnel—as well as National Guard and Armed Forces Reserves units—should already have the training and experience to address the strategic and tactical issues outlined here.

These checklists were developed to assist first responders in the first hours of an attack. In the chaos of the moment, the lists will quickly remind you of what to do and when.

REMEMBER
If you are the first to arrive at the scene of a terrorism incident, *you* are the on-scene commander until relieved.

OPERATIONAL CONSIDERATIONS

ASSESS SECURITY—RESPONSE AND INITIAL APPROACH

INDICATORS

- Is the response to a target hazard or target event?
- Has there been a threat?
- Are there multiple trauma and/or nontrauma-related victims?
- Are responders victims?
- Are hazardous substances involved?
- Has there been an explosion?
- Has there been a secondary attack/explosion?

IF THERE IS ONE INDICATOR ...

- Respond with a heightened level of awareness

IF THERE ARE MULTIPLE INDICATORS ...

- You may be on the scene of a terrorist incident
- Initiate response operations with extreme caution
- Be alert for actions against responders
- Evaluate and implement personal protective measures
- Consider the need for maximum respiratory protection
- Make immediate contact with law enforcement for coordination
- Response route considerations:

WARNING
Approach cautiously, from uphill/upwind direction.

- Consider law enforcement escort
- Avoid choke points (i.e., congested areas)
- Designate rally points *(usually predetermined locations to which all people near the scene of a terrorism incident can evacuate, and at which first responders can regroup and a revised plan can be established)*
- Establish command post and identify safe staging area(s) *(where responders assemble to be deployed to the scene)* for incoming units

PRIMARY COMMAND CONSIDERATIONS

- Establish initial command post
- Isolate area/deny entry
- Ensure scene security
- Initiate on-scene size-up and hazard/risk assessment

REMEMBER

If you are the first to arrive at the scene of a terrorism incident, *you* are the on-scene commander until relieved.

- Provide, identify, and designate safe staging location(s) *(where responders assemble to be deployed to the scene)* for incoming units
- Ensure the use of personal protective measures and shielding
- Assess emergency egress routes
  - Position apparatus to facilitate rapid evacuation
  - If you must use emergency egress, reassemble at designated rally point(s)
- Ensure personnel accountability
- Designate incident safety officer
- Assess command post security
- Consider assignment of liaison and public information positions
- Assess decontamination requirements (gross, mass, etc.)
- Consider the need for additional/specialized federal, state, county, and local resources:
  - Fire
  - EMS
  - Hazmat
  - Law enforcement/explosive ordnance disposal (bomb squad)
  - Emergency management
  - Public health
  - Public works
  - Environmental
  - Others
- Consider as a potential crime scene:
  - Consider everything at the site as potential evidence
  - Ensure coordination with law enforcement

- Make appropriate notifications:
  - Dispatch center (update situation report)
  - Hospitals
  - Utilities
  - Law enforcement
  - State point of contact as appropriate
- Prepare for transition to unified command
- Ensure coordination of communications and identify needs
- Consider the need for advance/response of a regional, state, or national incident management team

ON-SCENE SIZE-UP

- Review dispatch information
- Look for physical indicators and other outward warning signs of biological, nuclear, incendiary, chemical, and explosive events—including armed assault:
  - Unusual odors, color of smoke, vapor clouds
  - Dead animals and vegetation
  - Severe structural damage without an obvious cause
  - Mass casualty/fatality with minimal or no trauma
  - Debris field
  - Responder casualties
  - System(s) disruptions (utilities, transportation, etc.)
- Victims' signs and symptoms of hazardous substance exposure:
  - Are there unconscious victims with minimal or no trauma?
  - Are there victims exhibiting **SLUDGEM** signs/seizures?

SLUDGEM

✓ **S**alivation (drooling)
✓ **L**acrimation (tearing of eyes)
✓ **U**rination
✓ **D**efecation
✓ **G**astrointestinal distress (stomach cramps)
✓ **E**mesis (vomiting)
✓ **M**iosis (very small pupils in eyes)

  - Is there blistering, reddening of skin, discoloration, or skin irritation?

Figure 1. Organizing the scene of a terrorism incident.

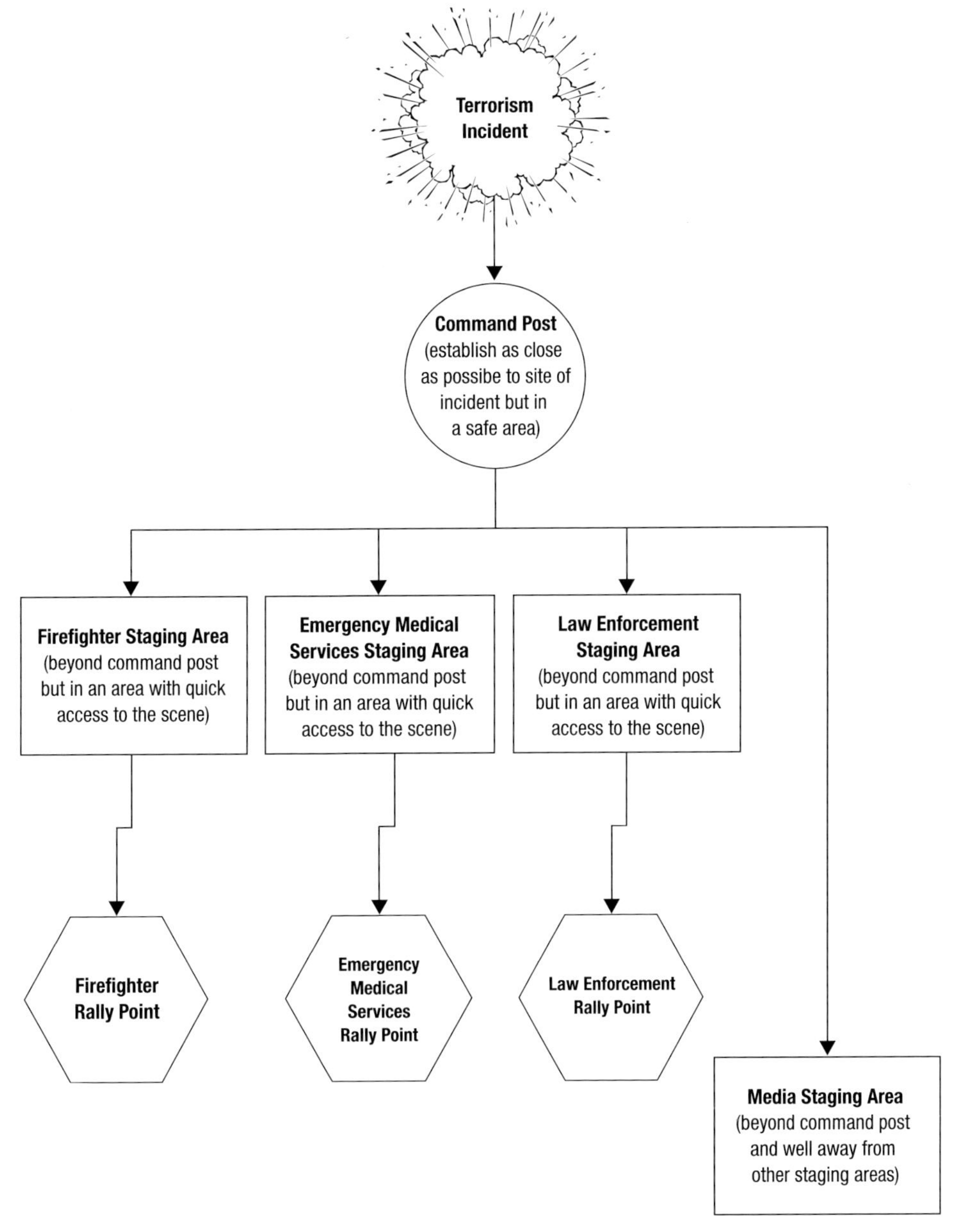

Terrorism Incident

Command Post
(establish as close as possibe to site of incident but in a safe area)

Firefighter Staging Area
(beyond command post but in an area with quick access to the scene)

Emergency Medical Services Staging Area
(beyond command post but in an area with quick access to the scene)

Law Enforcement Staging Area
(beyond command post but in an area with quick access to the scene)

Firefighter Rally Point

Emergency Medical Services Rally Point

Law Enforcement Rally Point

Media Staging Area
(beyond command post and well away from other staging areas)

- Are victims having difficulty breathing?
- Identify apparent sign/symptom commonality
- Interview victims and witnesses (if possible):
  - Is everyone accounted for?
  - What happened (information on delivery system)?
  - When did it happen?
  - Where did it happen?
  - Who was involved?
  - Did they smell, see, taste, hear, or feel anything out of the ordinary?
- Identify type of event(s):

B-NICE

✓ **B**iological
✓ **N**uclear/radiation
✓ **I**ncendiary
✓ **C**hemical
✓ **E**xplosive

  - Also be alert for an armed assault
    ✓ Are any combatants still on scene?
    ✓ Beware of secondary explosive devices
- Weather report considerations:
  - Downwind exposures
  - Monitor forecast
- Determine life safety threats to:
  - Self
  - First responders
  - Victims
  - The public
- Determine mechanism(s) of injury:

TRACEM-P

✓ **T**hermal (heat)
✓ **R**adiological (radiation)
✓ **A**sphyxiant (suffocating)
✓ **C**hemical (blister, choking, nerve)
✓ **E**tiological (disease)
✓ **M**echanical (machinery or tools)
✓ **P**sychological (mental)

- Estimate number of victims:
  - Those who are able to walk
  - Those who are not able to walk
  - Number of ambulances needed to transport victims
- Identify damaged/affected surroundings:
  - Environmental exposures
  - Downwind exposures
  - Structural exposures
  - Below-grade occupancies
  - Below-grade utilities
  - Aviation/air space hazards
- Consider potential for secondary attack:
  - Booby traps
  - Secondary explosive devices
  - Chemical dispersal devices
- Determine available and needed federal, state, county, and local resources:
  - Fire
  - Hazmat
  - Law enforcement/explosive ordnance disposal (bomb squad)
  - Emergency management
  - Public health
  - Public works
  - Environmental
  - Others
  - E-mails

INCIDENT SITE MANAGEMENT, SAFETY, AND SECURITY

- Reassess initial isolation/standoff distances:
  - Establish an outer perimeter *(an outmost area from a hazard that is secure)*
  - Establish an inner perimeter *(a secured inner area of operations)*
- Initiate public protection actions:
  - Remove endangered victims from high-hazard areas
- Establish safe refuge area *(an area within the contamination reduction zone for assembling people who witness the incident, separating those who are contaminated from those who aren't)*
  - Evacuate
  - Protect in place
- Identify appropriate personal protection equipment options prior to committing personnel
- Dedicate EMS needed for responders
- Prepare for gross decontamination *(initial decontamination to remove large amounts of*

contaminants) operations for first responders
- Coordinate with law enforcement to provide security and control of perimeters
- Ensure force protection
- Designate an emergency evacuation signal

TACTICAL CONSIDERATIONS

- Life safety:
  - Isolate/secure and deny entry
  - Public protection (evacuate/protect in place)
  - Implementation of self-protection measures
  - Commit only essential personnel/minimize exposure
  - Confine/contain all contaminated and exposed victims
  - Establish gross decontamination *(initial decontamination to remove large amounts of contaminants)* capabilities
- Rescue considerations:
  - Is the scene safe for operations?
  - Can I make it safe to operate?
  - Are victims alive?
  - Are they able to walk?
  - Can they self-evacuate?
  - Are they contaminated?
  - Do they require extrication (as in a bombing event)?
  - Is a search safe and possible?
  - Is specialized personal protection equipment required?
- Incident stabilization (consider defensive operations):
  - Hazmat control
  - Fire suppression
  - Exposure protection
  - Utility control
  - Water supply

MASS DECONTAMINATION

- Separate the victims into groups of:
  - Those exhibiting signs/symptoms of exposure
  - Those not exhibiting signs/symptoms of exposure
  - Those able to walk
  - Those not able to walk
- Properly protected medical personnel may access the victims in the holding area to initiate triage, administer antidotes, and provide basic care in accordance with local protocols
- The type of decontamination system is dependent on the number of victims, the severity of their injuries, and the resources available
- Several victims may be handled with a single hose line, while numerous patients will require the use of a mass decontamination corridor
- Large numbers of victims may require engine companies to use the "side-by-side" system as well as numerous showers to move multiple lines of victims through the process

SYMPTOMATIC VICTIMS

- Begin emergency gross decontamination *(initial decontamination to remove large amounts of contaminants)* immediately on victims who:
  - Exhibit signs/symptoms of exposure
  - Have visible liquid product on their clothing
  - Were in close proximity to the discharge

REMEMBER

In a mass casualty setting, life safety takes precedence over containing runoff.

- Set up decontamination in an area such that contaminated water will flow away from your operation and into the grass or soil, if possible
- Provide privacy only if it will not delay the decontamination process
- Remove all of the victims' clothing down to their underwear.
- Separate lines may be required to process patients who can't walk
- As resources become available, separate decontamination lines may be established for male and female victims, as well as families
- Provide emergency covering (i.e., emergency blankets and sheets for the victims)
- Transfer victims to EMS for triage/treatment

CONTAMINATED OR EXPOSED VICTIMS WHO DO NOT YET SHOW SYMPTOMS

- Process victims through the gross decontamination *(initial decontamination to remove large amounts of contaminants)* showers with their clothes on
- Direct victims to holding area(s)
- Set up tents/shelters and provide showers or an improvised wash system
- Victims should be numbered and bags should be used to store their personal effects
- Provide emergency covering/clothing
- Transfer victims to a holding area for medical evaluation

REMOTE SITE OPERATIONS (I.E., HOSPITAL EMERGENCY ROOM)

- Stand-alone decontamination systems may have to be established outside of hospital emergency rooms for victims who self-present at the location:
  - Dispatch mobile units with decontamination capabilities to establish a system
  - Triage the victims and separate them into two groups:
    ✓ Those exhibiting signs/symptoms of exposure
    ✓ Those not exhibiting signs/symptoms of exposure
  - Give priority to victims who are symptomatic or who have visible product on their clothes
  - Remove clothes and flush thoroughly
  - Liaise with the hospital staff to determine where victims will be sent after decontam-ination
- Alert designated trauma center and county hospitals to their need for decontamination prior to influx of victims

EVIDENCE PRESERVATION

REMEMBER

The scene of a terrorism incident is a crime scene.

- Recognize potential evidence:
  - Unexploded device(s)
  - Portions of device(s)
  - Clothing of victims
  - Containers
  - Dissemination device(s)
  - The victim(s)
- Note location of potential evidence
  - Do not touch or contaminate
- Report findings to appropriate authority
- Move potential evidence only for life safety/incident stabilization

---

LAW ENFORCEMENT PERSONNEL

Establish and maintain chain of custody for evidence preservation.

INCIDENT-SPECIFIC ACTIONS

CHEMICAL

GENERAL INFORMATION

- Victims' signs and symptoms of hazardous substance exposure:
  - Are there unconscious victims with minimal or no trauma?
  - Are there victims exhibiting **SLUDGEM** signs/seizures?

SLUDGEM

✓ **S**alivation (drooling)
✓ **L**acrimation (tearing of eyes)
✓ **U**rination
✓ **D**efecation
✓ **G**astrointestinal distress (stomach cramps)
✓ **E**mesis (vomiting)
✓ **M**iosis (very small pupils in eyes)

  - Is there blistering, reddening of skin, discoloration or skin irritation?
  - Are the victims having difficulty breathing?

- Look for physical indicators and other outward warning signs:
  - Medical mass casualty/fatality with minimal or no trauma
  - Dead animals and vegetation
  - Responder casualties
  - Unusual odors, color of smoke, or vapor clouds in the area
- Types of dispersal method(s):
  - Air handling system
  - Misting or aerosolizing device
  - Sprayer
  - Gas cylinder
  - Dirty bomb

For signs and symptoms, personal protection, and administering first aid for biological agents, see Part Three: Terrorism Agents in Brief.

RESPONSE RECOMMENDATIONS

- Approach from uphill and upwind

URGENT!
Victims exposed to chemical agents require *IMMEDIATE* removal of clothing, gross decontamination *(initial decontamination to remove large amounts of contaminants),* and definitive medical care.

- Law enforcement should establish an outer perimeter to completely secure the scene
- If a particular agent is known or suspected, this information should be forwarded to EMS personnel and hospitals so that sufficient quantities of antidotes can be obtained
- Upon arrival, establish command post and staging areas *(where responders assemble to be deployed to the scene)* at a safe distance from the site
- Secure and isolate the area/deny entry
- Complete a hazard and risk assessment to determine if it is acceptable to commit responders to the site

- Be aware of larger secondary chemical devices

WARNING!
Even personnel in structural personal protection equipment/self-contained breathing apparatus should *NOT* enter areas of high concentration, unventilated areas, or below-grade areas for any reason.

- Personnel in structural personal protection equipment/self-contained breathing apparatus may enter the hot zone near the perimeter *(outside of areas of high concentration)* to perform life-saving functions
- Confine all contaminated and exposed victims to a restricted/isolated area at the outer edge of the hot zone
- Victims exhibiting signs/symptoms of exposure should be segregated into one area and those not exhibiting signs/symptoms should be placed in another area
- Move victims who can walk away from the area of highest concentration or source
- Hospitals should be notified immediately that contaminated victims of the attack may arrive or self-present at the hospital
- Begin emergency gross decontamination *(initial decontamination to remove large amounts of contaminants)* procedures starting with the most severe symptomatic victims. Use soap-and-water decontaminant, liquid detergent, and bleach
- Decontamination capabilities should be provided at the hospital to assist with emergency gross decontamination prior to victims' entering the facility
- If available, hazmat personnel in chemical personal protection equipment may be used for rescue, reconnaissance, and agent identification
- Victims not exhibiting signs/symptoms of exposure should be decontaminated in a private area (i.e., a tent or shelter) and then forwarded to a holding area for medical evaluation

BIOLOGICAL

GENERAL INFORMATION

- Biological agents may produce delayed reactions
- Unlike exposure to chemical agents, exposure

to biological agents does not require immediate removal of victims' clothing or gross decontamination in the street
- Inhalation is the primary route of entry
- Self-contained breathing apparatus and structural firefighting clothing provides adequate protection for first responders

RESPONSE RECOMMENDATIONS

- Position uphill and upwind and away from building exhaust systems
- Isolate/secure the area (initial isolation distance of 80 feet is recommended)
- Do not allow unprotected individuals to enter area
- Be alert for small explosive devices designed to disseminate the agent

---

REMEMBER
The scene of a terrorism incident is a crime scene.

- Gather information:
  - Type and form of agent (liquid, powder, aerosol)
  - Method of delivery
  - Location in structure

OPERATIONAL PROCEDURES

EVALUATE SOURCE—IS IT A WET AGENT OR A DRY AGENT?

REMEMBER
A wet agent—i.e., pneumonic plague—is spread by droplets in the air, often by victims coughing.
A dry agent—i.e., inhalational anthrax—is spread by powder and inhaled.

- Isolate area
- Personnel entering area must wear full personal protection equipment, including self-contained breathing apparatus

- Avoid contact with puddles, wet surfaces, powdery substances, etc.
- Keep all potentially exposed individuals—but who do not yet show signs/symptoms—in close proximity, but out of the high-hazard area
- If indoors, shut down heating, ventilation, and air conditioning systems that service the area as soon as possible
- If victims have visible agent on them:
  - You must wear personal protection equipment to avoid self-contamination
  - Wash exposed skin with soap and water
  - If highly contaminated (i.e., splashed) and the facility is equipped with showers, victims may take a shower and change clothes as a precaution
  - Hazmat team may be able to conduct a bioassay field test (limited number of agents)
- If possible, a sample of the material may be collected for testing:
  - If test results are positive, decontaminate in shower facility with warm water/soap
  - Provide emergency covering/clothing and bag personal effects
  - Refer to medical community for treatment

IF YOU SUSPECT A DRY AGENT (I.E., ANTHRAX, RICIN) PLACED INTO A HEATING, VENTILATION, OR AIR CONDITIONING SYSTEM, OR IF YOU FIND A PACKAGE WITH NO OTHER PHYSICAL EVIDENCE ...

- Isolate the building:
  - Keep all potentially exposed victims in the building
  - Shut down all heating, ventilation, and air conditioning systems in the building
- Collect information regarding the threat, target, or any previous activity to gauge the credibility of the threat
- Initiate a search of the building
- Personnel entering area must wear full personal protection equipment, including self-contained breathing apparatus
- Avoid contact with puddles, wet surfaces, etc.
- Investigate all heating, ventilation, and air conditioning intakes, returns, etc., for evidence of agent or dispersal equipment

- If evidence of an agent is found in/near the heating, ventilation, or air conditioning system, remove occupants from the building and isolate them in a secure and comfortable location
- If a suspicious package is found, handle as a point-source event
- Contaminated victims should shower and change. No decontamination should take place unprotected and in the open. Tents or other sites should be used
- Exposed victims may shower and change at their discretion
- Refer to medical community for treatment

IF A CONFIRMED AGENT WAS PLACED INTO A HEATING, VENTILATION, OR AIR CONDITIONING SYSTEM (AS INDICATED BY A VISIBLE FOGGER, SPRAYER, OR AEROSOLIZING DEVICE) ...

- Personnel entering must wear full personal protection equipment and self-contained breathing apparatus
- Avoid contact with puddles, wet surfaces, etc.
- Remove occupants from building/area, and isolate in a secure and comfortable location.
- Shut down heating, ventilation, and air conditioning system(s)
- Hazmat team may be able to conduct a bioassay field test (limited number of agents)
- If possible, a sample of the material may be collected for testing
- If test results are positive, contaminated victims should shower and change. No decontamination should take place unprotected and in the open. Tents or other sites should be used
- Gather all decontaminated victims in a specific holding area for medical evaluation

> **For signs and symptoms, personal protection, and administering first aid for biological agents, see Part Three: Terrorism Agents in Brief.**

NUCLEAR/RADIATION
GENERAL INFORMATION

- Radiation agents may produce both immediate and delayed reactions
- In most cases, self-contained breathing apparatus and structural firefighting clothing provide adequate protection for first responders
- Unlike exposure to chemical agents, exposure to radiation agents does not require immediate removal of victims' clothing or gross decontamination in the street
- Inhalation is the primary route of entry for particulate radiation
- Consider how strong the source is. If it's strong, minimize exposure time and maintain an appropriate distance

> **REMEMBER**
>
> Self-protection is not selfish. It is necessary if you are continue to help others and not become a victim yourself.

- Exposed/contaminated victims may not exhibit obvious injuries

RESPONSE RECOMMENDATIONS

- Position upwind of any suspected event
- Isolate/secure the area (a minimum distance of 80 to 160 feet is recommended)
- Be alert for small explosive devices designed to disseminate radioactive agent(s)

> **REMEMBER**
>
> Use time, distance, and shielding as self-protection measures.

- Use full personal protection equipment, including self-contained breathing apparatus
- Avoid contact with agent. Stay out of any visible smoke or fumes

- Establish background levels outside of suspected area
- Monitor radiation levels
- Remove victims from high-hazard area to a safe holding area
- Triage, treat, and decontaminate trauma victims as appropriate
- Detain or isolate uninjured persons or equipment. Delay decontamination for such persons/equipment until instructed by radiation authorities
- Use radiation detection devices, if possible, to determine if victims are contaminated with radiation material

EXPLOSIVES

GENERAL INFORMATION

- Explosive devices may be designed to disseminate chemical, biological, or radiation agents
- Explosives may produce secondary hazards, such as unstable structures, damaged utilities, hanging debris, void spaces, and other physical hazards
- Devices may contain antipersonnel features such as nails, shrapnel, fragmentation design, or other materials.

WARNING!

Always be alert for the possibility of secondary devices.

- Outward warning signs:
  - Oral or written threats
  - Container/vehicle that appears out of place
  - Devices attached to compressed gas cylinders, flammable liquid containers, bulk storage containers, pipelines, and other chemical containers (dirty bomb)
  - Oversized packages with oily stains, chemical odors, excessive postage, protruding wires, excessive binding, no return address, etc.

RESPONSE RECOMMENDATIONS

UNEXPLODED DEVICE/PRE-BLAST OPERATIONS

- Command post should be located away from areas where improvised secondary devices may have been placed (e.g., mailboxes, trash cans, etc.)
- Stage incoming units:
  - Away from line of sight of target area
  - Away from buildings with large amounts of glass
  - In such a way as to utilize distant structural and/or natural barriers to assist with protection
- Isolate/deny entry
- Secure perimeter based on the size of the device

REMEMBER

Non-law enforcement first responders should coordinate activities with law enforcement and be prepared for operations if the device activates.

- Attempt to identify device characteristics:
  - Type of threat
  - Location
  - Time
  - Package
  - Device
  - Previous threats (letters, envelopes, e-mails, etc.)
  - Associated history
- Standoff distance should be commensurate with the size of the device:
  - Car bomb=1,500 feet (increase distance for larger vehicles)
  - Package bomb (one to 25 pounds)=1,000 feet
  - Pipe bomb=500 feet
- Use extreme caution if caller identifies a time for detonation. It is very possible that the device will activate prior to the announced time
- Discontinue use of all radios, mobile data terminals, and cell phones in accordance with local protocols
- Evaluate scene conditions:
  - Potential number of affected people
  - Exposure problems

- Potential hazards: utilities, structures, fires, chemicals, etc.
- Water supply
- Evaluate available resources (EMS, hazmat, technical rescue, etc.)
- Review preplans for affected buildings
- Make appropriate notifications
- Develop action plan that identifies incident priorities, key strategies, tactical objectives, potential tactical assignments, and key positions in the incident command system unified command *(a unified team effort allowing all agencies responsible for the incident to establish a common set of objectives and strategies without losing or abdicating agency authority, responsibility, or accountability)*

EXPLODED DEVICE/POST-BLAST OPERATIONS

REMEMBER
A memorandum of understanding has been agreed upon designating who is in charge.

- Command post should be located away from areas where improvised secondary devices may be placed (e.g., mailboxes, trash cans, etc.)
- Initial arriving unit(s):
  - Stage a safe distance from reported incident (or where you first encounter debris)
    - ✓ Away from line of sight of target area
    - ✓ Away from buildings with large amounts of glass
  - Utilize distant structural and/or natural barriers to assist with protection

---

WARNING!
Be aware of the possibility of secondary devices and their possible location.

- Stage incoming units at a greater distance. Consider using multiple staging areas *(where responders assemble to be deployed to the scene)*
- Debris field may contain unexploded bomb material

WARNING!
Radios, mobile data terminals, and cell phones can trigger an explosive device. Discontinue their use in accordance with local protocols.

- Remove all citizens and ambulatory victims from the affected area.
- Determine on-scene conditions and evaluate resource requirements:
  - What type of explosion is it?
  - Is a fire still burning?
  - Is a building unstable and in danger of collapsing?
  - Are people trapped or unable to walk who require search/rescue?
  - Is it a chemical or radiation exposure?
  - Are utilities such as gas and electricity still on?
  - How many victims are there and what is the extent of their injuries?
  - Are there other hazards?
- Complete hazard and risk assessment

REMEMBER
If it is determined that entry/intervention (for the purpose of life safety) must occur, the following procedures should be implemented:

- Personnel should only be allowed to enter the blast area for life safety purposes
- Remove viable victims to safe refuge area
- Direct ambulatory victims to care

- Make notifications (law enforcement, hospitals, emergency management) as appropriate:
  - Local
  - State
  - Federal

- Limit number of personnel and minimize exposure time. Personnel entering the blast area should:
  - Wear full protective clothing, including self-contained breathing apparatus
  - Monitor atmosphere:
    - ✓ Radiation
    - ✓ Flammability
    - ✓ Toxicity
    - ✓ Chemical
    - ✓ pH
- Establish emergency gross decontamination *(initial decontamination to remove large amounts of contaminants)*

WARNING!

Area should be evacuated of all emergency responders if there is any indication of a secondary device.

- Remove victims from the initial blast site to a safe refuge area *(an area within the contamination reduction zone for assembling individuals who are witnesses to the incident, permitting the separation of contaminated and uncontaminated people)*
- Establish triage/treatment area at the casualty collection point *(a predefined location in which patients are assembled, triaged, and provided with initial medical care)*
- Once triage/treatment area is established:
  - Notify hospitals
  - Implement mass casualty plan
- Do not allow rescuers to enter unsafe buildings or high-hazard areas
- Control utilities and protect exposures from a defensive position
- Preserve and maintain evidence

AGENCY-RELATED ACTIONS

LAW ENFORCEMENT

IF FIRST ON SCENE:

- Isolate/secure the scene, establish control zones

- Establish command
- Stage incoming units

IF COMMAND HAS BEEN ESTABLISHED:

- Report to command post
- Evaluate scene safety/security:
  - Ongoing criminal activity
  - Consider victims to be possible terrorists
  - Secondary devices
  - Additional threats
- Gather witness statements/observations and document
- Initiate law enforcement notifications:
  - FBI (Federal Bureau of Investigation)
  - ATF (Bureau of Alcohol, Tobacco and Firearms)
  - EOD (Explosive Ordnance Disposal)/bomb squad
  - State police agency
  - Private security forces
- Request additional resources
- Secure outer perimeter
- Traffic control considerations:
  - Staging areas *(where responders assemble to be deployed to the scene)*
  - Entry/egress
- Use appropriate self-protective measures:
  - Time, distance, and shielding
  - Minimize number of personnel exposed to danger
  - Proper personal protection equipment—if provided
- Initiate public safety measures:
  - Evacuate
  - Protect in place
- Assist with control/isolation of victims
- Coordinate activities with other response agencies
- Evidence preservation:
  - Diagram the area
  - Photograph the area
  - Prepare a narrative description
  - Maintain an evidence log
- Participate in a unified command system with:
  - Fire/rescue services
  - EMS
  - Hospitals/public health
  - Emergency management
  - Public works

FIRE DEPARTMENT

- In a terrorist incident where fire is present any fire may present intense conditions:
  - Rapid spread
  - High heat
  - Multiple fires
  - Chemical accelerant

REMEMBER

Self-protection is not selfish. It is necessary if you are to continue to help others and not become a victim yourself.

- In a suspected terrorist incident, be aware that:
  - Terrorists may sabotage fire protection devices
  - Be alert for booby traps
  - Be aware of the possibility of multiple devices
- Isolate/secure the scene, deny entry, establish control zones
- Establish command
- Evaluate scene safety/security
- Stage incoming units
- Gather information regarding the incident, number of victims, etc.
- Assign incident command system positions as needed
- Initiate notifications (i.e., hospitals, law enforcement, state/federal agencies, etc.)
- Request additional resources
- Use appropriate self-protective measures:
  - Proper personal protection equipment
  - Time, distance, and shielding
  - Minimize number of personnel exposed to danger
- Initiate public safety measures:
  - Rescue
  - Evacuate
  - Protect in place
- Establish water supply:
  - Suppression activities
  - Decontamination
- Control and isolate victims (away from the hazard, at the edge of the hot/warm zone)
- Coordinate activities with law enforcement

- Begin and/or assist with triage, administering antidotes, and treatment
- Begin gross mass decontamination *(initial decontamination to removed large amounts of contaminants)* operations

AS THE INCIDENT PROGRESSES, PREPARE TO INITIATE UNIFIED COMMAND SYSTEM:

- Establish unified command post, including representatives from the following organizations:
  - Emergency medical services
  - Law enforcement
  - Hospitals/public health
  - Emergency management
  - Public works
- Establish and maintain chain of custody for evidence protection

EMERGENCY MEDICAL SERVICES

IF FIRST ON SCENE:

- Isolate/secure the scene, establish control zones
- Establish command
- Evaluate scene safety/security
- Stage incoming units

IF COMMAND HAS BEEN ESTABLISHED:

- Report to and/or communicate with command post/incident commander
- Gather information regarding:
  - Type of event
  - Number of patients
  - Severity of injuries
  - Signs and symptoms
- Establish the EMS group within the incident command system
- Notify hospitals
- Request additional resources as appropriate:
  - Basic life support/advanced life support
  - Medivac helicopter (trauma/burn only)
  - Medical equipment and supply caches
  - Metropolitan Medical Response System
  - National Medical Response Team
  - Disaster Medical Assistance Team
  - Disaster Mortuary Response Team

- Use appropriate self-protection measures:
  - Proper personal protective equipment
  - Time, distance, and shielding
  - Minimize number of personnel exposed to danger
- Initiate mass casualty procedure
- Evaluate the need for casualty collection point for ambulatory (walking wounded) victims and a victim treatment area
- Control and isolate victims (away from the hazard, at the edge of the hot/warm zone)
- Ensure victims are decontaminated prior to being forwarded to the cold zone
- Triage, administer antidotes (see "Terrorism Agents in Brief," page 000), treat, and transport victims
- Evidence preservation/collection is law enforcement's responsibility:
  - Recognize potential evidence
  - Report findings to appropriate authority
  - Consider embedded objects as possible evidence
  - Secure evidence found in ambulance or at hospital
- Establish and maintain chain of custody for evidence preservation
- Ensure participation in unified command system when implemented
- Establish the hazmat group within the incident command system
- Provide technical information/assistance to:
  - Command
  - EMS providers
  - Hospitals
  - Law enforcement
- Detect/monitor to identify the agent, determine concentrations, and ensure proper control zones
- Continually reassess control zones
- Enter the hot zone (wearing chemical personal protection equipment) to perform rescue, product confirmation, and reconnaissance
- Product control/mitigation may be implemented in conjunction with expert technical guidance
- Improve hazardous environments:
  - Ventilation
  - Control heating, ventilation, air conditioning
  - Control utilities
- Implement a technical decontamination corridor for Hazardous Materials Response Team personnel

- Coordinate and assist with mass decontamination
- Provide specialized equipment as necessary, such as tents for operations, shelter, etc.
- Assist law enforcement personnel with evidence preservation/collection, decontamination, etc.

ASSISTING AGENCIES

- Federal Bureau of Investigation
  - WMD Coordinator
  - Hazmat Response Unit

For the telephone number(s) of local or regional FBI offices in your area, call FBI headquarters in Washington, DC:

202-324-3000

- U.S. Army Medical Research Institute of Chemical Defense
- U.S. Army Medical Research Institute of Infectious Disease
- U.S. Army Medical Research Institute of Chemical Causality Care Division
- U.S. Army Tech Escort Unit
- Soldier and Biological Chemical Command
- Public works
- Public health
- Centers for Disease Control and Prevention
- Agency for Toxic Substance Disease Registry
- Federal Emergency Management Agency
- Disaster Medical Assistance Team
- Disaster Mortuary Response Team
- Chemical/Biological Incident Response Force
- Bureau of Alcohol, Tobacco, and Firearms
- Department of Energy
- Nuclear Emergency Search Team
- Local emergency managers
- Assorted state agencies (local law enforcement, state police, etc.)

This list is not all-encompassing. Different types of incidents will generate different responses by assisting agencies. Supplement this list with local/state resources as needed.

VICTIM CARE MAINSTAYS WORKSHEET

DURING DECONTAMINATION	AFTER DECONTAMINATION

VICTIM EXPOSURE CONSIDERATIONS

SUPPORTIVE CARE CONSIDERATIONS

DECONTAMINATION CONSIDERATIONS

PERSONAL PROTECTION CONSIDERATIONS
(potential infectious diseases or secondary contamination)

MEDICAL INTERVENTION

BLS TREATMENT	ALS TREATMENT

VICTIM TRANSPORT AND TRANSFER CONSIDERATIONS

PART TWO

SIGNS AND SYMPTOMS

SIGNS & SYMPTOMS

PRIMARY/DISTINCTIVE SYMPTOM	SUSPECTED AGENT	OTHER SYMPTOMS
BODY AS A WHOLE		
Bleeding (mouth, eyes, ears, under the skin, internal organs, vomiting of blood)	**Viral hemorrhagic fever** (see page 45)	Fever, fatigue, exhaustion, dizziness, muscle aches, loss of strength, bloody diarrhea
Flu-like symptoms	**Anthrax, inhalational** (see page 37)	**Anthrax:** Fever, fatigue, cough, chest discomfort, shortness of breath, muscle aches
	Brucellosis (see page 151)	**Brucellosis:** Fever, sweats, sick feeling, appetite loss, back pain, headache
	Eastern equine encephalitis (EEE) (see page 154)	**EEE:** Fever, headache, nausea, chills vomiting
	Q Fever (see page 161)	**Q Fever:** Fever (104°-105° F), headache, muscle aches, chills, confusion, non-productive cough, sore throat, vomiting, diarrhea, abdominal pain, and chest pain
	Ricin (see page 41)	Weakness, fever, cough (aerosol exposure), death of muscle tissue, enlarged lymph glands (such as in the neck and armpits) (injection); GI bleeding (ingestion)
	Smallpox (see page 43)	**Smallpox:** Fever (above 102° F), headache, chills, vomiting, body aches, exhaustion, followed by rash (begins on inside of mouth and face, then spreads to arms, legs, hands, and feet), and progresses to raised bumps and pus-filled blisters
	Staphylococcus enterotoxin B (see page 166)	**Staphylococcus enterotoxin B:** Fever, cough, chest pain, and difficulty breathing (inhalation); vomiting, abdominal pain with or without diarrhea (ingestion)
	Typhus (see page 167)	**Typhus:** Fever, headache, chills, muscle aches, rash (faint and rose colored and fades with pressure)
	Venezuelan equine encephalitis (VEE) (see page 168)	**VEE:** No fever but chills, muscle aches, headache, intolerance to light, unusual sensitivity of the skin, vomiting
	Western equine encephalitis (WEE) (see page 169)	**WEE:** Fever, headache, chills, nausea, vomiting, dizziness, respiratory symptoms
Muscle aches	**Viral hemorrhagic fever** (see page 45)	Bleeding, fever, fatigue, exhaustion, dizziness, bloody diarrhea

PRIMARY/DISTINCTIVE SYMPTOM	SUSPECTED AGENT	OTHER SYMPTOMS
CENTRAL NERVOUS SYSTEM		
Altered mental status (impaired reasoning, hallucinations)	**BZ** (see page 55)	Loss of muscle coordination, low body temperature (after 4 to 20 hours), delirium (after 20 to 96 hours), paranoid thoughts, deep sleep, uncontrollable crawling behavior (late symptoms), enlarged pupils, dry skin
Auditory hallucinations	**Sodium monofluoroacetate** (see page 82)	Facial sensations of prickling, tingling, or creeping on the skin, vomiting, low blood pressure, muscle twitching, increased heart rate, rapid eyeball movement (odorless)
Convulsions, paralysis	**NERVE AGENTS**	Pinpoint pupils, urination, defecation, bronchial secretions, nausea, vomiting, abdominal pain, muscle weakness
	Sarin (see page 80)	**Sarin:** Mild/Fruity Odor
	Tabun (see page 86)	**Tabun:** Faint/Fruity Odor
	VX (see page 88)	**VX:** Odorless
Facial sensations of prickling, tingling, or creeping on the skin	**Sodium monofluoroacetate** (see page 82)	Auditory hallucinations, vomiting, low blood pressure, muscle twitching, increased heart rate, rapid eyeball movement
Paralysis	**Botulism** (see page 38)	Neurological syndrome (clear mental state but double vision, altered voice production, slurred speech, difficulty swallowing), mouth, muscle weakness, dry no fever
DERMATOLOGIC (Skin)		
Blisters	**VESICANTS (BLISTER AGENTS)**	
	Sulfur mustard (see page 242)	**Sulfur mustard:** Yellow blistering, eye pain/irritation, tearing, swelling eyes, shortness of breath, airway irritation, cough, abdominal pain, diarrhea, dizziness, nausea, vomiting (garlic-mustard-onion odor)
	Lewisite (see page 68)	**Lewisite:** Immediate pain on contact, skin pain/irritation/redness, skin blistering, eye pain, tearing, swelling

PRIMARY/DISTINCTIVE SYMPTOM	SUSPECTED AGENT	OTHER SYMPTOMS
DERMATOLOGIC (Skin) cont.		
Chemical burns (3rd degree)	**Phosphorus** (see page 79)	Choking, coughing, wheezing, difficulty breathing, eye burning, abdominal pain, vomiting/stool (garlic odor), confusion, delirium
Dry skin (lack of sweat)	**BZ** (see page 55)	Altered mental status (impaired reasoning, hallucinations), loss of muscle coordination, very high fever (after 4 to 20 hours), delirium (after 20 to 96 hours), paranoid thoughts, deep sleep, uncontrollable crawling behavior (late symptoms), enlarged pupils
Swollen, tender lymph glands (such as in the neck and armpits)	**Anthrax, oropharyngeal** (see page 37)	**Anthrax:** Fever (sudden onset), chills, headache, exhaustion
Convulsions, paralysis	**Bubonic plague** (see page 40)	**Plague:** Fever, chills, severe throat pain, difficulty swallowing, mouth sores, sores under the tongue
	Tularemia, ulceroglandular (see page 44)	**Tularemia:** Fever, skin sores
Rash (begins on chest and spreads to rest of trunk and extremities but not to palms and soles)	**Typhus** (see page 167)	**Typhus:** Fever, headache, chills, muscle aches, rash (faint and rose colored and fades with pressure)
Rash (begins in the mouth and face spreads to arms, legs, hands and feet; progresses to raised bumps and pus-filled blisters)	**Smallpox** (see page 43)	Preceded by high fever (above 102°), headache, chills, vomiting, body aches, exhaustion
Reddish or purplish spot containing blood	**Viral hemorrhagic fever** (see page 45)	Fever, fatigue, exhaustion, dizziness, muscle aches, bloody diarrhea, bleeding
Skin eruption (painful, itchy, welt-like lesions)	**Phosgene oxime** (see page 77)	Eye irritation, excessive tearing, runny nose, sinus pain
Skin irritation	**RIOT CONTROL AGENTS (TEAR GASES)**	Eye irritation, excessive tearing, throat irritation/burning, nausea vomiting, headache
	Bromobenzylcyanide (CA) (see page 54)	**CA:** Sour fruit odor
	Chloroacetophenone (CN) (see page 57)	**CN:** Apple blossom odor
	Dibenzoxazepine (CR) (see page 62)	**CR:** See general signs and symptoms for Riot Control Agents above

PRIMARY/DISTINCTIVE SYMPTOM	SUSPECTED AGENT	OTHER SYMPTOMS
DERMATOLOGIC (Skin) cont.		
Skin irritation	**Chlorobenzylidenemalonitrile (CS)** (see page 58)	**CS:** Pepper odor
	Oleoresin capsicum (OC)/capsaicin (see page 73)	**OC:** See general signs and symptoms for Riot Control Agents on previous page
	Chloropicrin (PS) (see page 59)	**PS:** Strong, pungent odor
Skin irritation/chemical burn	**Hydrofluoric acid** (see page 66)	Eye irritation, airway irritation/ burning (strong, irritating odor)
Skin lesions (pustular, suggest smallpox)	**Glanders** (see page 158)	**Glanders:** Fever, muscle aches, chest pain, muscle tightness, and headache
Skin lesion (raised bump that develops into a painless ulcer; with a characteristic black, dying area in the center)	**Anthrax, cutaneous** (see page 37)	Bodily swelling, swollen lymph glands (such as in the neck and armpits)
Skin ulcer	**Tularemia, ulceroglandular** (see page 44)	Fever, swollen lymph glands (such as in the neck and armpits)
Skin sensitivity	**Venezuelan equine encephalitis (VEE)** (see page 168)	No fever but chills, muscles aches, headache, intolerance to light, vomiting
GASTROINTESTINAL (Stomach)		
Abdominal pain (severe)	**Anthrax, gastrointestinal** (see page 37)	Fever, nausea, loss of appetite, vomiting, severe diarrhea
Abdominal pain/side pain	**Arsine** (see page 50)	Frontal headache, vomiting, feeling of bodily discomfort or fatigue, yellowish skin, discoloration of urine (garlic odor)
Abdominal pain with or without diarrhea	**Staphylococcus enterotoxin B** (see page 166)	**Staphylococcus enterotoxin B:** Fever, cough, chest pain, and difficulty breathing (inhalation); vomiting (ingestion)
Diarrhea (watery)	**Cholera** (see page 152)	Vomiting, fever, leg cramp
Diarrhea (watery, mild, continuous, large volume)	**Cryptosporidum** (see page 153)	
Diarrhea (watery/bloody)	**Escherichia Coli 0157-H7 (E. coli)** (see page 157)	**E. coli:** No fever
	Shigella (see page 165)	**Shigella:** Fever, abdominal cramps
Diarrhea	**Salmonella** (see page 164)	Fever, abdominal cramps
GI bleeding (ingestion)	**Ricin** (see page 41)	Weakness, fever, cough (aerosol exposure); death of muscle tissue, enlarged lymph glands (such as in the next and armpits) (injection)

PRIMARY/DISTINCTIVE SYMPTOM	SUSPECTED AGENT	OTHER SYMPTOMS
GASTROINTESTINAL (Stomach) cont.		
Nausea/vomiting	**BLOOD AGENTS**	
	Arsine (see page 50)	**Arsine:** Abdominal pain/side pain, frontal headache, feeling of bodily discomfort or fatigue, yellowish skin, discoloration of urine (garlic odor)
	Cyanide (see page 60)	**Cyanide:** Headache, dizziness, drowsiness, mucous membrane irritation, rapid breathing, altered mental status (faint, bitter almond odor)
	Sodium monofluoroacetate (see page 82)	**Sodium monofluoroacetate:** Auditory hallucinations; facial sensations of pricking, tingling, or creeping on the skin; low blood pressure; muscle twitching; increased heart rate; rapid eyeball movement (odorless)
	INCAPACITATING AGENTS	
	Adamsite (see page 46)	**Adamsite:** Eye irritation, bodily discomfort or fatigue, diarrhea, abdominal cramps, severe headache, chest tightness, sneezing
Nausea/vomiting	**Fentanyl** (see page 64)	**Fentanyl:** Extremely labored breathing or inability to breathe, low blood pressure, reduced heart rate, chest wall rigidity, seizures
	ORGANIC SOLVENTS	
	Benzene (see page 52)	**Benzene:** Eye pain, drowsiness, dizziness, light headedness, headache, skin breakdown (sweet odor)
Nausea/vomiting/abdominal pain	**NERVE AGENTS**	Watery eyes, salivation, urination, defecation, bronchial secretions, small or pinpoint pupils, muscle weakness, muscle paralysis
	Sarin (see page 80)	**Sarin:** Mild/fruity Odor
	Tabun (see page 86)	**Tabun:** Faint/fruity Odor

PRIMARY/DISTINCTIVE SYMPTOM	SUSPECTED AGENT	OTHER SYMPTOMS
GASTROINTESTINAL (Stomach) cont.		
Nausea/vomiting/abdominal pain	**NERVE AGENTS, cont.** **VX** (see page 88)	**VX:** Odorless
Vomiting/stool (garlic odor)	**Phosphorus** (see page 79)	Chemical burns (3rd degree), choking, coughing, wheezing, eye burning, abdominal pain, confusion, delirium vomiting/stool (garlic odor)
OPHTHALMIC (Eye)		
Enlarged pupils	**BZ** (see page 55)	Altered mental status (impaired reasoning, hallucinations, loss of muscle coordination, very high temperature (after 4 to 20 hours), delirium (after 20 to 96 hours), paranoid thoughts, deep sleep, uncontrollable crawling behavior (late symptoms), dry skin
Double/blurred vision	**Botulism** (see page 38)	Neurological syndrome (mental clarity but paralysis, altered voice production, slurred speech, difficulty swallowing), dry mouth, muscle weakness, no fever
Eye Irritation/excessive tearing	**RIOT CONTROL AGENTS (TEAR GASES)** **Bromobenzylcyanide (CA)** (see page 54)	Skin irritation, throat irritation/burning, nausea, vomiting, headache **CA:** Sour fruit odor
Eye irritation/excessive tearing	**Chloroacetophenone (CN)** (see page 57) **Dibenzoxazepine (CR)** (see page 62) **Chlorobenzylidenemalonitrile (CS)** (see page 58) **Oleoresin capsicum (OC)/capsaicin** (see page 73) **Chloropicrin (PS)** (see page 59)	**CN:** Apple blossom odor **CR:** See general signs and symptoms for Riot Control Agents above **CS:** Pepper odor **OC:** See general signs and symptoms for Riot Control Agents above **PS:** Strong, pungent odor
Eye pain	**Benzene** (see page 52)	Drowsiness, dizziness, lightheadedness, nausea, vomiting, headache, skin breakdown (sweet odor)
Eye Irritation/pain	**Hydrofluoric Acid** (see page 66)	Skin irritation, chemical burn, airway irritation/burning (strong, irritating odor)

PRIMARY/DISTINCTIVE SYMPTOM	SUSPECTED AGENT	OTHER SYMPTOMS
OPHTHALMIC (Eye) cont.		
Intolerance to light	**Venezuelan Equine Encephalitis (VEE)** (see page 168)	No fever but chills, muscle aches, headache, skin sensitivity, vomiting
Pinpoint pupils	**NERVE AGENTS**	Watery eyes, salivation, urination, defecation, bronchial secretions, nausea, vomiting, abdominal pain, muscle aches, muscle paralysis
	Sarin (see page 80)	**Sarin:** Mild/fruity odor
	Tabun (see page 86)	**Tabun:** Faint/fruity odor
	VX (see page 88)	**VX:** Odorless
Rapid eye movement (side to side)	**Sodium Monofluoroacetate** (see page 82)	Facial sensations of prickling, tingling, or creeping on the skin; auditory hallucinations; vomiting; low blood pressure; muscle twitching; increased heart rate (odorless)
Watery eyes	**NERVE AGENTS**	Pinpoint pupils, urination, defecation, bronchial secretions, nausea, vomiting, abdominal pain, muscle weakness, salivation, muscle paralysis
	Sarin (see page 80)	**Sarin:** Mild/fruity odor
Watery eyes	**Tabun** (see page 86)	**Tabun:** Faint/fruity odor
	VX (see page 88)	**VX:** Odorless
ORAL (Mouth/Throat)		
Salivation	**NERVE AGENTS**	Pinpoint pupils, watery eyes, urination, defecation, bronchial secretions, nausea, vomiting, abdominal pain, muscle weakness
	Sarin (see page 80	**Sarin:** Mild/fruity odor
	Tabun (see page 86)	**Tabun:** Faint/fruity odor
	VX (see page 88)	**VX:** Odorless
Throat irritation	**RIOT CONTROL AGENTS (TEAR GASES)**	Eye irritation, skin irritation, excessive tearing, nausea, vomiting, headache

PRIMARY/DISTINCTIVE SYMPTOM	SUSPECTED AGENT	OTHER SYMPTOMS
ORAL (Mouth/Throat) cont.		
Throat irritation	**RIOT CONTROL AGENTS (TEAR GASES)**	
	Bromobenzylcyanide (CA) (see page 54)	**CA:** Sour fruit odor
	Chloroacetophenone (CN) (see page 57)	**CN:** Apple blossom odor
	Dibenzoxazepine (CR) (see page 62)	**CR:** See general signs and symptoms Riot Control Agents on previous page
	Chlorobenzylidenemalonitrile (CS) (see page 58)	**CS:** Pepper odor
	Oleoresin capsicum (OC)/capsaicin (see page 73)	**OC:** See general signs and symptoms for Riot Control Agents on previous page
	Chloropicrin (PS) (see page 59)	**PS:** Strong, pungent odor
Severe throat pain, difficulty swallowing	**Anthrax, Oropharyngeal** (see page 37)	Fever, marked swelling on one or both sides of the neck, mouth sores, sores under the tongue
RESPIRATORY (Lung)		
Airway irritation/burning	**Hydrofluoric Acid** (see page 66)	Eye irritation, skin irritation, chemical burn (strong, irritating odor)
Chest tightness/shortness of breath	**Chloropicrin (PS)** (see page 59)	Eye irritation (redness, vision), excessive tearing, throat irritation, coughing, sense of suffocation, nausea, vomiting, hoarseness, wheezing, skin irritation (redness, burn, rash) (strong, pungent odor)
Choking/coughing/wheezing/ difficulty breathing	**CHOKING/PULMONARY AGENTS**	
	Ammonia (see page 47)	**Ammonia:** Mild eye, nose, throat irritation (strong, pungent odor)
	Bromine (see page 53)	**Bromine:** Eye/nose inflammation, sore throat, bronchial spasm dizziness, dry rash resembling eczema (bleach odor)
	Chlorine (see page 56)	**Chlorine:** Burning sensation in nose and throat, chest pain, vomiting (distinctive odor)

PRIMARY/DISTINCTIVE SYMPTOM	SUSPECTED AGENT	OTHER SYMPTOMS
RESPIRATORY (Lung) cont.		
	Hydrochloric acid (see page 65)	**Hydrochloric acid:** Mouth/throat burning, nausea, vomiting, diarrhea, skin irritation (redness, pain) (acid-like odor)
	Methyl bromide (see page 69)	**Methyl bromide:** Muscle weakness, visual disturbance, dizziness, nausea, vomiting, tremors (chloroform odor)
	Methyl isocyanate (see page 71)	**Methyl isocyanate:** Eye burning, excessive tearing, nausea, vomiting (sharp/distinctive odor)
	Osmium tetroxide (see page 75)	**Osmium tetroxide:** Eye irritation, throat burning, headache, impaired vision (appearance of halos), skin discoloration
	Phosgene (see page 76)	**Phosgene:** Fatigue, headache, nausea, sore throat (green corn or moldy hay odor)
	Phosphine (see page 78)	**Phosphine:** Nausea, vomiting, dizziness, abdominal pain, diarrhea, chills (fishy, garlicky odor)
Choking/coughing/wheezing/ difficulty breathing	**Phosphorus** (see page 79)	**Phosphorus:** 3rd degree burns, eye burning, abdominal pain, confusion, delirium, vomiting/ stool (garlic odor)
	Sulfuryl fluoride (see page 85)	**Sulfuryl Fluoride:** Nausea, vomiting, diarrhea, skin/eye irritation (odorless)
Extreme difficulty breathing or inability to breathe	**Fentanyl** (see page 64)	Nausea, vomiting, low blood pressure, very slow heart rate (to less than 60 beats per minute), chest wall rigidity, seizures
Fluid accumulation in the lungs	**Epsilon-Toxin** (see page 156)	Kidney failure, shock
Pneumonia-like symptoms	**Glanders** (see page 158)	**Glanders:** Fever, muscle aches, chest pain, muscle tightness, and headache, skin lesions (pustular, suggest smallpox)
Pneumonia-like symptoms with nonproductive cough (dry cough)	**Psittacosis** (see page 160)	**Psittacosis:** Fever, sore throat, swollen, lymph nodes (such as in the neck and armpits)

PRIMARY/DISTINCTIVE SYMPTOM	BIOTERRORISM AGENT	OTHER SYMPTOMS
RESPIRATORY (Lung) cont.		
	Tularemia, Pneumonic (see page 44)	**Tularemia:** Fever; shortness of breath or difficult, labored breathing; chills; headache; profound physical exhaustion; mental impairment; pulse-temperature disassociation; swollen lymph nodes (such as in the neck and armpits), pleural effusion (excess fluid between the lining of the lungs and the lining of the inside chest wall) (later stages)
Pneumonia-like symptoms with productive cough (bloody sputum)	**Pneumonic plague** (see page 40)	Fever, difficulty breathing, weakness, chest pain
Pneumonia-like symptoms with nonproductive or productive cough	**Meliodosis** (see page 159)	**Meliodosis:** Fever, sputum, headache, muscle aches, chest pain
Sneezing	**Adamsite** (see page 46)	Eye irritation, a feeling of bodily discomfort or fatigue, nausea, diarrhea, abdominal cramps, severe headache, chest tightness, vomiting
URINARY		
Discoloration of urine	**Arsine** (see page 50)	Abdominal pain/side pain, frontal headache, vomiting, a feeling of bodily discomfort or fatigue, yellowish skin (garlic odor)

See next page for full-color images of the presentation of cutaneous anthrax, plague, mustard gas, and smallpox.

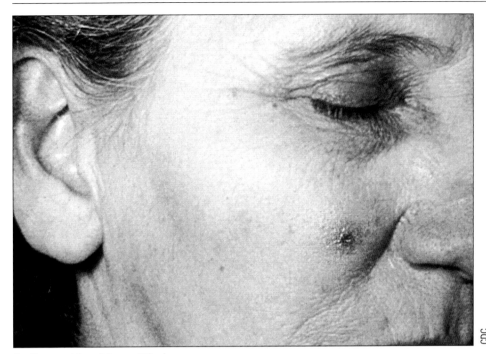

Anthrax, skin of face, 4th day.

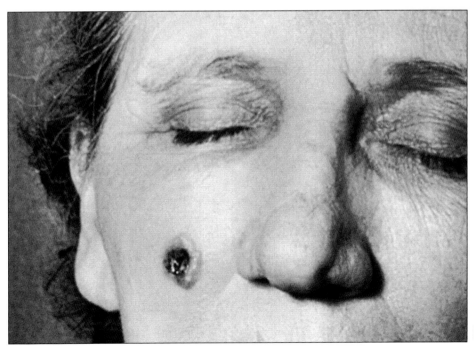

Anthrax, skin of face, 5th day.

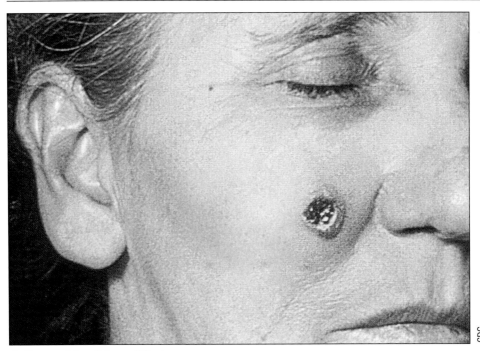

Anthrax, skin of face, 6th day.

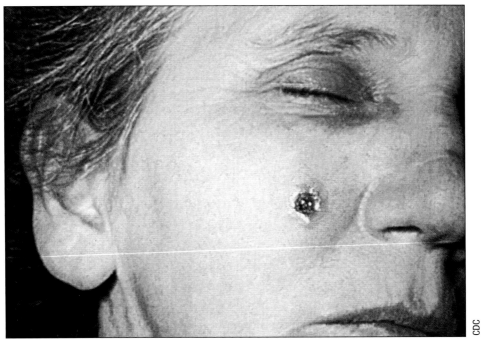

Anthrax, skin of face, 8th day.

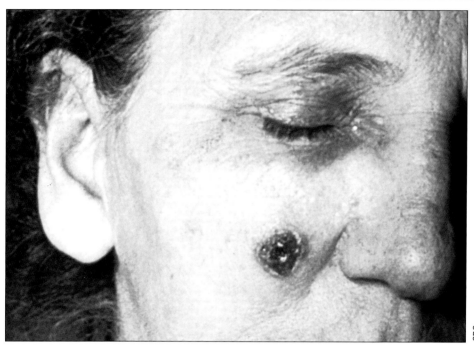

Anthrax, skin of face, 11th day.

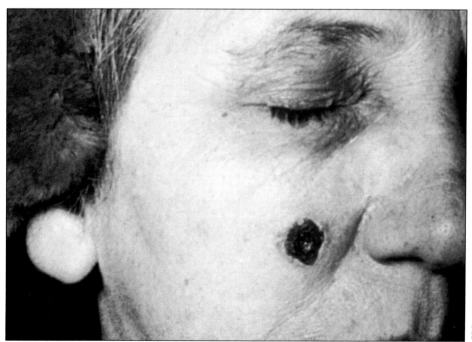

Anthrax, skin of face, 13th day.

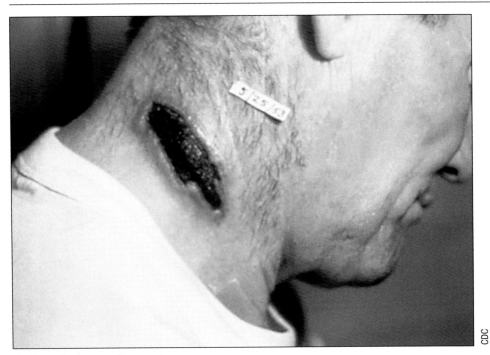

Anthrax lesion on the neck.

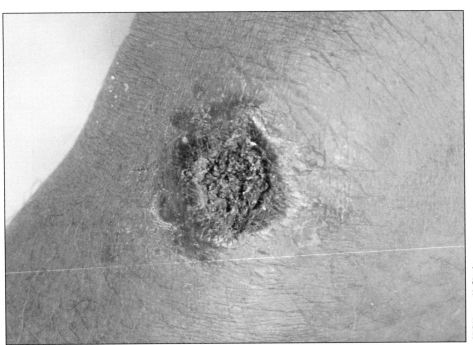

Anthrax lesion on the skin of the forearm.

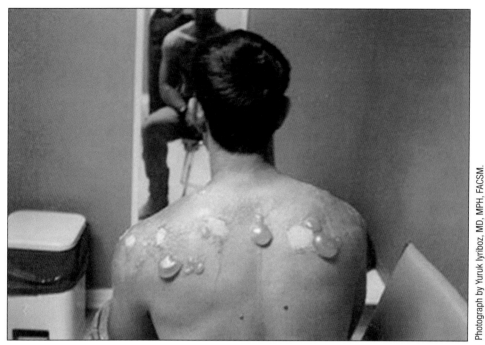

Photograph by Yuruk Iyriboz, MD, MPH, FACSM.

Second day after mustard gas exposure: typical pendulous bullae.
On the third day, burns extended to 10% of the body's surface.

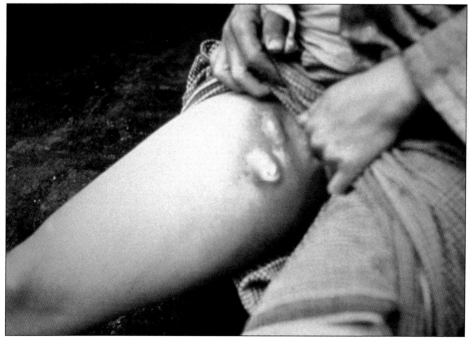

CDC

This plague patient is displaying a swollen, ruptured inguinal lymph node,
or buboe.

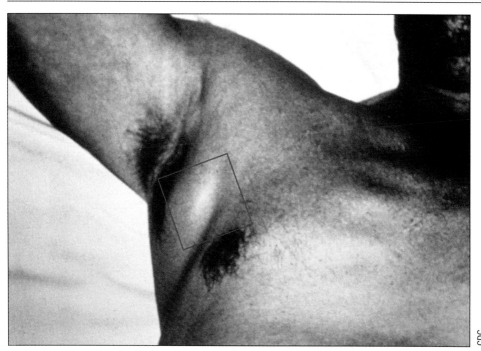

Plague patient displaying a swollen axillary lymph node.

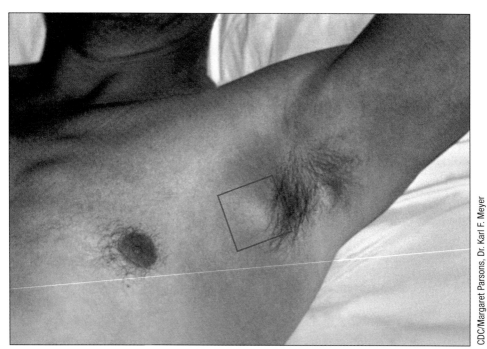

Plague patient displaying an axillary buboe and edema.

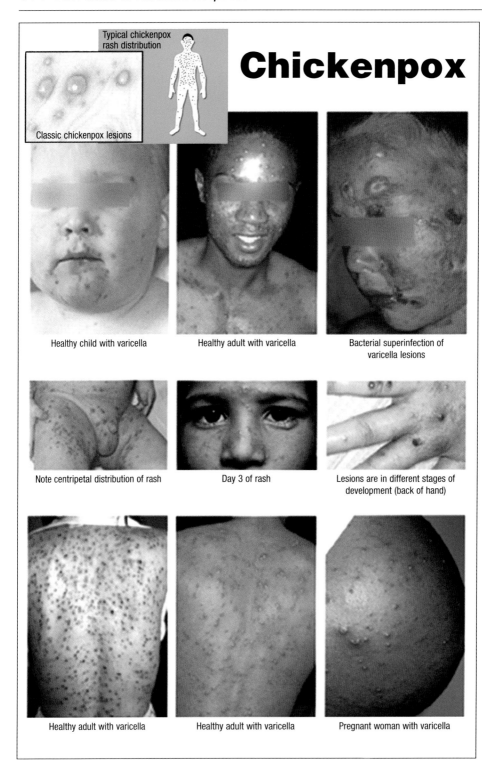

Chickenpox

Typical chickenpox rash distribution

Classic chickenpox lesions

Healthy child with varicella

Healthy adult with varicella

Bacterial superinfection of varicella lesions

Note centripetal distribution of rash

Day 3 of rash

Lesions are in different stages of development (back of hand)

Healthy adult with varicella

Healthy adult with varicella

Pregnant woman with varicella

CDC

Images of Chickenpox (Varicella)

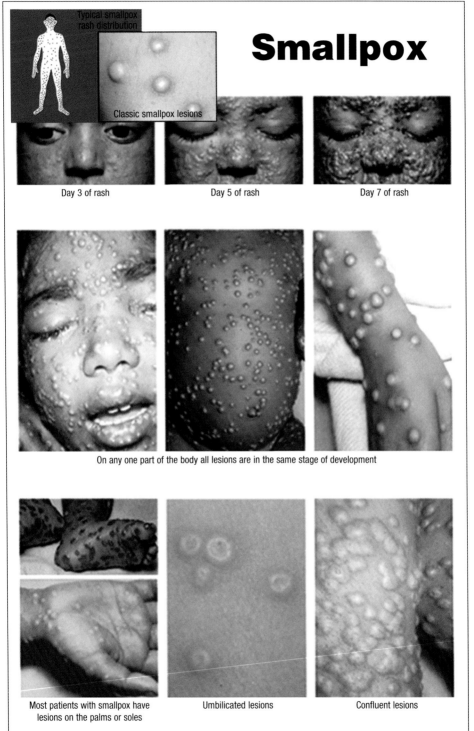

Typical smallpox rash distribution

Classic smallpox lesions

Smallpox

Day 3 of rash

Day 5 of rash

Day 7 of rash

On any one part of the body all lesions are in the same stage of development

Most patients with smallpox have lesions on the palms or soles

Umbilicated lesions

Confluent lesions

CDC

Images of Smallpox (Variola)

TERRORISM AGENTS IN BRIEF

Continued...

EXPLOSIVE AGENTS

INCENDIARY AGENTS

NUCLEAR/RADIATION AGENTS

ANTHRAX (BIOLOGICAL AGENT)

OVERVIEW (FOR FURTHER DETAILS, SEE PAGE 97)

- Photographs of anthrax victims can be found at the end of this section.

- A serious disease caused by infection with the bacterium *Bacillus anthracis*.

- Not spread from person to person. Spread by infected animals (rarely) and weapons containing the bacteria (such as powders or aerosols).

- Three forms: cutaneous (enters through the skin), inhalation (enters through the lungs), gastrointestinal (enters through the digestive tract).

- Cutaneous anthrax: most common and mildest form. Treatment with antibiotics can cure most cases. Slight chance of spreading to other areas of the body.

- Potential risk of person-to-person transmission if direct contact occurs with open skin sores or blisters. Use gloves and protective clothing.

- Inhalation anthrax: most severe form. Can destroy lung tissue and spread to the brain. Often fatal even with antibiotic treatment.

- Gastrointestinal anthrax: extremely rare; never documented in the U.S. Caused by handling animal products or eating undercooked meat from an infected animal.

STEP ONE: IDENTIFY ACUTE HAZARDS/SIGNS/SYMPTOMS

- Effects usually appear within 7 days after exposure but can take up to 45 days

- First sign: raised bump; looks like insect bite; sometimes itchy

- 1-2 days later: bump turns into blister

- Blister then turns into skin ulcer (open sore) with black center; usually painless

- Early signs: cold or flu symptoms for first 3-4 days

- Sore throat

- Cough

- Mild fever

- Chills or night sweats

- Muscle aches

- Chest discomfort

- Shortness of breath

- Tiredness

- Nausea

- Vomiting

- Loss of appetite

- Stomach pain

- Severe diarrhea

- Vomiting blood

- Symptoms quickly worsen after a few days, leading to high fever, breathing problems, and shock

- Runny nose or sneezing are not usually symptoms

STEP TWO: PROTECT YOURSELF

- Do not breathe contaminated air.

- Hold breath until self-contained breathing apparatus can be put on.

- Without protection, avoid the area.

- Wear gloves and protective clothing.

- Do not touch broken skin such as cuts, rashes, or blisters, especially if they are oozing.

STEP THREE: ADMINISTER FIRST AID

- Remove victim from source of exposure.

- If breathing is labored, give oxygen.

- If breathing has stopped, give artificial respiration. Give mouth to mouth only when facial contamination is absent.

- Immediately remove contaminated clothing and wash exposed area thoroughly with soap and water

- Contaminated clothing can expose others through direct contact. Triple-seal in plastic bags.

- Seek medical help at once

BOTULISM (BIOLOGICAL AGENT)

OVERVIEW (FOR FURTHER DETAILS, SEE PAGE 107)

- A muscle-paralyzing disease caused by a bacterial toxin (poison).

- Three forms: foodborne, wound, and intestinal (infant and adult). All can occur naturally from absorption of bacteria through the gut or a wound. The toxin does not penetrate intact skin.

- Not spread from person to person.

- As a weapon, the toxin can be delivered by inhalation (aerosols) and through food or water.

STEP ONE: IDENTIFY ACUTE HAZARDS/SIGNS/SYMPTOMS

- Signs tend to occur 3-4 days after exposure

- Mucus in throat

- Difficulty swallowing

- Dry mouth

- Nausea and vomiting

- Abdominal cramps

- Dizziness

- Difficulty moving eyes

- Enlarged pupils or pupils that react slowly to stimuli

- Involuntary eye movements

- Blurred or double vision

- Drooping eyelids

- Difficulty speaking or slurred speech

- Difficulty walking

- Muscle weakness and paralysis. Paralysis starts at shoulders, then moves down to upper arms, lower arms, thighs, calves, etc.

- Paralysis of breathing muscles can occur and cause breathing to stop. Death will occur unless assistance with breathing (ie, mechanical ventilation) is provided

STEP TWO: PROTECT YOURSELF

- If aerosol delivery is suspected, cover mouth and nose with clothing such as an undershirt, shirt, scarf, or handkerchief, or, ideally, put on a self-contained breathing apparatus.

- When caring for victims, use standard precautions.

- Contagion is not a problem. Botulism is not spread from person to person.

- After exposure to botulinum toxin, clothing and skin should be washed with soap and water.

- Contaminated objects or surfaces should be cleaned with 0.1% hypochlorite bleach solution if they cannot be avoided for the hours to days required for natural degradation.

STEP THREE: ADMINISTER FIRST AID

- If an aerosol attack, remove victim from source of exposure.

- If breathing is labored, provide mechanical ventilation.

- Seek medical help at once.

PLAGUE (BIOLOGICAL AGENT)

OVERVIEW (FOR FURTHER DETAILS, SEE PAGE 115)

- Photographs of plague victims can be found at the end of this section.

- Plague is a bacterial disease that occurs naturally but is usually controlled by standard public health measures.

- Three forms: bubonic, septicemic, and pneumonic.

- Pneumonic plague most likely candidate for bioterrorism agent; it can be delivered by aerosol spray and infect the lungs.

- Highly contagious and can quickly spread through airborne particles caused by coughing or sneezing.

- Fatal without antibiotic treatment.

- Must be caught early and treated within 24 hours of the first symptoms.

- When released into the air, plague bacteria can survive for up to 1 hour, depending on the conditions. The bacteria are easily destroyed by sunlight and drying.

STEP ONE: IDENTIFY ACUTE HAZARDS/SIGNS/SYMPTOMS

- Highly contagious; spreads easily by coughing and sneezing

- Signs appear within 1-6 days.

- Fever

- Weakness

- Rapidly developing pneumonia:

  - Shortness of breath

  - Chest pain

  - Coughing: can produce bloody or watery mucus

- Nausea and vomiting

- Abdominal pain

- Without treatment, leads to loss of breathing, shock, and death

STEP TWO: PROTECT YOURSELF

- Without protection, avoid the area. Pneumonic plague is highly contagious.

- Do not breathe contaminated air. Hold breath until self-contained breathing apparatus can be put on. In absence of SCBA, wear a surgical mask.

- Without protection, do not stand within 3 feet of infected persons unless they have been treated with antibiotics for at least 48 hours.

- Wear gloves and protective clothing.

- Do not eat, drink, or smoke when treating victims. Afterward, wash hands thoroughly.

- After being around plague victims, if you develop a new cough or temperature of 101° F, you should promptly receive antibiotic treatment.

- If you are exposed to a plague victim but show no symptoms yourself, the risk of getting sick can be greatly reduced if you begin antibiotic treatment within 7 days.

STEP THREE: ADMINISTER FIRST AID

- Seek medical help immediately. The sooner victims receive antibiotic therapy, the better their chances of recovery.

RICIN (BIOLOGICAL AGENT)

OVERVIEW (FOR FURTHER DETAILS, SEE PAGE 162)

- A toxin (poison) made from waste left over from processing castor beans.

- Poisoning most likely due to bioterrorism. Accidental exposure is highly unlikely.

- Poisoning can occur by breathing in mist or powder. Ricin can also be added to water or food. Pellets of ricin dissolved in solution can be injected into the body.

- Very small amounts can be fatal if inhaled or injected. Larger amounts would be needed if swallowed.

- Ricin poisoning could cause death within 36 to 72 hours after exposure, depending on the dose received and route of exposure (inhalation, ingestion, or injection).

- If death has not occurred within 3 to 5 days, the victim usually recovers.

- There is no antidote for ricin poisoning. Avoid exposure, if possible. If exposure cannot be avoided, the most important factor is getting the poison off or out of the body.

- Ricin poisoning does not spread from person to person.

STEP ONE: IDENTIFY ACUTE HAZARDS/SIGNS/SYMPTOMS

- After exposure to mist or powder, effects are usually immediate; otherwise, signs occur within 8 hours of exposure

- Redness

- Pain

- Fever

- Nausea

- Cough

- Vomiting and diarrhea that may become bloody

- Blood in urine

- Heavy sweating

- Severe dehydration could result from excessive fluid loss, leading to low blood pressure

- Hallucinations

- Seizures

- Difficulty breathing (skin might turn blue)

- Tightness in chest

- Fluid buildup in the lungs

- Within several days, liver, spleen, and kidneys might fail, leading to death.

STEP TWO: PROTECT YOURSELF

- Wear self-contained breathing apparatus in area of suspected contamination.

- Wear goggles to shield eyes.

- Wear gloves, booties, and other protective clothing to shield skin.

- If you are helping other people remove their clothing, avoid touching contaminated areas.

- Do not eat, drink, or smoke while assisting victims.

- If exposure occurs:

  - Quickly move to an area with fresh air.

  - Remove clothing quickly. Do not pull clothing over your head. Cut it off body.

  - Quickly wash entire body with soap and water.

  - Remove contact lenses if worn and dispose of them in a plastic bag.

  - Rinse eyes thoroughly with warm water for 10 to 15 minutes.

  - Wash eyeglasses thoroughly with soap and water. After washing, you can put your glasses back on.

  - Seek medical help immediately.

STEP THREE: ADMINISTER FIRST AID

- Quickly move victim to an area with fresh air.

- If breathing is labored, give oxygen.

- Perform CPR if necessary. Do not give mouth-to-mouth resuscitation if area around mouth is contaminated.

- Quickly remove the victim's clothing, avoiding contaminated areas as much as possible. Do not pull clothing over the head. Cut it off the body.

- Thoroughly wash entire body with soap and water.

- Rinse mouth if ingested but do not induce vomiting.

- Rinse eyes thoroughly with warm water for 10 to 15 minutes.

- Remove contact lenses, if worn, and dispose of them in a plastic bag.

- Remove eyeglasses and wash thoroughly with soap and water. After washing, victim can put glasses back on.

- Administer activated charcoal to bind the poison in the stomach.

- Seek medical help immediately.

SMALLPOX (BIOLOGICAL AGENT)

OVERVIEW (FOR FURTHER DETAILS, SEE PAGE 125)

- In its early stages, smallpox resembles chickenpox. Photographs of the progressive stages of each disease can be found at the end of this section.

- A very serious, contagious, and sometimes fatal infectious disease.

- Victims—and people in contact with victims—should be quarantined until assessed by medical specialists.

- There is no specific treatment; the only prevention is vaccination.

- Can be transmitted through face-to-face contact, direct contact with infected bodily fluids or contaminated objects, or exposure to aerosol release.

- If released as an aerosol, the virus can be killed relatively easily by sunlight and heat.

- Incubation period averages 12 to 14 days before symptoms appear.

- Blindness can occur. Fatality rate is approximately 30%.

STEP ONE: IDENTIFY ACUTE HAZARDS/SIGNS/SYMPTOMS

- Fever (usually 101° F to 104° F)

- Tiredness

- Severe headache and backache

- Vomiting

- Rash appears on the face and spreads to the arms and legs and then to the hands and feet; patient is most contagious at this point

- Rash becomes raised bumps which fill with fluid

- Bumps eventually scab

- Scabs fall off leaving pitted scars

- Small red spots appear on the tongue and mouth

STEP TWO: PROTECT YOURSELF

- Avoid face-to-face contact with victims suspected of smallpox infection.

- Do not touch clothes or objects that may have been contaminated

STEP THREE: ADMINISTER FIRST AID

- Seek immediate medical treatment for victim and people who may have had contact with victim.

TULAREMIA (BIOLOGICAL AGENT)

OVERVIEW (FOR FURTHER DETAILS, SEE PAGE 113)

- Also known as "rabbit fever," a potentially serious illness that is caused by a bacterium found in animals.

- Not known to spread from person to person, but can be fatal if not treated with antibiotics.

- If used as a biological weapon, tularemia would probably be aerosolized for exposure by inhalation.

- Release in a densely populated area would be expected to result in many victims with acute feverish symptoms beginning 3 to 5 days later.

STEP ONE: IDENTIFY ACUTE HAZARDS/SIGNS/SYMPTOMS

- Sudden fever

- Chills

- Dry cough

- Headache

- Sore throat

- Mouth sores

- Skin ulcers

- Swollen and painful lymph glands

- Muscle aches

- Joint pain

- Inflamed eyes

- Diarrhea

- Progressive weakness

- Severe respiratory illness, including life-threatening pneumonia

STEP TWO: PROTECT YOURSELF

Tularemia is not known to be contagious.

STEP THREE: ADMINISTER FIRST AID

Seek medical treatment at once.

VIRAL HEMORRHAGIC FEVERS (BIOLOGICAL AGENTS)

OVERVIEW (FOR FURTHER DETAILS, SEE PAGE 141)

- Viral hemorrhagic fevers (VHFs) refer to a group of illnesses that are caused by several distinct families of viruses.

- VHFs are initially transmitted by infected animals.

- Some viruses that cause hemorrhagic fever can spread from one person to another. Ebola, Marburg, Lassa, and Crimean-Congo hemorrhagic fever viruses are examples.

- This type of secondary transmission can occur directly, through close contact with infected people or their body fluids. It can also occur indirectly, through contact with objects contaminated with infected body fluids. For example, contaminated syringes and needles have played an important role in spreading infection in outbreaks of Ebola and Lassa hemorrhagic fevers.

- The overall vascular system is typically damaged and the body's ability to regulate itself is impaired.

- While some types of VHF viruses cause relatively mild illnesses, many of these viruses cause severe, life-threatening disease.

STEP ONE: IDENTIFY ACUTE HAZARDS/SIGNS/SYMPTOMS

- Sore throat

- Mouth sores

- Pneumonia

- Skin ulcers

- Swollen and painful lymph glands

- Inflamed eyes

- Bloody diarrhea

- Bleeding from mucous membranes

STEP TWO: PROTECT YOURSELF

- VHFs can be highly contagious. Do not approach victims suspected of being infected by a VHF without wearing personal protection equipment.

- The wearing of flexible plastic hoods equipped with battery-powered blowers provides excellent protection of the mucous membranes and airways.

- Mask, gown, glove and needle precautions should be exercised.

STEP THREE: ADMINISTER FIRST AID

Seek immediate medical treatment.

ADAMSITE (INCAPACITATING AGENT)

OVERVIEW (FOR FURTHER DETAILS, SEE PAGE 201)

- At room temperature, light green or yellow crystals; turns to vapor/yellow smoke when heated.

- Odorless.

- Dispersed as an aerosol.

- Most exposure occurs by inhalation, but also toxic through ingestion or skin contact.

- Effects begin within minutes and may last for hours.

STEP ONE: IDENTIFY ACUTE HAZARDS/SIGNS/SYMPTOMS

- Irritation of the eyes and mucous membranes

- Coughing, sneezing

- Severe headache

- Acute pain and tightness in the chest

- Nausea, vomiting

- Irritation of the skin

STEP TWO: PROTECT YOURSELF

- Wear a respiratory protective mask/respirator in spite of any coughing, sneezing, salivation, or nausea; lift mask as necessary to permit any of the above.

STEP THREE: ADMINISTER FIRST AID

- Remove the victim to fresh air.

- Rinse the nose and throat with saline water or bicarbonate of soda solution.

- Wash exposed skin and scalp with soap and water and allow to dry on the skin.

- Dust skin with borated talcum.

- Seek medical attention immediately.

AMMONIA (CHOKING/PULMONARY AGENT)

OVERVIEW (FOR FURTHER DETAILS, SEE PAGE 183)

- Colorless gas that dissolves easily in water to form caustic solutions.

- As a terrorist agent, most likely to be released as a gas.

- Strong, pungent odor.

- Can be extremely irritating to any surface, but especially to mucous membranes.

- Exposure by inhalation, skin exposure, eye exposure, or ingestion.

- **NOTE:** Rescuers should be trained and use appropriate protective gear when dealing with ammonia as a terrorism agent. If proper equipment or attire is not available, or if rescuers have not been properly trained, seek assistance from hazmat personnel or other properly equipped response teams.

STEP ONE: IDENTIFY ACUTE HAZARDS/SIGNS/SYMPTOMS

- Low concentrations:
  - Internal burning in the nose or throat
- Higher concentrations:
  - Nausea
  - Vomiting
  - Abdominal pain
  - Esophageal burns
- Wheezing
- Coughing
- Shortness of breath
- Corneal ulcers
- Conjunctivitis
- Airway destruction

- Fluid in lungs

- Seizure

- Blindness (may be temporary or permanent)

- Coma

- Exposure of more than a few minutes: pain and corrosive injury

- Exposure to concentrated vapor or solution: inflammation, blisters, deep burns

- Exposure to compressed liquid ammonia: frostbite

- Large exposure may result in death.

STEP TWO: PROTECT YOURSELF

- Wear self-contained breathing apparatus

- Wear chemical-protective clothing.

- Avoid direct contact with clothing or skin of victims contaminated with liquid ammonia.

STEP THREE: ADMINISTER FIRST AID

- Remove victim from contaminated area

- Remove contaminated clothing; double-bag contaminated clothing and belongings

- Administer humidified oxygen

- Treat with inhaled bronchodilators

- Contaminated skin should be flushed with copious tap water for 5-15 minutes

- Remove contact lenses, if worn; be careful not to cause additional trauma to eyes

- **DO NOT** induce vomiting

- **DO NOT** administer activated charcoal

- If victim is able to swallow, administer 4 to 8 ounces of water or milk

- Prepare ambulance with towels and open plastic bags in case victim vomits toxic material

- Transport victim for medical care

- Asymptomatic victims: Take names and contact information; release with instructions to seek medical care if symptoms develop

ARSENIC (METAL)

OVERVIEW (FOR FURTHER DETAILS, SEE PAGE 209)

- A naturally occurring element existing in several forms: organic, gaseous, elemental, and inorganic. The inorganic form is the most prevalent and the gaseous form (arsine) is the most potentially harmful.

- Soil, water, and food contaminated with arsenic are the primary sources for arsenic exposure in the general population.

- Acute toxicity may occur within 10 minutes to hours after exposure.

- Patients will typically complain of nausea, vomiting, abdominal pain, and severe diarrhea that has been described as "cholera-like."

- Arsenic is strongly associated with lung and skin cancer in humans.

STEP ONE: IDENTIFY ACUTE HAZARDS/SIGNS/SYMPTOMS

- Sore throat or irritated lungs

- Headaches, confusion, and drowsiness

- May cause redness and swelling

- Darkening of the skin

- Severe diarrhea

- Nausea and vomiting

- Abdominal pain

- Abnormal heart rhythm

- A sensation of "pins and needles" in hands and feet

- Appearance of small "corns" or "warts" on the palms, soles, and torso

STEP TWO: PROTECT YOURSELF

- Wear self-contained breathing apparatus.

- Wear goggles, gloves, and protective clothing.

STEP THREE: ADMINISTER FIRST AID

- In acute arsenic poisoning, vomiting should be induced by ipecac syrup in an alert victim.

- Gastric lavage may be useful.

- Activated charcoal may be tried.

- Seek immediate medical treatment.

ARSINE (BLOOD AGENT)

OVERVIEW (FOR FURTHER DETAILS, SEE PAGE 177)

- Colorless, flammable toxic gas. Can have a garlic-like odor, but smell can only be detected at levels greater than those necessary to cause poisoning.

- Formed when arsenic comes into contact with an acid.

- As a weapon, most likely route of exposure is inhalation after gas has been released into the air. Absorption through the eyes and skin has not been known to occur.

- An arsine attack would have few warning signs. The gas is not irritating and would not cause potential victims to leave the scene.

- Arsine vapor is heavier than air and would be more likely to settle in low-lying areas.

- Extent of poisoning depends on amount of arsine released and length of exposure time. Exposure to high doses can cause immediate death.

- There is no antidote for arsine poisoning. The toxic gas damages red blood cells after entering the bloodstream. Organ failure and death may result.

- Severe health effects are usually delayed, causing further difficulty in pinpointing the site and time of release.

STEP ONE: IDENTIFY ACUTE HAZARDS/SIGNS/SYMPTOMS

- After a low to moderate dose, signs appear within 2-24 hours:
  - Weakness and fatigue
  - Headache
  - Drowsiness
  - Confusion
  - Shortness of breath
  - Rapid breathing
  - Nausea, vomiting, and/or abdominal pain
  - Red or dark urine
  - Yellow skin and eyes (jaundice)
  - Muscle cramps

- After a large dose, signs may also include:

  - Loss of consciousness

  - Convulsions

  - Paralysis

  - Loss of breathing, possibly leading to death

- Little or no information is available on direct toxic effects to the eyes or skin

- Exposure to liquid arsine (the compressed gas) can cause frostbite

- Ingestion unlikely because arsine is a gas at room temperature

- Ingested metal arsenides (solids) can react with digestive acid and release arsine gas in the stomach

STEP TWO: PROTECT YOURSELF

- Do not breathe contaminated air. Hold breath until self-contained breathing apparatus can be put on. Without protection, avoid the area.

- Wear gloves, booties, and other protective clothing.

- Do not eat, drink, or smoke while assisting victims.

- If exposure occurs:

  - Quickly move to an area with fresh air

  - Remove clothing quickly. *Do not* pull clothing over your head. Cut it off the body and place in a plastic bag

  - Remove contacts and dispose of them in a plastic bag

  - Remove jewelry and thoroughly wash with soap and water, if possible; if not, jewelry should be placed in plastic bag with contaminated clothing

  - Quickly wash entire body with soap and water

  - Rinse eyes thoroughly with water for 10 to 15 minutes

  - Wash eyeglasses thoroughly with soap and water; after washing, you can put your glasses back on

  - Seek medical help immediately

STEP THREE: ADMINISTER FIRST AID

- Quickly move victim to an area with fresh air

- If breathing is labored, give oxygen

- If breathing has stopped, give artificial respiration. *Give mouth to mouth only when facial contamination is absent.*

- Follow instructions in Step Two.

BENZENE (ORGANIC SOLVENT)

OVERVIEW (FOR FURTHER DETAILS, SEE PAGE 225)

- Colorless or light yellow liquid at room temperature. It has a sweet odor and is highly flammable.

- Highly volatile, flammable liquid. Benzene vapor is heavier than air and may accumulate in low-lying areas.

- Most exposures occur by inhalation, after which absorption is rapid.

- Immediate effects occur after exposure to high concentrations of benzene. Symptoms include headache, lightheadedness, and dizziness.

STEP ONE: IDENTIFY ACUTE HAZARDS/SIGNS/SYMPTOMS

- Immediate symptoms upon inhalation of high concentrations:
  - Headache
  - Light-headedness
  - Confusion

- Irritation of the respiratory tract and fluid accumulation in lungs

- Degreases skin after prolonged or repeated contact

- Redness and burning sensation

- Eye irritation and visual blurring

- Burning/eye pain

- Irritation of the stomach causing nausea, vomiting, and diarrhea

STEP TWO: PROTECT YOURSELF

- Self-contained breathing apparatus is recommended.

- Chemical protective clothing is not required when only vapor is suspected.

- Chemical protective clothing is required when contact with liquid benzene is a danger.

- If exposed, seek medical help at once.

STEP THREE: ADMINISTER FIRST AID

- Remove clothing that may be exposed to chemical.

- Flush liquid-exposed skin and hair with copious amounts of tap water.

- Remove contact lenses, if worn.

- For eye exposures, continue water irrigation for 15 minutes.

- Seek immediate medical attention.

BROMINE (CHOKING/PULMONARY AGENT)

OVERVIEW (FOR FURTHER DETAILS, SEE PAGE 184)

- Brownish-red liquid at room temperature.
- Emits an odor similar to bleach.
- Exposure possible via contaminated water or food, or by contact with bromine gas or liquid.
- Bromine gas is heavier than air and will settle in low-lying areas.

STEP ONE: IDENTIFY ACUTE HAZARDS/SIGNS/SYMPTOMS

- Eye and nose inflammation
- Sore throat
- Chest tightness
- Bronchial spasm
- Dizziness
- Headaches
- Coughing
- Difficulty breathing
- Irritation of mucous membranes
- Watery eyes
- Burning or irritation at point of contact
- Stomach pain

STEP TWO: PROTECT YOURSELF

- If gas is suspected, put on self-contained breathing apparatus.
- Avoid touching contaminated skin or clothing of victim without wearing protective gloves.

STEP THREE: ADMINISTER FIRST AID

- Transport the victim out of contaminated area, preferably to higher ground.
- Administer oxygen, if needed.
- Rinse eyes with plain water for 10 to 15 minutes.
- Glasses can be reused after washing with soap and water.

- Remove victim's clothing. Do not pull clothing over victim's head; cut clothing off if necessary.
- Double-bag contaminated clothing.
- Wash entire body thoroughly with soap and water.
- Remove contact lenses and store with contaminated clothing.
- **DO NOT** induce vomiting.
- **DO NOT** give the victim anything to drink.
- Seek immediate medical attention.

BROMOBENZYLCYANIDE (RIOT CONTROL AGENT)

OVERVIEW (FOR FURTHER DETAILS, SEE PAGE 229)

- Bromobenzylcyanide (CA) is clear to white crystalline substance with the odor of sour fruit.
- A tear gas which can be used as an incapacitating agent.
- Can be absorbed into the body via inhalation and mucous membrane contact.
- Targets eyes, skin, mucous membranes, and lungs.
- Most effects are of limited duration and usually resolve within 30 to 60 minutes following evacuation and decontamination.
- With longer and more intense exposure, noncardiogenic pulmonary edema may occur.

STEP ONE: IDENTIFY ACUTE HAZARDS/SIGNS/SYMPTOMS

- Irritation of the throat occurs rapidly
- Cough, hoarseness, chest tightness, sensation of suffocation
- Nausea, vomiting and headache are commonly reported
- Irritation on moist and sensitive areas of the skin
- Redness, pain, and blistering of exposed skin
- Irritation and tearing of the eyes occurs rapidly
- Redness, blurred vision, and corneal burns

STEP TWO: PROTECT YOURSELF

- Do not breath fumes. Hold breath until self-contained breathing apparatus can be put on.
- Avoid touching any contaminated areas.

- Wear rubber gloves.

- Use protective goggles.

STEP THREE: ADMINISTER FIRST AID

- Quickly move to an area where fresh air is available.

- Supplemental oxygen should be provided for hypoxic or dyspneic (labored breathing) patients.

- Remove contacts lenses, if worn.

- Rinse CA-exposed skin with copious water and soap.

- Rinse eyes with tap water for 10 to 15 minutes.

- Eyes can also be liberally irrigated with sterile saline or Lactated Ringers solution.

- Remove any clothing that may have CA on it. Any clothing that must be pulled over the head should be cut off the body instead.

BZ (INCAPACITATING AGENT)

OVERVIEW (FOR FURTHER DETAILS, SEE PAGE 202)

- Most likely to be inhaled as an aerosolized solid or dissolved for ingestion or absorption through the skin.

- Effects may appear within a few minutes or up to 36 hours after exposure, depending on route of absorption.

- Symptoms may last up to 96 hours.

STEP ONE: IDENTIFY ACUTE HAZARDS/SIGNS/SYMPTOMS

- Hallucinations

- Impaired reasoning or judgment

- Agitation

- Dilated pupils

- Blurred vision

- Urinary retention

- Bowel obstruction

- Elevated temperature and blood pressure

- Rapid heart beat

- Dry mucous membranes

- Dry skin

- Rapid heart beat

STEP TWO: PROTECT YOURSELF

- If aerosolized BZ is suspected, put on self-contained breathing apparatus before entering contaminated area.

STEP THREE: ADMINISTER FIRST AID

- Seek immediate medical attention.

CHLORINE
(CHOKING/PULMONARY AGENT)

OVERVIEW (FOR FURTHER DETAILS, SEE PAGE 186)

- One of the 10 most produced industrial chemicals in the U.S.

- At room temperature, greenish-yellow gas.

- Reacts with water to form hydrochloric acid and hypochlorous acid.

- Distinctive, irritating odor usually prompts victims to flee contaminated area.

- Heavier than air.

- As a terrorism agent, most likely to be dispersed as a gas from a transport vessel or large facility.

STEP ONE: IDENTIFY ACUTE HAZARDS/SIGNS/SYMPTOMS

- Mucous membrane irritation within approximately one hour of exposure

- Respiratory tract irritation

- Chest pain

- Coughing

- Wheezing

- Vomiting

- Irritation

- Conjunctivitis

- Corneal abrasion

- Massive exposure to high concentrations may result in death

STEP TWO: PROTECT YOURSELF

- Wear self-contained breathing apparatus when entering an area where chlorine gas is suspected.

STEP THREE: ADMINISTER FIRST AID

- Transport victim from contaminated area.
- Give supportive treatment of airway.
- Administer oxygen as needed.
- Irrigate with most available neutral fluid (e.g., water).
- Transport victim to medical care.

CHLOROACETOPHENONE (RIOT CONTROL AGENT)

OVERVIEW (FOR FURTHER DETAILS, SEE PAGE 230)

- Chloroacetophenone (CN)) is a white to grayish crystalline solid.
- In vapor form, emits an odor resembling apple blossoms.
- A tear gas that tends to collect in low-lying areas.
- Can be absorbed into the body via inhalation and mucous membrane contact.
- Targets eyes, skin, mucous membranes, and lungs.
- Most effects are of limited duration and usually resolve within 30 to 60 minutes following evacuation and decontamination.
- With longer and more intense exposure, noncardiogenic pulmonary edema may occur.

STEP ONE: IDENTIFY ACUTE HAZARDS/SIGNS/SYMPTOMS

- Irritation of the throat occurs rapidly
- Cough, hoarseness, chest tightness, and sensation of suffocation
- Nausea, vomiting, and headache are commonly reported
- Irritation on moist and sensitive areas of the skin
- Redness, pain, and blistering of exposed skin
- Irritation and tearing of the eyes occurs rapidly
- Redness, blurred vision, and corneal burns

STEP TWO: PROTECT YOURSELF

- Do not breathe fumes. Hold breath until self-contained breathing apparatus can be put on.

- Avoid touching any contaminated areas.

- Wear rubber gloves.

- Use protective goggles if eyes are not otherwise shielded.

STEP THREE: ADMINISTER FIRST AID

- Quickly move to an area where fresh air is available.

- Remove any clothing that may have CN on it. Any clothing that must be pulled over the head should be cut off the body instead.

- Wash any agent from the skin with copious soap and water.

- Remove contact lenses, if worn.

- Rinse eyes with plain water for 10 to 15 minutes.

- Eyes can be liberally irrigated with sterile saline or Lactated Ringers solution.

- Supplemental oxygen should be provided for hypoxic or dyspneic (labored breathing) patients.

- Seek immediate medical attention.

CHLOROBENZYLIDENEMALONONITIRILE (RIOT CONTROL AGENT)

OVERVIEW (FOR FURTHER DETAILS, SEE PAGE 232)

- A white to grayish crystalline solid that is typically dispersed as an aerosol or in conjunction with an incendiary device.

- As a vapor at low concentrations, its odor has been described as resembling that of pepper.

- Targets eyes, skin, mucous membranes, and lungs.

- Most effects are of limited duration and usually resolve within 30 to 60 minutes following evacuation and decontamination.

- With longer and more intense exposure, noncardiogenic pulmonary edema may occur.

STEP ONE: IDENTIFY ACUTE HAZARDS/SIGNS/SYMPTOMS

- Irritation of the nose and throat occurs rapidly

- Cough, hoarseness, chest tightness, and sensation of suffocation

- Nausea, vomiting, and headache are commonly reported

- Irritation on moist and sensitive areas of the skin

- Redness, pain, and blistering of exposed skin

- Irritation and tearing of the eyes occurs rapidly

- Redness, blurred vision, and corneal burns

STEP TWO: PROTECT YOURSELF

- Do not breathe fumes. Hold breath until self-contained breathing apparatus can be put on.

- Avoid touching any contaminated areas.

- Wear rubber gloves.

- Use protective goggles if eyes are not otherwise protected.

STEP THREE: ADMINISTER FIRST AID

- Quickly move to an area where fresh air is available.

- Supplemental oxygen should be provided for hypoxic or dyspneic (labored breathing) patients.

- Remove any clothing that may have agent on it. Any clothing that must be pulled over the head should be cut off the body instead.

- Wash any agent from the skin with large amounts of soap and water.

- Remove contact lenses, if worn.

- Rinse eyes with plain water for 10 to 15 minutes.

- Eyes can be liberally irrigated with sterile saline or Lactated Ringers solution.

- Seek immediate medical attention.

CHLOROPICRIN (RIOT CONTROL AGENT)

OVERVIEW (FOR FURTHER DETAILS, SEE PAGE 234)

- A colorless liquid with an oily consistency and a strong, pungent odor.

- Can be absorbed into the body via inhalation, ingestion, and mucous membrane contact.

- Targets eyes, skin, mucous membranes, and lungs.

- Most effects are of limited duration and usually resolve within 30 to 60 minutes following evacuation and decontamination.

- With longer and more intense exposure, lung injury and pulmonary edema may occur. Death from acute pulmonary edema has been reported.

STEP ONE: IDENTIFY ACUTE HAZARDS/SIGNS/SYMPTOMS

- Irritation of the nose and throat occurs rapidly.

- Cough, hoarseness, chest tightness, and sensation of suffocation.

- Nausea, vomiting, and headache are commonly reported.

- Irritation on moist and sensitive areas of the skin.

- Redness, pain, and blistering of exposed skin.

- Irritation and tearing of the eyes occurs rapidly.

- Redness, blurred vision, and corneal burns.

STEP TWO: PROTECT YOURSELF

- Do not breathe fumes. Hold breath until self-contained breathing apparatus can be put on.

- Avoid touching any contaminated areas.

- Wear rubber gloves.

- Use protective goggles if eyes are not otherwise protected.

STEP THREE: ADMINISTER FIRST AID

- Quickly move to an area where fresh air is available.

- Supplemental oxygen should be provided for hypoxic or dyspneic (labored breathing) patients.

- Remove contact lenses, if worn.

- Rinse eyes with plain water for 10 to 15 minutes.

- Eyes can be liberally irrigated with sterile saline or Lactated Ringers solution.

- Remove any clothing that may have agent on it. Any clothing that must be pulled over the head should be cut off the body instead.

- Wash any agent from the skin with liberal amounts of soap and water.

- Seek immediate medical attention.

CYANIDE (BLOOD AGENT)

OVERVIEW (FOR FURTHER DETAILS, SEE PAGE 178)

- Fast-acting and potentially deadly chemical. Can be a colorless gas or in crystal (salt) form.

- Sometimes said to have a bitter almond smell. Does not always give off an odor and cannot be detected by everyone.

- As a bioweapon, may be released as a gas or vapor or used in conjunction with various explosive devices. May also be used to taint consumer products or food. Not likely to be used to contaminate water supplies due to logistical problems.

- Exposure occurs by breathing air, drinking water, eating food, or touching soil that contains cyanide. Extent of poisoning depends on amount released, route of exposure, and length of exposure time.

- Breathing the gas causes the most harm and is most dangerous when trapped in enclosed places. Swallowing cyanide can be toxic as well.

- The gas is less harmful outdoors. It is less dense than air and will rise and disperse quickly in open spaces.

- Cyanide prevents cells from using oxygen and is most harmful to the heart and brain. Death can occur rapidly (within minutes) following inhalational exposure.

- Antidotes to cyanide poisoning do exist, but immediate treatment is essential. Potential for survival is good if victim arrives at the hospital with intact vital signs.

STEP ONE: IDENTIFY ACUTE HAZARDS/SIGNS/SYMPTOMS

- Signs may occur within minutes. Symptoms of mild poisoning include:
  - Rapid breathing
  - Restlessness
  - Dizziness
  - Headache
  - Nausea and vomiting
  - Mucosal irritation
- Severe effects may include:
  - Low blood pressure
  - Difficulty breathing
  - Rapid heartbeat
  - Slow heart rate
  - Loss of consciousness
  - Seizures
  - Death

STEP TWO: PROTECT YOURSELF

- Wear face mask or shield.

- Do not breathe contaminated air. Hold breath until gas mask can be put on. Without protection, avoid the area. (Cyanide is lighter than air, so its volatility limits its toxicity in the open air).

- Wear gloves, booties, and other protective clothing.

- If you are helping other people remove their clothing, avoid touching contaminated areas.

- Afterward, remove your clothing quickly and follow procedures listed below.

- If exposure occurs:

  - Quickly move to an area with fresh air

  - Remove clothing quickly. Do not pull clothing over your head. Cut it off the body and place in a plastic bag

  - Remove jewelry and thoroughly wash with soap and water, if possible. If not, it should be placed in a plastic bag with contaminated clothing

  - Quickly wash entire body with soap and water

  - Seek medical help immediately

- If exposure occurs:

  - Rinse eyes thoroughly with water for 10 to 15 minutes

  - Remove contacts and dispose of them in a plastic bag

  - Wash eyeglasses thoroughly with soap and water. After washing, you can put your glasses back on

  - Seek medical help immediately

STEP THREE: ADMINISTER FIRST AID

- Quickly move victim to an area with fresh air.

- If breathing is labored, give oxygen.

- If breathing has stopped, give artificial respiration. *Give mouth to mouth only when facial contamination is absent.*

- See Step Two for decontamination procedures.

DIBENZOXAZEPINE (RIOT CONTROL AGENT)

OVERVIEW (FOR FURTHER DETAILS, SEE PAGE 236)

- A micro-particulate solid that is usually dispersed as an aerosol.

- Could be dispersed via an incendiary device (tear gas bomb or grenade).

- Can be absorbed into the body via inhalation, ingestion, and mucous membrane contact.

- Targets eyes, skin, mucous membranes, and lungs.

- Most effects are of limited duration and usually resolve within 30 to 60 minutes following evacuation and decontamination.

- Can cause asphyxiation and pulmonary edema in higher concentrations.

STEP ONE: IDENTIFY ACUTE HAZARDS/SIGNS/SYMPTOMS

- Burning eyes and tearing.

- Irritation of the nose and throat.

- Itching, pain, irritation, and redness of the skin.

- Cough, hoarseness, chest tightness, sensation of suffocation.

- Nausea, vomiting, and headache are commonly reported.

STEP TWO: PROTECT YOURSELF

- Do not breathe fumes. Hold breath until gas mask can be put on.

- Avoid touching any contaminated areas.

- Wear rubber gloves.

- Use protective goggles.

STEP THREE: ADMINISTER FIRST AID

- Quickly move to an area where fresh air is available.

- Supplemental oxygen should be provided for hypoxic or dyspneic patients.

- Remove any clothing that may have contacted the agent. Do not pull clothing over head; cut it off the body instead.

- Wash any agent from the skin with large amounts of soap and water. Note: this agent is not inactivated by washing, so make sure any decontamination waste water does not come in contact with patients, health care providers, or you.

- Remove contact lenses, if worn.

- Rinse eyes with plain water for 10 to 15 minutes.

- Eyes can be liberally irrigated with sterile saline or Lactated Ringers solution.

FENTANYL
(INCAPACITATING AGENT)

OVERVIEW (FOR FURTHER DETAILS, SEE PAGE 203)

- An intravenous anesthetic containing an analgesic potency 80 times that of morphine.

- Exposure typically occurs through ingestion, but potentially can result from inhalation.

- Clinical effects include lethargy or coma, decreased respiratory rate, pupil contraction, and possibly apnea (cessation of breathing).

- The biological effects of fentanyl are indistinguishable from those of heroin, with the exception that fentanyl may be hundreds of times more potent.

STEP ONE: IDENTIFY ACUTE HAZARDS/SIGNS/SYMPTOMS

- Large numbers of people from the same general location (such as a mall or theater) with similar symptoms, which may include:

  - Nausea and vomiting

  - Severe respiratory depression

  - Low blood pressure

  - Slow heart rate

  - Chest-wall rigidity

  - Seizures

STEP TWO: PROTECT YOURSELF

- Administer standard protective measures.

STEP THREE: ADMINISTER FIRST AID

- Remove victims from suspected area of contamination.

- Promptly administer naloxone, a specific antidote for opioid toxicity.

- Naloxone can be given IV, IM, under the tongue, or endotracheally, depending upon the clinical situation.

HYDROCHLORIC ACID
(ACID/CHOKING/PULMONARY AGENT)

OVERVIEW (FOR FURTHER DETAILS, SEE PAGE 173)

- Usually found as a colorless liquid with a pungent odor.

- May be dispersed as an aerosolized mist.

- May be mixed with bleach or other chemicals to liberate chlorine gas.

- Exposure possible by inhalation, ingestion; dermal and ocular damage also possible.

- Heavier than air.

STEP ONE: IDENTIFY ACUTE HAZARDS/SIGNS/SYMPTOMS

- Irritation of mucous membranes and airways

- Coughing or choking

- Hoarseness

- Ulceration of nose, throat, respiratory tract

- In severe cases, signs include:
  - Noncardiogenic pulmonary edema
  - Circulatory failure
  - Accumulation of fluid in lungs
  - Death

- If ingested, hydrochloric acid may induce:
  - Pain and burns in mouth, throat, esophagus, and GI tract
  - Nausea, vomiting, and diarrhea

- Skin contact will cause:
  - Redness
  - Pain

STEP TWO: PROTECT YOURSELF

- **NOTE:** Rescuers should be trained and use appropriate protective gear. If proper equipment or attire is not available, or if rescuers have not been properly trained, seek assistance from hazmat personnel or other properly equipped response teams.

- Wear self-contained breathing apparatus.

- Wear chemical protection clothing.

- Avoid contact with contaminated clothing or skin of victim.

STEP THREE: ADMINISTER FIRST AID

- Transport victim from contaminated area to medical facility, but *only after decontamination*.

- Decontaminate with copious amounts of soap and water.

- Administer supportive care, with special attention to airway.

- Administer humidified oxygen.

- Administer advanced life support protocols for patients who are comatose, hypotensive, or seizing.

- If applicable, irrigate eyes with tepid water or saline.

- Remove contact lenses, if worn. Avoid causing further trauma to eye.

- If ingestion is suspected:

  - DO NOT induce vomiting.

  - DO NOT administer activated charcoal.

  - If victim is able to swallow, give 4 to 8 ounces water or milk (2 to 4 ounces for children).

  - Administer advanced life support protocols for patients who are comatose, hypotensive, or seizing.

  - Prepare ambulance with towels and plastic bags to clean up and isolate vomitus.

  - Transport victim to medical care.

HYDROFLUORIC ACID (ACID)

OVERVIEW (FOR FURTHER DETAILS, SEE PAGE 174)

- Can be a colorless gas or fuming liquid. Has a strong, irritating odor.

- Exposure generally occurs by inhalation. However, ingestion and exposure to skin and eyes are also a concern.

- As a bioweapon it could be released into the air as a gas by damaging an industrial storage facility or transport vehicle.

- Can be absorbed easily and quickly through the skin and into body tissues. Once absorbed, it can damage cells and interfere with their function, leading to serious complications and possibly death.

- Severity depends on amount, route, and length of exposure, as well as age and pre-existing medical conditions.

- Breathing hydrofluoric acid can burn lung tissue and cause buildup of fluid in the lungs.

- Skin contact may cause severe burns that develop after several hours and eventually form skin ulcers (open sores).

- Pain that occurs with hydrofluoric acid exposure is often described as a deep, burning pain, possibly due to cell and nervous system dysfunction.

- Treatment consists of neutralizing the effects of poisoning by giving calcium gluconate gels, solutions, and medications, along with other supportive measures.

STEP ONE: IDENTIFY ACUTE HAZARDS/SIGNS/SYMPTOMS

- Exposure to eyes may cause:
  - Rapid onset of eye irritation and pain
  - Conjunctival injection, corneal abrasion, opaque corneas
- Inhalation may cause:
  - Difficulty breathing with airway irritation and burning.
  - Fluid buildup in the lungs, leading to loss of breathing and death.
  - Irregular or fast heartbeat, or extremely low blood pressure, possibly leading to death.
- Skin contact may cause:
  - Local irritation and chemical burns.

STEP TWO: PROTECT YOURSELF

- **NOTE:** Rescuers should be trained and use appropriate protective gear. If proper equipment or attire is not available, or if rescuers have not been properly trained, seek assistance from hazmat personnel or other properly equipped response teams.

- Wear self-contained breathing apparatus.

- Wear chemical protection clothing.

- Avoid contact with contaminated clothing or skin of victim

STEP THREE: ADMINISTER FIRST AID

- Transport victim from contaminated area to medical facility, but *only after decontamination*.

- Decontaminate with copious amounts of soap and water.

- Administer supportive care, with special attention to airway.

- Quickly remove victims' clothing, avoiding contaminated areas as much as possible. Do not pull clothing over the head. Cut it off the body.

- Administer humidified oxygen.

- Administer advanced life support protocols for patients who are comatose, hypotensive, or seizing.

- Treat bronchospasm with inhaled beta agonists or parenteral steroids.

- Treat skin exposure with calcium gluconate or calcium carbonate gel 2.5% to 3.3% concentration.

- Do not give mouth to mouth resuscitation unless you are sure facial and oral contamination are not present .

- If agent is in victim's eyes:

  - Rinse eyes thoroughly with water for 10 to 15 minutes.

  - Remove contacts and dispose of them in a plastic bag.

  - Remove eyeglasses and wash thoroughly with soap and water. After washing, victim can put the glasses back on.

  - Seek ophthalmic consultation immediately.

LEWISITE (BLISTER AGENT)

OVERVIEW (FOR FURTHER DETAILS, SEE PAGE 241)

- Blister agent that causes blistering of the skin and mucous membrane on contact. Can cause systemic poisoning leading to shock and death.

- Pure form is an oily, colorless, and odorless liquid. It can appear amber to black in its impure form. It has a strong geranium odor.

- Can be absorbed into the body by all routes.

- Short-term exposure: large skin burns and possibly lung edema, diarrhea, restlessness, subnormal temperature, and low blood pressure.

- Long-term or repeated exposure: chronic lung impairment.

STEP ONE: IDENTIFY ACUTE HAZARDS/SIGNS/SYMPTOMS

- Immediate burning pain and irritation

- Skin redness within 30 minutes with pain and itching for 24 hours

- Blisters within 12-18 hours

- Gray-appearing areas of dead skin may be visible

- Intense eyelid spasms

- Eye pain

- Restlessness, weakness

- Subnormal temperature

- Low blood pressure

- Shock

STEP TWO: PROTECT YOURSELF

- Do not breathe fumes. Hold breath until self-contained breathing apparatus is put on.

- Use protective gloves, chemical goggles, and face shield to avoid injury.

STEP THREE: ADMINISTER FIRST AID

- If breathing is labored, administer oxygen.

- If breathing has stopped, administer artificial respiration.

- Do not give mouth to mouth resuscitation unless you are sure facial and oral contamination are not present.

- Immediately flush contaminated area with water for 10-15 minutes.

- Washing with soap and water is the primary mode for decontamination.

- 0.5% hypochlorite solution can be used.

- Transport to medical facility immediately.

- If agent is in victim's eyes:

  - Rinse eyes thoroughly with water for 10 to 15 minutes.

  - Remove contact lenses, if worn, and dispose of them in a plastic bag.

  - Remove eyeglasses, if worn, and wash thoroughly with soap and water. After washing, the person can put glasses back on.

  - Seek ophthalmic consultation immediately.

METHYL BROMIDE (CHOKING/PULMONARY AGENT)

OVERVIEW (FOR FURTHER DETAILS, SEE PAGE 191)

- Colorless and odorless, a gas at room temperature.

- At high concentrations, it may have odor similar to chloroform.

- Poisoning occurs usually through inhalation, but concurrent dermal exposure is possible.

- Onset of symptoms may be delayed up to 48 hours.

- Heavier than air.

STEP ONE: IDENTIFY ACUTE HAZARDS/SIGNS/SYMPTOMS

- Irritation of eyes, skin, respiratory tract, and mucous membranes
- Shortness of breath
- Muscle weakness
- Lack of muscular coordination
- Slurred speech
- Visual problems
- Nausea and vomiting
- Impaired gate
- Impaired sense of touch
- Dizziness
- Headache
- Tremors
- Seizures
- Respiratory failure

STEP TWO: PROTECT YOURSELF

- Wear self-contained breathing apparatus (SCBA) with full face piece.
- Wear chemical protection clothing, including boots and gloves.
- Avoid contact with contaminated skin or clothing of victim.

STEP THREE: ADMINISTER FIRST AID

- Transport victim from contaminated area to medical facility *after decontamination*.
- Remove contaminated clothing, including footwear, and double-bag.
- Flush skin and hair with copious water.
- Administer supportive care (airway maintenance, ventilation, cardiac monitoring).
- Administer oxygen as needed.
- Administer pulse oximetry, as needed.
- Treat patients who are comatose, hypotensive, seizing, or in arrhythmia with advanced life support protocols.
- Remove contact lenses, if worn, avoiding additional eye trauma.

METHYL ISOCYANATE (CHOKING/PULMONARY AGENT)

OVERVIEW (FOR FURTHER DETAILS, SEE PAGE 192)

- Colorless liquid with sharp, pungent odor.

- Exposure usually occurs through inhalation; dermal absorption and ocular exposure are also possible.

- Effects may progress over 72 hours.

- Vapor is heavier than air.

- Most likely to be dispersed as an aerosol as a chemical weapon.

STEP ONE: IDENTIFY ACUTE HAZARDS/SIGNS/SYMPTOMS

- Burning eyes and tearing

- Coughing

- Nausea

- Vomiting

- Abdominal pain

- Diarrhea

STEP TWO: PROTECT YOURSELF

- Wear self-contained breathing apparatus (SCBA) with full face piece

- Wear chemical-protection clothing

- Wear protective eye gear

- Avoid contact with contaminated skin or clothing of victim.

- **NOTE:** Rescuers should be trained and use appropriate protective gear. If proper equipment or attire is not available, or if rescuers have not been properly trained, seek assistance from hazmat personnel or other properly equipped response teams.

STEP THREE: ADMINISTER FIRST AID

- Transport victim from contaminated area to medical facility *after decontamination*.

- Remove contaminated clothing, including footwear, and double-bag.

- Flush skin and hair with copious water and soap.

- Administer oxygen as needed.

- Administer mechanical ventilation as needed.

- Treatment patients who are comatose, hypotensive, or seizing according to advanced life support protocols.

- Remove contact lenses, if worn, avoiding additional trauma.

- Treat bronchospasm with beta agonists.

- Eye exposures should be irrigated, then treated with topical anesthetics and mydratics for comfort.

MUSTARD GAS (BLISTER AGENT)

OVERVIEW (FOR FURTHER DETAILS, SEE PAGE 242)

- A photograph of a mustard gas victim can be found at the end of this section.

- Can be a vapor or liquid. Severe irritant. Contact may be fatal.

- Pure liquid is colorless and odorless. Forms yellow prisms on cooling. Agent grade material is yellow to dark brown or black and the odor may be reminiscent of burning garlic, onions, or mustard.

- Can be absorbed into the body by all routes. Tender skin, mucous membranes, and perspiration-covered skin are more sensitive to the effects.

- Blister agent (chlorinated compound) that damages tissues of eyes, skin, and respiratory tract. Skin healing process is very slow. Exposure to nearly lethal doses can injure the bone marrow, lymph nodes, and spleen, causing a drop in white blood cell counts and increasing infection risk.

- Detoxification rate is very slow. Repeated or long-term exposure causes chronic lung impairment (cough, shortness of breath, chest pain); cancer of the mouth, throat, respiratory tract, and skin; and leukemia. Birth defects possible.

STEP ONE: IDENTIFY ACUTE HAZARDS/SIGNS/SYMPTOMS

- Foreign-body sensation in eyes

- Eye pain, redness, and swelling

- Tearing

- Light sensitivity

- Reddening, swelling, and yellow blisters (small to very large) in 4-24 hours

- Warm, moist, thin-skinned areas most sensitive to this agent

- Dry/barking cough

- Asthma

- Hemorrhage and necrosis of lung tissue resulting in coughing up blood

- Difficulty breathing

- Nausea and vomiting

- Diarrhea and abdominal pain

- Dizziness

- Malaise

- Lethargy

STEP TWO: PROTECT YOURSELF

- Do not breathe fumes. Hold breath until self-contained breathing apparatus and (ideally) oxygen tank can be put on. Without protection, avoid the area.

- Use special gloves, clothing, and boots to avoid injury.

- Use chemical goggles and face shield to avoid injury.

- Do not eat, drink, or smoke during work. Afterward, wash hands well before eating.

STEP THREE: ADMINISTER FIRST AID

- Remove victim from source of exposure.

- If breathing is labored, give oxygen.

- If breathing has stopped, give artificial respiration.

Do not give mouth to mouth resuscitation unless you are sure facial and oral contamination are not present.

- Immediately remove contaminated clothing and wash exposed area thoroughly with soap and water.

- Contaminated clothing can expose others through direct or off-gassing vapor and should be triple-bagged.

- Do not cover with bandages.

- Affix dark or opaque goggles to victims to ease lightsensitivity and irritation.

- Do not induce vomiting.

- Give milk to drink.

- Transport to medical facility immediately

OLEORESIN CAPSICUM AND CAPSAICIN (INCAPACITATING AGENTS)

OVERVIEW (FOR FURTHER DETAILS, SEE PAGE 204)

- Most commonly referred to as "pepper spray."

- Amber orange to light orange brown liquid.

- Exposure causes irritation to skin, eyes, and mucous membranes of the upper respiratory tract; may cause inflammation. Repeated contact may cause allergic dermatological reaction.

- Induces coughing, gagging, and shortness of breath, as well as a small but significant increase in blood pressure.

- Exposure and inhalation do not result in significant risk for respiratory compromise or asphyxiation.

STEP ONE: IDENTIFY ACUTE HAZARDS/SIGNS/SYMPTOMS

- – Rapid onset of eye and throat irritation

- – Severe burning sensation in the eyes with copious tears

- – Nausea and vomiting

- – Headache

- – Irritation of moist and sensitive skin areas

- The above effects are of limited duration and usually resolve within 30-60 minutes following evacuation and decontamination:

- Asthmatics may be more sensitive and have stronger reactions to this agent.

- Asphyxia due to throat closing may occur.

STEP TWO: PROTECT YOURSELF

- Wear protective gloves.

- Use protective glasses.

STEP THREE: ADMINISTER FIRST AID

- Remove victim to well-ventilated area.

- Ask victim to remain still, breath normally, and relax as much as possible.

- Decontaminate with soap and water.

- Remove contact lenses, if worn, before flushing the eyes with water, and then thoroughly clean and soak the lenses with an appropriate cleaning solution.

- Flush victim's eyes with sterile saline or Lactated Ringers solution.

- Do not allow victim to rub eyes.

- Administer supplemental oxygen, if needed.

- Administer mechanical ventilation as needed.

OSMIUM TETROXIDE (CHOKING/PULMONARY AGENT)

OVERVIEW (FOR FURTHER DETAILS, SEE PAGE 192)

- Colorless crystalline substance or yellow solid at room temperature.
- Dispersal would most likely result from detonation of an explosive device.
- Could be used to contaminate food or water.

STEP ONE: IDENTIFY ACUTE HAZARDS/SIGNS/SYMPTOMS

- Burning sensation
- Irritation to mucus membranes and lungs
- Cough
- Headache
- Wheezing
- Shortness of breath
- Visual disturbances or vision loss
- Redness
- Pain
- Dark discoloration
- Blisters
- Blurred vision
- Abdominal cramps
- Shock
- Collapse

STEP TWO: PROTECT YOURSELF

- Put on self-contained breathing apparatus before entering an area where agent may have been dispersed.
- Wear protective clothing and gloves.
- Wear goggles if eyes are not otherwise protected.

STEP THREE: ADMINISTER FIRST AID

- Remove victim to fresh air.

- Settle victim in half-upright position.

- Administer artificial respiration as needed.

- Remove contaminated clothing.

- Decontaminate with large amounts of water and, if available, soap.

- If worn, contact lenses should be carefully removed to prevent further trauma.

- Seek immediate medical care.

PHOSGENE (CHOKING/PULMONARY AGENT)

OVERVIEW (FOR FURTHER DETAILS, SEE PAGE 193)

- Colorless gas with an odor similar to moldy hay or green corn.

- Exposure most likely to occur by inhalation.

- Heavier than air.

- Onset of symptoms may be delayed for several hours.

- Lung swelling may occur up to a day following exposure.

STEP ONE: IDENTIFY ACUTE HAZARDS/SIGNS/SYMPTOMS

- Nose irritation

- Throat irritation

- Lower respiratory irritation

- Headache

- Nausea

- Irritation

- Burning

STEP TWO: PROTECT YOURSELF

- Don self-contained breathing apparatus before entering area where agent is suspected.

STEP THREE: ADMINISTER FIRST AID

- Remove victim to fresh air.

- Administer oxygen as needed.

- Remove contaminated clothing.

- Decontaminate with copious amounts of water.

- Transport to medical care.

PHOSGENE OXIME (URTICANT/NETTLE AGENT)

OVERVIEW (FOR FURTHER DETAILS, SEE PAGE 239)

- Colorless in its solid form.

- As a liquid, yellowish-brown with a disagreeable odor.

- Readily absorbed by skin, causing immediate corrosive lesion.

- Severe pain and irritation occur immediately on eye contact.

STEP ONE: IDENTIFY ACUTE HAZARDS/SIGNS/SYMPTOMS

- Immediate irritation to the upper respiratory tract

- Runny nose, hoarseness, and sinus pain

- May result in fluid accumulation in the lungs, shortness of breath, and cough

- Immediate pain and local tissue destruction on contact

- Whitening of the skin surrounded by red rings within 30 seconds

- Within 15 minutes, skin develops hives

- Severe pain and local tissue destruction on contact

- Tearing and temporary blindness

- Inflammation on cornea resulting in burning pain and blurry vision

STEP TWO: PROTECT YOURSELF

- Do not breathe fumes. Hold breath until self-contained breathing apparatus can be put on.

- To avoid injury, personal protection equipment and special gloves must be worn at all times.

- Chemical goggles and face shield are needed if face is not otherwise protected.

STEP THREE: ADMINISTER FIRST AID

- Self-contained breathing apparatus for victim is recommended.

- Gas mask for victim is recommended.

- Seek medical help at once.

- Immediately remove contaminated clothing.

- Wash exposed area with liberal amounts of soap and water for 15 minutes.

- Remove contact lenses, if worn, and dispose.

- Do not induce vomiting. Treat nausea and vomiting with antiemetics.

- Give milk or water to swallow.

- Seek medical help at once.

PHOSPHINE (CHOKING/PULMONARY AGENT)

OVERVIEW (FOR FURTHER DETAILS, SEE PAGE 195)

- Colorless gas, usually odorless, but may have a fishy or garlicky odor.

- Exposure most likely to be via inhalation.

- Some symptoms (e.g., pulmonary edema) may be delayed by as much as a day.

- Heavier than air.

- **NOTE:** Rescuers should be trained and use appropriate protective gear. If proper equipment or attire is not available, or if rescuers have not been properly trained, seek assistance from hazmat personnel or other properly equipped response teams.

STEP ONE: IDENTIFY ACUTE HAZARDS/SIGNS/SYMPTOMS

- Chest tightness

- Cough

- Shortness of breath

- Nausea

- Abdominal pain

- Vomiting

- Diarrhea

- Dizziness

- At high concentration, death

STEP TWO: PROTECT YOURSELF

- Off-gassing from victims to first responders a major concern.

- Wear self-contained breathing apparatus.

- Wear rubber gloves.

- Wear rubber apron, if available.

STEP THREE: ADMINISTER FIRST AID

- Transport victim from contaminated area.

- Treat patients who are comatose, hypotensive, or seizing with advanced life support protocols.

- Flush exposed skin with water for 3 to 5 minutes, then wash with mild soap.

- Continue irrigating as needed.

- Transport to medical care *only after decontamination.*

PHOSPHORUS (CHOKING/PULMONARY AGENT)

OVERVIEW (FOR FURTHER DETAILS, SEE PAGE 196)

- Colorless or slightly yellow solid.

- Extremely flammable.

- May be inhaled, absorbed through the skin, or ingested.

STEP ONE: IDENTIFY ACUTE HAZARDS/SIGNS/SYMPTOMS

- Burns to skin

- Burns to mucous membranes

- Burns to lungs

- Anxiety

- Restlessness

- Confusion

- Severe abdominal pain

- Vomiting (vomitus may be smoking or luminescent)

- Diarrhea (stool may be smoking)

- Coma

- Death

STEP TWO: PROTECT YOURSELF

- Wearing self-contained breathing apparatus, personal protection equipment, and gloves is essential.

STEP THREE: ADMINISTER FIRST AID

- Transport victim from contaminated area.

- Administer oxygen as needed.

- Remove clothing and wash exposed skin with soap and water.

- Flush eyes with copious water.

- Continue irrigation as needed.

- Administer topical anesthetics and mydriatics for comfort.

- Administer charcoal if agent was ingested.

- Seek immediate medical attention.

SARIN (NERVE AGENT)

OVERVIEW (FOR FURTHER DETAILS, SEE PAGE 215)

- Nerve agents as a group are the most toxic of the known chemical warfare agents.

- Sarin the most volatile nerve agent. Reacts with steam or water to produce toxic and corrosive vapors.

- Colorless liquid.

- Odorless in pure form.

- Can be absorbed in the body by all routes.

- Only a slight difference between a fatal dose and a dose that produces more mild health effects.

- Death usually occurs within 15 minutes after absorption of a fatal dose.

- **NOTE:** Off-gassing agent for about 30 minutes after victim contact poses hazard to first responders.

STEP ONE: IDENTIFY ACUTE HAZARDS/SIGNS/SYMPTOMS

- Symptoms may occur within minutes or hours depending on dose.

- Runny nose and tightness in the chest begin within seconds to minutes after exposure.

- Gastrointestinal symptoms may occur immediately or shortly after exposure.

- Mild exposure:

  – Runny nose

  – Chest tightness

  – Difficulty breathing

  – Eye pain

- Moderate exposure:

  – Eye symptoms such as pinpoint pupils with blurred vision

  – Drooling

  – Excessive sweating

  – Nausea

  – Vomiting

  – Severe nasal congestion

  – Headache

  – Confusion

  – Twitching of large muscle groups

- Severe exposure:

  – Involuntary defection and urination

  – Twitching

  – Jerking

  – Convulsions

  – Cessation of breathing

  – Death

STEP TWO: PROTECT YOURSELF

- Do not breathe fumes. Hold breath until self-contained breathing apparatus can be put on.

- Be aware that you can be exposed to agent via off-gassing from victim.

- Chemical goggles and face shield are needed to avoid injury if face is not otherwise protected.

- Special gloves and protective clothing are needed to avoid injury.

- Skin contact should be avoided at all times.

- Do not eat, drink, or smoke while assisting victims.

- Wash hands thoroughly before eating or smoking.

STEP THREE: ADMINISTER FIRST AID

- Give artificial respiration if breathing has stopped.

- Use mouth-to-mouth when mask-bag or oxygen delivery systems not available. *Do not use mouth-to-mouth if face is contaminated.*

- Administer oxygen if breathing is difficult.

- Do not induce vomiting. First symptoms are likely to be gastrointestinal.

- The primary mode for decontamination is soap and water. A 0.5% hypochlorite solution can be used.

- Immediately flush eyes with water for 10-15 minutes, then affix respiratory protective mask to victim.

- Immediately evacuate victims to hospital.

SODIUM MONOFLUOROACETATE (BLOOD AGENT)

OVERVIEW (FOR FURTHER DETAILS, SEE PAGE 179)

- A compound that occurs naturally in certain plants in South America, South Africa, and Australia, sodium monofluoroacetate (SMFA) can be made into an odorless, white powder.

- Easily dissolves in water.

- Normally used as rat poison and to poison livestock predators (e.g., coyotes).

- Poisoning most likely to occur by ingestion. Could also occur by exposure to the skin (through a cut or open wound), eyes, or lungs (inhalation).

- As a bioweapon, could be released into water supplies. SMFA would be potentially less harmful if released into large reservoirs due to dilution. If added to smaller water supplies, could result in mass casualties.

- SMFA affects the heart and central nervous system. Even low doses can be deadly.

STEP ONE: IDENTIFY ACUTE HAZARDS/SIGNS/SYMPTOMS

- Signs occur within 30 to 150 minutes; one report of signs occurring 36 hours after exposure

- Auditory hallucinations (hearing imaginary voices or sounds)

- Vomiting

- Low blood pressure

- Facial paralysis

- Muscle twitching

- Rapid heartbeat

- Fluid in the lungs

- Shock

- Heart failure, seizures, or coma, possibly leading to death.

STEP TWO: PROTECT YOURSELF

- Although exposure usually occurs via ingestion, eye, skin, and inhalation exposures are also a concern. If in doubt about nature of exposure, wear self-contained breathing apparatus, personal protection equipment, and gloves.

STEP THREE: ADMINISTER FIRST AID

- Quickly move victim to an area with fresh air.

- If breathing is labored, administer oxygen.

- If breathing has stopped, give artificial respiration. *Give mouth to mouth only when facial contamination is absent.*

- Decontaminate with copious amounts of water and, if available, soap.

- Seek medical help immediately.

SOMAN (NERVE AGENT)

OVERVIEW (FOR FURTHER DETAILS, SEE PAGE 217)

- Nerve agents are the most toxic of the known chemical warfare agents.

- When pure, Soman is a colorless liquid with a fruity odor. With impurities, amber or dark brown in color with a camphor odor.

- Can be absorbed in the body by all routes.

- Reacts with steam or water to produce toxic and corrosive vapors. Liquids or vapors can be fatal.

STEP ONE: IDENTIFY ACUTE HAZARDS/SIGNS/SYMPTOMS

- Symptoms may occur within minutes or hours depending on dose.

- Runny nose and tightness in the chest begin within seconds to minutes after exposure.

- Gastrointestinal symptoms may occur immediately or shortly after exposure.

- Mild exposure:

  - Runny nose

  - Chest tightness

- Difficulty breathing

- Eye pain

- Moderate exposure:

  - Eye symptoms such as pinpoint pupils with blurred vision

  - Drooling

  - Excessive sweating

  - Nausea

  - Vomiting

  - Severe nasal congestion

  - Headache

  - Confusion

  - Twitching of large muscle groups

- Severe exposure:

  - Involuntary defection and urination

  - Twitching

  - Jerking

  - Convulsions

  - Cessation of breathing

  - Death

STEP TWO: PROTECT YOURSELF

- Do not breathe fumes. Hold breath until self-contained breathing apparatus can be put on.

- Be aware that you can be exposed to agent via off-gassing from victim.

- Chemical goggles and face shield are needed to avoid injury if face is not otherwise protected.

- Special gloves and protective clothing are needed to avoid injury.

- Skin contact should be avoided at all times.

- Do not eat, drink, or smoke while assisting victims.

- Wash hands thoroughly before eating or smoking.

STEP THREE: ADMINISTER FIRST AID

- Give artificial respiration if breathing has stopped.

- Use mouth-to-mouth when mask-bag or oxygen delivery systems not available.
  Do not use mouth-to-mouth if face is contaminated.

- Administer oxygen if breathing is difficult.

- Do not induce vomiting. First symptoms are likely to be gastrointestinal.

- The primary mode for decontamination is soap and water. A 0.5% hypochlorite solution can be used.

- Immediately flush eyes with water for 10-15 minutes, then affix respiratory protective mask to victim.

- Immediately evacuate victims to hospital.

SULFURYL FLUORIDE (CHOKING/PULMONARY AGENT)

OVERVIEW (FOR FURTHER DETAILS, SEE PAGE 198)

- Colorless, odorless gas.

- Exposure usually occurs via inhalation, but may also effect skin and eyes.

- Intentional release would likely involve aerosolization.

- Heavier than air. Collects in low-lying areas.

STEP ONE: IDENTIFY ACUTE HAZARDS/SIGNS/SYMPTOMS

- Respiratory irritation

- Irritation of eyes, nose, and throat

- Cough

- Excessive tearing

- Nausea, vomiting

- Diarrhea

- Altered mental status (i.e., depression)

- Seizure

- In severe exposure, cardiac dysrhythmias and possibly cardiac arrest

STEP TWO: PROTECT YOURSELF

- If entering potentially contaminated area, put on self-contained breathing apparatus.

- Wear goggles and face shield if face is not otherwise protected.

STEP THREE: ADMINISTER FIRST AID

- Transport victim from contaminated area.

- Administer oxygen as needed.

- Remove clothing and wash exposed areas with soap and water.

- Administer topical anesthetics and mydriatics for comfort.

- Seek immediate medical assistance.

TABUN (NERVE AGENT)

OVERVIEW (FOR FURTHER DETAILS, SEE PAGE 219)

- Nerve agents are the most toxic of the known chemical warfare agents.

- Tabun is a colorless to brown liquid with faintly fruity odor. Odorless in pure form.

- Can be absorbed in the body by all routes.

- Liquid or vapor can be fatal.

- Contaminated clothing releases agent for about 30 minutes after contact with vapor.

- **NOTE:** Off-gassing agent after victim contact poses hazard to first responders.

STEP ONE: IDENTIFY ACUTE HAZARDS/SIGNS/SYMPTOMS

- Symptoms may occur within minutes or hours depending on dose.

- Runny nose and tightness in the chest begin within seconds to minutes after exposure.

- Gastrointestinal symptoms may occur immediately or shortly after exposure.

- Mild exposure:

  - Runny nose

  - Chest tightness

  - Difficulty breathing

  - Eye pain

- Moderate exposure:

  - Eye symptoms such as pinpoint pupils with blurred vision

  - Drooling

  - Excessive sweating

  - Nausea

  - Vomiting

  - Severe nasal congestion

- Headache

- Confusion

- Twitching of large muscle groups

- Severe exposure:

  - Involuntary defecation and urination

  - Twitching

  - Jerking

  - Convulsions

  - Cessation of breathing

  - Death

STEP TWO: PROTECT YOURSELF

- Do not breathe fumes. Hold breath until self-contained breathing apparatus can be put on.

- Be aware that you can be exposed to agent via off-gassing from victim.

- Chemical goggles and face shield are needed to avoid injury if face is not otherwise protected.

- Special gloves and protective clothing are needed to avoid injury.

- Skin contact should be avoided at all times.

- Do not eat, drink, or smoke while assisting victims.

- Wash hands thoroughly before eating or smoking.

STEP THREE: ADMINISTER FIRST AID

- Give artificial respiration if breathing has stopped.

- Use mouth-to-mouth when mask-bag or oxygen delivery systems not available.
  Do not use mouth-to-mouth if face is contaminated.

- Administer oxygen if breathing is difficult.

- Do not induce vomiting. First symptoms are likely to be gastrointestinal.

- The primary mode for decontamination is soap and water. A 0.5% hypochlorite solution can be used.

- Immediately flush eyes with water for 10-15 minutes, then affix respiratory protective mask to victim.

- Immediately evacuate victims to hospital.

THALLIUM (METAL)

OVERVIEW (FOR FURTHER DETAILS, SEE PAGE 213)

- A trace mineral that is bluish-white in color and is both odorless and tasteless.

- Pesticide that can be potentially harmful to humans.

- Can be absorbed into the body by all routes. Exposure occurs mainly from ingesting contaminated food or water.

STEP ONE: IDENTIFY ACUTE HAZARDS/SIGNS/SYMPTOMS

- Finger and toe numbness

- Even light touching of victim may be painful

- Nausea and vomiting

- Constipation

- Temporary hair loss

- Seizure

- Delirium

- Sleep disturbances

- Stomach pain

- Coma

- Respiratory paralysis

- Death

STEP TWO: PROTECT YOURSELF

- Avoid eating food or drinking water that may be the source of thallium poisoning.

STEP THREE: ADMINISTER FIRST AID

- Seek immediate medical attention.

VX (NERVE AGENT)

OVERVIEW (FOR FURTHER DETAILS, SEE PAGE 221)

- Nerve agents are the most toxic of the known chemical warfare agents.

- Colorless to straw-colored liquid and odorless, similar in appearance to motor oil. It has low volatility unless temperatures are high.

- Can be absorbed in the body by all routes.

- Only a slight difference between a fatal dose and a dose that produces more mild health effects.

- Death usually occurs within 15 minutes after absorption of a fatal dose.

- **NOTE:** Off-gassing agent for about 30 minutes after victim contact poses hazard to first responders.

STEP ONE: IDENTIFY ACUTE HAZARDS/SIGNS/SYMPTOMS

- Symptoms may occur within minutes or hours depending on dose.

- Runny nose and tightness in the chest begin within seconds to minutes after exposure.

- Gastrointestinal symptoms may occur immediately or shortly after exposure.

- Mild exposure:

  - Runny nose

  - Chest tightness

  - Difficulty breathing

  - Eye pain

- Moderate exposure:

  - Eye symptoms such as pinpoint pupils with blurred vision

  - Drooling

  - Excessive sweating

  - Nausea

  - Vomiting

  - Severe nasal congestion

  - Headache

  - Confusion

  - Twitching of large muscle groups

- Severe exposure:

  - Involuntary defection and urination

  - Twitching

  - Jerking

  - Convulsions

  - Cessation of breathing

  - Death

STEP TWO: PROTECT YOURSELF

- Do not breathe fumes. Hold breath until self-contained breathing apparatus can be put on.

- Be aware that you can be exposed to agent via off-gassing from victim.

- Chemical goggles and face shield are needed to avoid injury if face is not otherwise protected.

- Special gloves and protective clothing are needed to avoid injury.

- Skin contact should be avoided at all times.

- Do not eat, drink, or smoke while assisting victims.

- Wash hands thoroughly before eating or smoking.

STEP THREE: ADMINISTER FIRST AID

- Give artificial respiration if breathing has stopped.

- Use mouth-to-mouth when mask-bag or oxygen delivery systems not available.
  Do not use mouth-to-mouth if face is contaminated.

- Administer oxygen if breathing is difficult.

- Do not induce vomiting. First symptoms are likely to be gastrointestinal.

- The primary mode for decontamination is soap and water. A 0.5% hypochlorite solution can be used.

- Immediately flush eyes with water for 10-15 minutes, then affix respiratory protective mask to victim.

- Immediately evacuate victims to hospital.

EXPLOSIONS

OVERVIEW (FOR FURTHER DETAILS, SEE PAGE 281)

- Bombs and explosions can cause unique patterns of injury seldom seen outside combat.

- The predominant post explosion injuries among survivors involve the standard penetrating and blunt trauma.

- Blast lung is the most common fatal injury among initial survivors.

- Half of all initial casualties will seek medical care over a one-hour period.

- Explosions in confined spaces (mines, buildings or large vehicles) and/or structural collapse are associated with greater morbidity and mortality.

SELECTED BLAST INJURIES

- Should be suspected for anyone with dyspnea (labored breathing), cough hemoptysis (blood spittle), or chest pain following blast exposure.

- Should be suspected in anyone with abdominal pain, nausea, vomiting, rectal pain, or testicular pain following blast exposure.

- Clinical signs of blast-related abdominal injuries can be initially silent until signs of acute abdomen or sepsis are advanced.

- Up to 10% of all blast survivors have significant eye injuries. Symptoms include eye pain or irritation, foreign body sensation, altered vision, periorbital swelling, or contusions.

- Signs of ear injury are usually present at time of initial evaluation and should be suspected for anyone with hearing loss, tinnitus, otalgia, vertigo, or bleeding from the external canal.

- Consider the proximity of the victim to the blast, particularly when given complaints of headache, fatigue, poor concentration, depression, or lethargy.

- A prophylactic chest tube (thorascostomy) is recommended before general anesthesia or air transport is indicated.

EMEGENCY MANAGEMENT OPTIONS

- Expect "upside-down" triage—the most severely injured arrive after the less-injured.

- If structural collapse occurs, expect increased severity and delayed arrival of casualties.

- Double the first hour's casualties for a rough prediction of total "first wave" of casualties.

- Consider the possibility of exposure to inhaled toxins and poisonings in both industrial and criminal explosions.

BURNS

OVERVIEW (FOR FURTHER DETAILS, SEE PAGE 245)

- Types of burns include thermal burns, chemical burns, and electrical burns.

- Burns are usually caused by heat (thermal burns), such as fire, steam, tar, or hot liquids.

- Burn classification include first-degree burns (involve only the top layer), second-degree burns (involve two layers of skin), and third-degree burns (penetrates the entire thickness of the skin).

STEP ONE: IDENTIFY ACUTE HAZARDS/SIGNS/SYMPTOMS

- First-degree burns:
  - Red, moist, swollen, and painful.
  - Burned area whitens (blanches) when lightly touched but does not develop blisters.
- Second-degree burns:
  - Red, swollen, and painful
  - Blisters develop that may ooze a clear fluid

- Third-degree burns:

    - Painless and involve all layers of skin

    - Areas may be charred black or appear dry and white

    - Does not whiten when lightly touched

STEP TWO: PROTECT YOURSELF

- First responders can be burned by residue from chemical burn victims. Wear gloves when touching affected areas.

- First responders can be electrocuted by electrical burn victims who are still in contact with the source. Turn off the source of electricity if possible. If that is not possible, move the source away from you and the victim by using cardboard, plastic, or wood.

STEP THREE: ADMINISTER FIRST AID

- Immediate treatment for burn victims: "Stop, Drop, and Roll" to smother flames.

- Removed all burned clothing. If clothing adheres to the skin, cut or tear around burned area.

- Remove all jewelry, belts, and tight clothing from over the burned areas and from around the victim's neck. *This is very important; burned areas swell immediately.*

- Look first. Don't touch. The person may still be in contact with the electrical source. By touching the person, it may pass to you.

- Turn off the source of electricity if possible. If it's not possible, move the source away from you and the affected person by using cardboard, plastic, or wood.

- Check for breathing once person is not contact with the electrical source. If breathing has stopped, begin CPR.

- If person is breathing, cover burned areas with sterile gauze or clean cloth. Do not use a blanket or towel.

- Flush chemicals off the skin with cool, running water for 20 minutes or longer.

- Wrap burned area with dry, sterile dressing.

- Seek medical assistance at once.

NUCLEAR/RADIATION

OVERVIEW (FOR FURTHER DETAILS, SEE PAGE 297)

- Radiation cannot be detected by the human senses.

- Exposure occurs when a victim is near a radiation source. Victim can suffer radiation illness if dose is high enough.

- Contamination occurs externally when loose particles of radioactive material are deposited on skin or clothing.

- Acute radiation syndrome is caused by high doses of radiation rapidly delivered to large portions of the body.

- Cutaneous radiation injury is acute radiation injury to the skin.

STEP ONE: IDENTIFY ACUTE HAZARDS/SIGNS/SYMPTOMS

- Acute Radiation Syndrome

  - Nausea, vomiting, possibly diarrhea (can occur minutes to days after exposure)

  - Symptoms can be immediate or delayed or mild to severe, depending on radiation dose

- Cutaneous radiation injury

  - Itching, tingling, redness, and heat sensation can occur within hours of exposure.

STEP TWO: PROTECT YOURSELF

- Wear a protective face mask with a HEPA filter to reduce inhalation of radioactive dust.

- Clothing will collect radioactive dust. Remove and discard after you leave the area. You will continue to expose others if you fail to remove clothing.

- Do not eat, drink, or smoke while exposed to radioactive dust or smoke.

- Open wounds or abrasions must be protected from radioactive contamination.

STEP THREE: ADMINISTER FIRST AID

- Survey patient with radiation meter:

  - Use consistent technique and trained personnel

  - Note exceptionally large amounts of radioactive material

  - Handle radioactive objects with forceps and store in lead containers

  - Record location and level of any contamination found

- Remove patient clothing:

  - Cut and roll clothing away from the face to contain the contamination

  - Use radioactive hazardous waste guidelines

  - Double-bag and label clothing

  - Repeat patient survey and record levels

- Cleanse contaminated areas:

  - Wash wounds with saline or water

  - Flush eyes, nose, and ears, and rinse mouth, if facial contamination occurs

- Do not irritate the skin. Gently wash intact skin with soap and water (start outside the contaminated skin and wash inward)

- Resurvey victim and note radiation levels

- Repeat washing until radiation remains unchanged or is no more than twice the background

- Use waterproof dressing to cover wounds

• Seek immediate medical attention.

NOTES

NOTES

NOTES

PART FOUR

BIOLOGICAL TERRORISM AGENTS IN DEPTH

By:
John G. Bartlett, MD
Chief, Division of Infectious Diseases
Johns Hopkins University School of Medicine
Baltimore, MD
Founding Co-Director, Center for Civilian Biodefense Strategies
Pittsburgh, PA

CDC CATEGORY A BIOTERRORISM AGENTS*

CDC CATEGORY B BIOTERRORISM AGENTS**

*Category A agents are most likely to be used by terrorists.
**Category B agents are less likely but still possible to be used by terrorists.

CDC CATEGORY A BIOLOGICAL TERRORISM AGENTS

ANTHRAX (BACILLUS ANTHRACIS)

IMPORTANT POINTS

- There are two forms of anthrax: cutaneous, usually resulting from surface contamination, and inhalation, resulting from inhalation of a fine particle aerosol.
- All anthrax cases must be immediately reported to public health officials.
- Inhalation anthrax is essentially diagnostic of bioterrorism; the last case of naturally occurring inhalation anthrax in the U.S. was in 1978.
- It is much easier to prevent anthrax with antibiotics than to treat it.
- There is no person-to-person transmission.
- Inhalation anthrax has a high mortality rate even with highly active antibiotics and good facilities for intensive care. This emphasizes the important role for prophylaxis and early antibiotic treatment.
- The lab is a great help—blood cultures are positive and CT scans show very characteristic changes.
- Antibiotic recommendations are based on the experience with the pan-sensitive Aims stain. They may change based on use of another stain.

BACKGROUND

Bacillus anthracis is the prototype agent for bioterrorism because it has ideal properties:
- Lab may show typical GPB on gram stain.
- It is easily produced, stored, and delivered.
- The spores will last in environments for decades
- Inhalation anthrax is highly lethal and all persons are highly susceptible

This agent also has precedent as the only major bioweapon in the past decade. There were 22 cases of anthrax from four contaminated letters, including 20 people who were mail handlers or at work sites where the mail was received. Of the 22 cases, 11 were inhalational anthrax and 11 were cutaneous anthrax. The mortality for the inhalational form was five of 11 (45%). Approximately 10,000 people received prophylaxis, either ciprofloxacin or doxycycline; none of these patients subsequently acquired anthrax.

The threat of this agent is largely dependent on how it is weaponized in terms of particle size. Letters to New York, for example, were crudely milled so that, when released, the spores fell away and most of the cases were cutaneous. By contrast, spores mailed to the Hart Senate Office Building were finely milled to about 1 micron, and they filled the air in the room within minutes after the letter was opened. Some people in the room at that time had nasal cultures that showed "wall-to-wall" growth of *B anthracis*.

The innoculum size necessary to cause inhalation anthrax (on the basis of primate studies) is approximately 10 spores; there were about 1 billion spores in the Hart letter. Bioweapon stores in the former Soviet Union and Iraq included several metric tons of these spores. It is estimated by WHO that a 70 kg drop from an airplane over a large metropolitan area would cause an estimated 100,000 deaths due to inhalation anthrax.

HOSPITAL PREPARATION

With anthrax, hospitals must be prepared for several issues regarding a bioterrorism event:
- Any case of anthrax needs to be immediately reported. There have been only two cases of naturally occurring anthrax in the U.S. from 1990 to 2005, and no cases of inhalation anthrax since 1978. Any case is a bioterrorism concern.
- There may be a contaminated letter to a health care facility. These facilities consequently need

policies to deal with potentially contaminated mail (and most do have them).

- There may be an event in which a person or group reports concern about a potential anthrax exposure. The facility/health care worker must be able to direct this query to the proper health authority—a contact that must be easily accessible.
- There should be an established plan to know when to suspect anthrax, how to report it to public health authorities, and how to provide care.
- Crucial challenges in an individual case are making the diagnosis when the symptoms are quite nonspecific and then rapidly giving antibiotics. With large numbers of casualties, the challenge is triage to separate the real cases and those "worried" but uninfected.
- There needs to be an established plan for mass delivery of prophylactic antibiotics, but this should not take place in the hospital (see below).

IN THE EVENT OF MASS CASUALTIES

For mass casualties in a large-scale attack, there are likely to be two presentations: cutaneous and inhalation anthrax. The inhalation form is highly lethal and will require extensive resources for triage and medical care. The cutaneous form is usually treated on an outpatient basis, but it can be nevertheless severe.

- Initial cases are likely to be a diagnostic challenge until blood cultures are returned. Virtually all patients with inhalation anthrax have bacteremia; the organism usually grows within eight to 12 hours; and the microbiologist can usually make a fast report if alerted to this possibility.
- Patients with suspected inhalation anthrax should be immediately treated with standard antibiotics according to CDC recommendations using the 2001 guidelines (below), unless updated.
- There is no need for special protective isolation in the emergency department or on hospital wards, since the organism is not transferred from person to person. It is vital to assure all personnel that caring for patients with inhalation anthrax is safe for health care workers and their families.
- There must be a systematic method for rapidly administering prophylactic antibiotics to those exposed. This should *not* be done in the hospital facility but at some other location, such as a civic

center or other large facility in proximity to those needing this service (e.g., close to the attack site).

PERSONAL PROTECTION

- With inhalation anthrax, standard precautions for patients are appropriate, since there is no person-to-person transmission.
- With cutaneous anthrax, there is the potential risk of person-to-person transmission, so contact precautions should be followed in patients with draining skin lesions.
- The clinical laboratory should be warned if there is a suspicion of anthrax, since it poses a risk to lab personnel. This helps to expedite detection.
- Remember: Many of the materials likely to be handled are also likely to constitute evidence for a criminal investigation.

DECONTAMINATION

- Surrogate studies of anthrax show no significant threat to personnel in areas heavily contaminated with *B anthracis* spores. Nevertheless, current recommendations are to decontaminate areas of a spill or near the point of release.
- Exposed skin and clothing should be cleaned with soap and water.
- Any person in direct contact with anthrax should receive prophylaxis.

QUARANTINE PROCEDURES

- Since there is no person-to-person spread with anthrax, quarantine should not be necessary.

CLINICAL PRESENTATION
CUTANEOUS ANTHRAX

- The usual incubation period is one to seven days after exposure.
- The initial lesion is a small papule or vesicle that ulcerates and forms an eschar within two to three days. This may be associated with regional edema and local adenopathy.
- Mortality is <1% and most patients are managed

- as outpatients, but infections can be severe.
- Lab may show typical GPB on gram stain.
- Differential diagnosis includes: strep or staph soft tissue infection (tender and eschars are uncommon), brown recluse spider bite (very painful blister), or rickettsial pox (painless papule, then eschar and generalized rash).

INHALATION ANTHRAX

- The modest U.S. exposure in 2001 and the large outbreak in Sverdlovsk, Russia, in 1979, indicate an incubation period in most people of two to 45 days. The course is biphasic: First there is a nonspecific influenza-like illness, and then, after three to four days, there is sepsis and shock.
- Initial symptoms include a flu-like illness with fever (100%), fatigue (100%), and cough (90%) that might easily be confused with any common respiratory tract infection.
- Initial symptoms are followed by severe respiratory distress and sepsis with shock and death.
- Lab: Blood cultures are virtually always positive if obtained before antibiotics. Chest x-rays show a wide mediastinum, and the CT scan shows highly characteristic large, hyperdense mediastinal adenopathy, often with large pleural effusions. These pleural effusions are usually bloody—the average accumulation in the Sverdlovsk outbreak was 1700 cc!—and daily pleural drainage was an important component of treatment in the U.S. 2001 epidemic.
- Differential diagnosis: common forms of community-acquired pneumonia (although inhalation anthrax is not commonly an infection of the pulmonary parenchyma), influenza (usually shows rhinorrhea and pharyngitis), and other forms of bioterrorism — e.g., tularemia (rarely severe or fatal), inhalation plague (often with hemoptysis), and influenza.

DISEASE FEATURES

CUTANEOUS ANTHRAX

- Beyond defined exposure, a hallmark of cutaneous anthrax is the characteristic single cutaneous skin lesion, which starts as a painless papule that rapidly evolves into an ulcer and then into an eschar over two to three days.

- This lesion also has the characteristic surrounding edema and regional adenopathy.

INHALATIONAL ANTHRAX

- The initial illness is not particularly distinctive compared with many other flu-like illnesses, except for the paucity of symptoms related to the upper airways, such as rhinorrhea and pharyngitis.
- The second phase is one of fulminate progression, with lung compression, sepsis, shock, and death. There are relatively few infectious diseases that progress this rapidly, especially in previously healthy adults or children. The mortality rate in the Sverdlovsk epidemic is estimated at about 80%, and it was 45% in the U.S. even with an alerted health care community with extensive resources for critical care.
- Blood cultures rapidly become positive if obtained before antibiotics, the chest x-ray shows the wide mediastinum, and the CT scan shows the highly characteristic hyperdense hilar nodes.

DIAGNOSIS

CLINICAL FEATURES

- **Cutaneous**—skin lesion that rapidly progresses from papule to eschar in two to six days.
- **Inhalation**—pulmonary process that starts like a viral infection and then rapidly progresses to dyspnea and hypoxemia with an x-ray showing a wide mediastinum.
- **Intestinal**—severe abdominal pain followed by fever and sepsis.
- **Oropharyngeal**—oral mucosal lesions, cervical adenopathy, and fever.

CONFINED CASE

- A clinical syndrome (described above) accompanied by a positive culture for *B anthrasis*.

DISTINGUISHING COMMUNITY-ACQUIRED PNEUMONIA AND INFLUENZA

The usual initial impression with inhalation anthrax is bacterial pneumonia, a "viral

Table 1. Treatment of Anthrax—2001 CDC Guidelines

INHALATION ANTHRAX

Adults

IV therapy (until stable)	Oral therapy (60 days to complete)
Ciprofloxacin 400 mg q12h	**Ciprofloxacin** 500 mg PO bid
or	*or*
Levofloxacin 750 mg q24h	**Levofloxacin** 500 mg PO bid
or	*or*
Doxycycline 100 mg q12h	**Doxycycline** 100 mg PO bid
plus	
One or two of the following: • **Rifampin** • **Chloramphenicol** • **Imipenem** • **Clindamycin** • **Clarithromycin** • **Vancomycin** • **Penicillin** • **Ampicillin**	

Pregnant Women

IV therapy (until stable)	Oral therapy (60 days to complete)
As Above	As Above

Children

IV therapy (until stable)	Oral therapy (60 days to complete)
Ciprofloxacin 10 mg/kg to 15 mg/kg q 12h (max 1 gm/d)	**Ciprofloxacin** 10 mg/kg to 15 mg/kg PO q 12h
or	*or*
Doxycycline >8 yrs and >45 kg 100mg bid 8 yrs and <45 kg	**Doxycycline** Dose as with IV, but PO
or	
<8 yrs 2.2 mg/kg q 12h	
and	
1 or 2 additional antimicrobials (see agents listed under therapy for adults)	

CUTANEOUS ANTHRAX

Adults	Children

IV therapy (until stable)	Oral therapy (60 days to complete)
Ciprofloxacin 500 mg bid x 60 days	**Ciprofloxacin** 500 mg bid x 60 days
or	*or*
Doxycycline 500 mg bid PO x 60 days	**Doxycycline** 100 mg bid PO x 60 days

syndrome," or influenza. A scoring system has been developed for inhalation anthrax:

- Low serum albumin—two points
- Pulse greater than 90—two points,
- Lack of rhinorrhea—two points
- Low sodium—one point
- Lack of headache—one point
- Elevated hematocrit—one point
- Lack of myalgias—one point

A score of at least four points showed a sensitivity of 100% and specificity of 96%.

- Laboratory personnel should be forewarned when the above is a diagnostic consideration, because they need to take precautions and can expedite diagnostic procedures. Cultures can be performed on standard media (blood agar). Growth on agar is usually noted in 12 to 24 hours and may be detected in blood cultures in as early as eight hours.

TREATMENT

- The four drugs approved for anthrax by the FDA are ciprofloxacin, levofloxacin, doxycycline, and penicillin. It is possible that another attack might involve a more resistant strain that would require a different approach to empiric selection.
- When these drugs are used empirically for *inhalation anthrax*, there are two principles of antibiotic therapy:
  - One of these drugs should be given rapidly by IV, preferably in combination with a second agent.
  - Antibiotic treatment should be continued for a prolonged period, usually 60 to 100 days.

- The rationale for the long duration is that a delivery of spores to the primate model shows that these forms persist despite antibiotics for up to 60 days or longer.
- Particularly important is the frequent drainage of the bloody pleural effusions.
- With **cutaneous anthrax**, treatment is oral or

Table 2. Prophylaxis for Anthrax

Adults
Ciprofloxacin
500 mg PO bid x 60 days
Levofloxacin
500 mg PO bid x 60 days
Doxycycline
100 mg PO bid x 60 days
Pregnant Women
Amoxicillin
500 mg PO bid x 60 days (may be used if isolate from outbreak is sensitive)
Children
Ciprofloxacin and **doxycycline**
Pediatric doses as indicated in previous table.

parenteral using the same drugs. However, treatment is extended to 100 days based on the assumption that there was potential exposure to inhalation anthrax as well.

PREVENTION

- In the 2001 epidemic, all exposed persons were advised to take prophylactic antibiotics using ciprofloxacin or doxycycline for 60 to 100 days. This required a major public health effort that was needed to bypass most standard medical processing. The average "put-through" time in NYC for >1,000 exposures was 30 minutes (from the time of reporting for evaluation until the antibiotic was given or denied). The evaluation was a brief questionnaire for the 10% who needed help.
- The alternative strategy is vaccination. The anthrax vaccine licensed by the FDA has well-established efficacy. However, it requires six immunizations (since that is the schedule used for registration with the FDA), and there has been substantial controversy about potential complications. As a result, new forms of anthrax vaccine are currently undergoing testing.

Clinical Pathway: Anthrax Inhalational Exposure

High probability of anthrax exposure (see page 103)

- Ill with compatible symptoms (see bottom, right)

  - Call Infectious Disease Service immediately
  - Obtain blood cultures and LP
  - Thoracentesis (for Gram stain and culture) if pleural effusion is present
  - Obtain Gram stain of CSF and any skin lesions suggestive of cutaneous anthrax
  - Consider Gram stain of unspun peripheral blood
  - Notify laboratory that anthrax is suspected
  - Obtain CXR and lab tests as appropriate

  Begin 3-drug antibiotic therapy (IV) (see page 104)

  Hospitalize using Standard Precautions; consider Contact Precautions for any draining cutaneous lesions

  If *B anthracis* is isolated, send to level B/C laboratory for confirmation and assessment of in vitro sensitivities; adjust therapy as needed

  Report suspected and confirmed cases to local public health department immediately

  - Continue antibiotics for at least 60 days
  - Consider anthrax vaccine or more prolonged use of antibiotics if high-dose exposure occurred (see page 104)

- Not ill or no compatible illness

  Begin prophylactic antibiotics (see page 105)

  Notify local public health department

  - Continue prophylactic antibiotics for at least 60 days
  - Consider anthrax vaccine or more prolonged use of prophylactic antibiotics if high-dose exposure occurred (see page 105)

  - Educate patient regarding side effects of prophylactic therapy and symptoms of anthrax
  - Instruct patient to follow up if side effects or symptoms occur
  - Routine follow-up to assess symptoms, side effects, and psychological support

Low probability of anthrax exposure or no known exposure (see page 103)

- Ill with compatible symptoms (see bottom, right)

  Differential diagnosis (DDx):
  - Influenza
  - Mycoplasmal pneumonia
  - Legionnaires' disease
  - Tularemia
  - Psittacosis
  - Other viral pneumonias
  - Q fever
  - Acute bacterial mediastinitis
  - Fibrous mediastinitis caused by *Histoplasma capsulatum*
  - Coccidioidomycosis
  - Tuberculosis
  - Noninfectious causes

  - Obtain CXR/chest CT
  - Obtain blood cultures
  - Obtain LP if symptoms suggestive of meningitis are present
  - Obtain pleural fluid for culture if effusion present
  - Obtain other clinical specimens as indicated per DDx

  - Begin broad-spectrum antimicrobial therapy while awaiting diagnostic testing
  - If anthrax is highly suspected, assure antibiotic coverage for *B anthracis* (see page 104)

- Not ill or no compatible illness

  Reassure patient regarding anthrax

  Evaluate further as indicated by signs and symptoms

  If hospital lab identifies *Bacillus* species, specimen should be sent to a level B/C laboratory for full identification

  If anthrax is highly suspected or *B anthracis* is isolated, contact local public health department immediately to initiate an epidemiologic investigation

---

Inhalational Anthrax

Early-phase symptoms:
Fever or chills
Fatigue
Malaise
Minimal or nonproductive cough
Dyspnea
Profound sweating
Nausea, vomiting
Rhinorrhea usually *not* present
Pleuritic pain

Late-phase symptoms:
Fever
Severe respiratory distress
Symptoms of meningitis
Shock

Laboratory findings:
CXR shows widened mediastinum, pleural effusion, or infiltrates (effusions are hemorrhagic)
WBC high or normal with left shift
SGOT or SGPT may be elevated
Hypoxemia (alveolar-arterial O_2 gradient >30 Hg on room air; O_2 sat <94%)

CT findings:
Hilar and mediastinal lymph node enlargement and pleural effusions
Paucity of parenchymal infiltrates

Continued...

Assessing the Probability of Anthrax Exposure

High Probability	***During a known anthrax event:*** • Persons exposed to an air space where a suspicious material may have been aerosolized (eg, near a suspicious powder-containing letter during opening) • Persons who shared an air space likely to be the source of an inhalational anthrax case (eg, being exposed to a shared ventilation system) • Persons who may have been exposed to an item contaminated with *Bacillus anthracis* (eg, an envelope or other vehicle) along the transit path of the item (eg, a postal sorting facility in which an envelope containing *B anthracis* was processed) ***In situations where anthrax has not previously been identified*:*** • Persons who opened a suspicious letter or package that was found to contain a white powder suspected to be a source of *B anthracis* • Persons exposed to an air space where suspicious material may have been aerosolized (eg, near a suspicious powder-containing letter during opening) • Sudden appearance of multiple patients with acute onset of characteristic illness (suggests common source exposure such as would be seen with a bioterrorist attack)
Low Probability	• No history of exposure to an item (eg, an envelope or other vehicle) or powder confirmed or suspected to harbor *B anthracis* spores • No history of exposure to an air space where a suspicious material could have been aerosolized (eg, being present at the time a powder-containing letter was opened) • No history of exposure to an air space likely to have been the source for a confirmed case of inhalational anthrax

*In situations where anthrax exposure is suspected but no prior cases of anthrax have been confirmed, a risk assessment should be conducted by local public health and law enforcement officials. If the probability of anthrax exposure is considered high on the basis of the risk assessment, prophylactic antimicrobial therapy should be initiated for asymptomatic exposed persons while the suspect material is being tested for *B anthracis*. Any persons who have symptoms compatible with anthrax should be treated with appropriate antibiotics, according to the clinical pathway (see page 102), until anthrax can be confirmed or ruled out.

Continued...

Treatment Protocol for Inhalational, Gastrointestinal, and Oropharyngeal Anthrax*

Patient Category	Initial IV Therapy†‡	Oral Regimens (continue therapy for 60 days [IV and PO combined])
Adults	Ciprofloxacin, 400 mg every 12 hr *or* Doxycycline, 100 mg every 12 hr** *and* One or two additional antimicrobials (agents with *in vitro* activity include rifampin, vancomycin, penicillin, ampicillin, chloramphenicol, imipenem, clindamycin, and clarithromycin) ††	Patients should be treated with IV therapy initially.§ Treatment can be switched to oral therapy when clinically appropriate: Ciprofloxacin, 500 mg PO twice daily *or* Doxycycline, 100 mg PO twice daily
Children	Ciprofloxacin, 10-15 mg/kg every 12 hr, not to exceed 1g/day ‡‡ *or* Doxycycline**§§: >8 yr and >45 kg: 100 mg every 12 hr >8 yr and ≤45 kg: 2.2 mg/kg every 12hr ≤8 yr: 2.2 mg/kg every 12 hr *and* One or two additional antimicrobials (see agents listed under therapy for adults)††	Patients should be treated with IV therapy initially.§ Treatment can be switched to oral therapy when clinically appropriate: Ciprofloxacin, 10-15 mg/kg PO every 12 hr, not to exceed 1g/day ‡‡ *or* Doxycycline§§: >8 yr and >45 kg: 100 mg PO every 12 12 hr >8 yr and ≤45 kg: 2.2 mg/kg PO every 12 hr ≤8 yr: 2.2 mg/kg PO every 12 hr
Pregnant women***	Same as for nonpregnant adults (high death rate from the infection outweighs risk posed by antimicrobial agent)	Patients should be treated with IV therapy initially.§ Treatment can be switched to PO when clinically appropriate. Oral therapy regimens are the same as for nonpregnant adults.
Immunocompromised persons	Same as for nonimmunocompromised persons and children.	Same as for nonimmunocompromised persons and children.

Abbreviations: IV, intravenously; PO, orally.

*These treatment recommendations were made during US 2001 anthrax outbreak. In other situations, antimicrobial susceptibility testing should be used to guide therapy decisions.
†Ciprofloxacin or doxycycline should be considered an essential part of first-line therapy for inhalational anthrax.
‡Steroids may be considered an adjunct therapy for patients with severe edema (Doust et al. Corticosteriod in treatment of malignant edema of chest and neck [anthrax]. *Dis Chest* 1968;53:773-4) and for meningitis based on experience with bacterial meningitis of other etiologies.
§Initial therapy may be altered based on clinical course of patient; one or two antimicrobial agents (eg, ciprofloxacin or doxycycline) may be adequate as patient improves.
**If meningitis is suspected, doxycycline may be less optimal because of poor central nervous system penetration.
††Because of concerns of constitutive and inducible beta-lactamases in *Bacillus anthracis* isolates, penicillin and ampicillin should not be used alone. Consultation with an infectious disease specialist is advised.
‡‡If intravenous ciprofloxacin is not available, oral ciprofloxacin may be acceptable because it is rapidly and well absorbed from gastrointestinal tract with no substantial loss by first-pass metabolism. Maximum serum concentrations are attained 1-2 hours after oral doing but may not be achieved if vomiting or ileus is present.
§§ American Academy of Pediatrics recommends treatment of young children with tetracyclines for serious infections (eg, Rocky Mountain Spotted Fever).
***Although tetracyclines are not recommended for pregnant women, their use may be indicated for life-threatening illness. Adverse effects on developing teeth and bones are dose-related; therefore, doxycycline might be used for a short time (7-14 days) before 6 months of gestation.

Adapted from CDC. Investigation of bioterrorism-related anthrax and interim guidelines for exposure management and antimicrobial therapy, October 2001. MMWR 2001:50(42):909-19.

Continued...

Recommendations for Postexposure Prophylaxis for Prevention of Inhalational Anthrax Following Exposure to *Bacillus anthracis*

Patient Category	Initial Therapy	Duration*
Adults (including immunocompromised patients)	Ciprofloxacin, 500 mg PO twice daily *or* Doxycycline, 100 mg PO twice daily	60 days
Pregnant women and breastfeeding mothers	Ciprofloxacin, 500 mg PO twice daily *or* Doxycycline, 100 mg PO twice daily [Amoxicillin, 500 mg orally three times daily, may be used if isolate involved in exposure is determined to be susceptible to penicillin†‡§]	60 days
Children (including immunocompromised patients)	Ciprofloxacin, 10-15 mg/kg PO every 12 hr, not to exceed 1 gm/day *or* Doxycycline: >8 yr and >45 kg: 100 mg PO twice daily >8 yr and <45 kg: 2.2 mg/kg PO twice daily <8 yr: 2.2 mg/kg PO twice daily [Amoxicillin, 80 mg/kg/day divided every 8 hr, not to exceed 500 mg/dose, may be used if the isolate involved in exposure is determined to be susceptible to penicillin‡]	60 days

Abbreviations: PO, orally.

*Additional recommendations were made for those exposed to high levels of anthrax; see comments below.
†See comments below from American College of Obstetricians and Gynecologists regarding use of amoxicillin.
‡Amoxicillin is not approved by the FDA for postexposure prophylaxis or treatment of anthrax; however, CDC indicated that it could be used for pregnant women or children for postexposure prophylaxis if the isolate is determined to be susceptible (CDC: Interim recommendations for antimicrobial prophylaxis for children and breastfeeding mothers and treatment of children with anthrax (http://www.bt.cdc.gov/DocumentsApp/Anthrax/Protective/10242001Protect.asp); CDC: Updated recommendations for antimicrobial prophylaxis among asymptomatic pregnant women after exposure to *Bacillus anthracis*. MMWR 2001;50(43):960.
§American Academy of Pediatrics considers ciprofloxacin and tetracyclines to usually be compatible with breastfeeding because the amount of either drug absorbed by infants is small, but little is know about the safety of long-term use. Therefore, amoxicillin may be considered an alternative for breastfeeding mothers if the isolate causing exposure is known to be susceptible to penicillin. Alternatively, mothers could consider expressing and discarding breast milk during therapy with ciprofloxacin or doxycycline and resuming breastfeeding after therapy is complete.

Adapted from CDC. Update: Investigation of bioterrorism-related anthrax and interim guidelines for exposure management and antimicrobial therapy, October 19, 2001. MMWR 2001;50(41):889-93.

BOTULISM (CLOSTRIDIUM BOTULINUM)

IMPORTANT POINTS

- The delivery system will dictate the epidemiology. An aerosol release could cause an epidemic in a defined area of common exposure, whereas contaminated milk would follow the distribution route with potential for outbreaks in a zip code, city, state, or nation.
- Suspect botulism with descending symmetrical paralysis, cranial nerve involvement, afebrile, mentally alert, decreased reflexes, intact sensation, normal CSF and MRI. In an epidemic setting, potential victims should be alerted to the clinical clues of difficulty seeing, speaking, and/or swallowing.
- The specific diagnosis is made by toxin assay of clinical specimens in a public health lab.
- Treatment is trivalent antitoxin preferably given within 24 hours of onset.
- There is no person-to-person spread.
- Many cases will require ventilator support for three months. Any large attack would rapidly deplete the nation's supply of ventilators.
- Suspect bioterrorism when: outbreak of acute flaccid paralysis, unusual toxin type (C, D, F or G), outbreak from geographic source, or multiple outbreaks.

BACKGROUND

Botulinum toxin has ideal properties as an agent of bioterrorism:
- It is easily produced.
- The botulinum toxins are the most lethal toxins known; for toxin A, the lethal toxic dose delivered by aerosol for a 70 kg person is 0.7 μg and delivered by mouth is 70 μg.
- The toxin may be delivered in a variety of ways: by inhalation, in a municipal water supply, in food, or in beverages. It is estimated that 10 g of toxin in a milk supply could result in 500,000 cases of botulism. Contamination of a commercial food or beverage supply could result in thousands of cases distributed across the country or could involve multiple countries.
- The most effective treatment is trivalent ABE antitoxin. There are three important antitoxin facts: 1) it should be given within 24 hours of the onset of symptoms; 2) a bioterrorism attack could involve toxin types that are not included in the antitoxin that is currently available from the CDC; and 3) the antitoxin is an equine preparation that carries the risk of anaphylaxis.
- Supportive care is likely to require prolonged mechanical ventilation; any major attack would quickly totally deplete the nation's supply of ventilators.

Recognizing these properties, the U.S. had a massive supply of botulinum toxin for potential bioterrorism prior to abandonment to the program after the 1972 Biological Weapons Convention. The Soviet Union also produced a large supply. During the Gulf War, Iraq had 19,000 liters of concentrated botulinum toxin, including some that was weaponized. Despite these large stockpiles, there has been no successful use of botulinum toxin as a bioweapon.

One important feature of botulinum toxin is the multiple methods for dissemination. Options include aerosolization with inhalation anthrax, or the toxin could enter by the gastrointestinal tract through contamination of the water supply, food supply, or a commercial beverage. Contamination of municipal water supplies is possible but unlikely due to the large quantity of toxin required. The epidemiology of cases would be very different, depending on the distribution pattern, but clinical presentation is the same regardless of the site of entry (GI tract or lung), and the treatment would be the same as well.

HOSPITAL PREPARATION

Hospitals need to be able to deal with several unique facets of an outbreak of botulism.
- Particularly important will be establishing the diagnosis of a relatively rare but severe neurologic syndrome with clinical features described below.
- The hospital microbiological lab cannot make this diagnosis. It requires referral of appropriate specimens to a designated public health lab or the CDC.

- There are 100 to 150 cases of botulism in the U.S. each year, and infant botulism is the most common form. The average number of food-borne outbreaks in the U.S. is 10 to 15 per year; the average number of cases per outbreak is two to three. There are isolated cases of wound botulism, and occasional outbreaks from contaminated illegal drugs.
- A hospital or emergency department that encounters multiple cases of botulism must consider the possibility of a food-borne source or contaminated illicit drugs in addicts, since these would be the most common natural form of epidemics. The link to a food-borne source or involvement of illicit drugs users becomes an important clue.
- In the event that botulism is suspected, it is the responsibility of the physician to immediately notify the appropriate local county or state authorities and to provide care.

For management in the event of multiple cases, there needs to be substantial hospital planning, specifically:
- There needs to be a supply of botulism antitoxin that targets the toxin type, usually A, B, or rarely E. However, with bioterrorism, there is the possible risk of an unusual toxin type (C, D, F or G), for which the standard CDC trivalent antitoxin would not be effective.
- The type of toxin would not be known for several days, until testing has been done at a public health facility, so the standard recommendation is to use the trivalent vaccine until the type is specified, and then use type-specific antitoxin.
- Pentavalent antitoxin with antibody to types A through G was developed by the U.S. Army. Once the type is identified, it would be assumed that all subsequent cases involved the same type.
- Antitoxin is given by slow IV infusion, started as quickly as possible.
- Antitoxin supplies are available through state or local health departments and the CDC; supplies are maintained at quarantine stations in airports at major metropolitan areas, including New York, Atlanta, Chicago, Miami, Los Angeles, Seattle, San Francisco and Honolulu.
- Penicillin is the preferred drug for *C botulinum*, but it plays almost no important role in treatment. A bioterrorism attack is likely to be the toxin and not the organism. The most important

immediate treatment for either is antitoxin.
- The other important facet of therapy is supportive care. Most critical is the need for ventilation support and an anticipated problem is the adequacy of the supply of ventilators, critical care beds, and skilled personnel to provide this support for weeks or months for any large number of patients who require therapy. Most will require ventilatory support for about three months. In addition, these patients will require other forms of supportive care, including hyperalimentation.
- There is no concern about contagion of *C botulinum* or its toxin. The toxin is acquired from a common source, but it is not transmitted from person to person, and environmental sources are not important.

PERSONAL PROTECTION

There is no person-to-person transmission of either the organism or the toxin. The organism cannot enter via intact skin. Health care workers and their families need to be assured that this is not an issue. Any identified common food or water source should be the subject of rapid intervention by public health officials.

DECONTAMINATION

- The toxin is inactivated by heating to 85°C for five minutes.
- Spores are susceptible to chlorine, including chlorinated water or hypochlorite solutions. The spores survive ultraviolet light, alcohol, phenol, radiation, and boiling for up to three to four hours.

QUARANTINE PROCEDURES

- There is no person-to-person spread of botulism so quarantine should not be necessary.

CLINICAL PRESENTATION

The recognized forms of botulism are:
- **Food borne**—often results in small outbreaks averaging two to three persons per outbreak,

and is usually due to improperly home-canned foods, especially vegetables.

- **Wound botulism**—due to a contaminated wound associated with traumatic injury or injection drug use with contaminated drugs.
- **Infant botulism**—the most common naturally occurring form, which usually occurs in the first year with the median age of three months via a source that is usually not defined. It is caused by ingestion of the organism with in vivo toxin production in the gut.
- **Inhalation botulism**—this form has not been reported since 1962 when veterenarians in Germany were working with an aerosolized preparation in animals. Any aerosol delivery is likely to mean bioterrorism.

The clinical presentation is the same regardless of the route of infection. The patient is not febrile and presents with a neurologic syndrome consisting of:

- ✔ Clear sensorium
- ✔ Symmetric descending flaccid paralysis
- ✔ The four D's—dysphonia, diploplia, dysarthria, and dysphagia.

- The incubation period depends on the amount of toxin. For food-borne disease, it is two hours to eight days; for the inhalation form, it is estimated at 24 to 72 hours.
- Physical exam shows symmetrical weakness of arms and legs, extra-ocular muscle abnormalities, ptosis, reduced deep tendon reflexes, diminished gag, intact sensory exam, intact mental status, and normal temperature.
- Laboratory tests are generally normal, including CBC, cerebrospinal fluid analysis, and imaging of the brain. The EMG gives characteristic changes consisting of an incremental response or facilitation to repeated stimulation.

DISEASE FEATURES

- Botulism is an acute, afebrile, symmetrical, descending, flaccid paralysis that begins in the bulbar musculature.
- Important clinical features of the condition are the normal mental status, lack of fever, and the descending paralysis with cranial nerve involvement.

- The differential diagnosis includes, Guillain-Barré Syndrome, myasthenia gravis, tick paralysis, CNS mass lesion, stroke, Lambert-Eaton syndrome, paralytic shellfish poisoning, puffer fish poisoning, belladonna toxicity, and toxicity due to nerve gas, carbon monoxide, organophosphates, or hypermagnesemia.

DIAGNOSIS

- The diagnoses includes detection of the toxin by the mouse bioassay in a designated public health lab using serum (30 mL obtained before antitoxin), vomitus, gastric aspirate, stool, and epidemiologically implicated food samples or environmental samples. Standard methods are used for culture of *C botulinum* using specimens of stool, other intestinal content, tissue from wounds, environmental samples, and food or water sources.
- The standard assay for botulinum toxin is the mouse bioassay. Evidence of disease usually occurs in six to 24 hours. The type of toxin is identified by toxin neutralization with types-specific antitoxin. This seems archaic in the era of modern EIA, PCR, etc., but the mouse bioassay seems to persist as the preferred diagnostic method in terms of sensitivity and specificity.
- EMG with repetitive nerve stimulation at 20 Hz to 30 Hz helps distinguish botulism from other causes of paralytic syndromes.

TREATMENT

- The mainstay of treatment is equine antitoxin, which prevents progression but does not reverse existing neurologic deficits. It should be given as quickly as possible. The antitoxin is type-specific, but the clinician will not know the type unless it is part of an epidemic in which prior cases have provided this information. Consequently, the initial cases would probably be treated with trivalent vaccine until the specific type of toxin is known. Most cases in the U.S. are type A or type B, and the predominant type in Alaska is type E. There may be other types involved in the event of bioterrorism, in which case the pentavalent antitoxin preparation developed by the U.S. Army with antitoxin to types A through G might be required.

- The standard doses of antitoxin are indicated in the package insert, which recommends doses that are more than necessary to neutralize the likely amount of toxin. However, these are standardized for the amount of toxin acquired in naturally occurring disease, such as food-borne botulism; bioterrorism might involve an unusually large amount. In such cases, additional doses might be given at least two to four hours after the initial dose. The antitoxin is equine serum, which incurs the risk of anaphylaxis. The prior experience with antitoxin indicates acute or delayed reactions in approximately 10% of patients.

- Toxoid immunization might be attempted for susceptible populations where there might be ongoing potential exposures. The standard dose is 0.5 mL given SC at two and 12 weeks, with a booster dose at one year.

- Supportive care with ventilatory support, protection from aspiration, and hyperalimentation are the key facets for long-term management. The need for mechanical ventilation may be reduced by use of a rigid mattress at 20%. This usually is required for about three months.

PREVENTION

- Standard precautions are adequate. Contaminated surfaces can be treated with 1% hypochlorite, and contaminated clothes and skin should be cleaned with soap and water. As noted, there is no person-to-person transmission.

- In an outbreak, there should be substantial efforts to rapidly treat patients with antitoxin, since the benefit is largely dependent on the time delay for administration of the first dose.

- Antitoxin is not advocated for prophylactic use because it is scarce and because the rate of severe reactions is high.

- Persons exposed to the toxin should be followed carefully and warned to promptly report any problems with vision, speaking, or swallowing.

Clinical Pathway: Botulism

- Acute onset of symmetrical paralysis in patient whose mental status is generally intact
- Patient presents with paralysis, history of progression is unclear

↓

- Obtain dietary, travel, and activity history for previous 8 days
- Obtain drug history or history of potential toxic exposures (organophosphates, belladonna alkaloids [eg, atropine], carbon monoxide, aminoglycosides, shellfish or pufferfish ingestion in previous few hours)

→

Botulism ruled out on basis of drug exposure history

Low probability of botulism, or diagnosis unclear

↓

Perform additional diagnostic testing as urgently as possible (see page 112 for differential diagnosis):
- LP (normal in botulism; elevated protein 1-2 wk after onset with GBS (including Miller Fisher variant, which may be a descending paralysis)
- Brain CT or MRI to rule out stroke, mass lesion (normal in botulism)
- Edrophonium challenge test (marked response with myasthenia gravis; usually negative in botulism, although may see partial response in some cases)
- Careful physical exam (especially of scalp) to look for attached tick, which would indicate tick paralysis
- Chest x-ray for evidence of lung carcinoma (often associated with Lambert-Eaton syndrome)
- Consider EMG (see page 113 for characteristic findings)

Botulism ruled out

Botulism still suspected

Abbreviations

BT, bioterrorism
CT, computed tomography
EMG, electromyography
GBS, Guillain-Barre syndrome
LP, lumbar puncture
MRI, magnetic resonance imaging

High probability of botulism:
- Clear history of cranial nerve dysfunction followed by descending paralysis; autonomic dysfunction (dry mouth, trouble focusing eyes) present
- History of ingestion of high-risk foods (eg, home-canned products, fermented native foods from Alaska, Northern Canada)

Note: Sudden appearance of multiple patients with acute onset of characteristic illness suggests common source exposure such as would be seen with a bioterrorist attack

↓

Contact state of local Health Department immediately to:
- Obtain botulinum antitoxin
- Arrange for laboratory testing of specimens
- Notify public health officials so epidemiologic investigation can be initiated

↓

- Collect serum (>30 mL of blood in "tiger"-top or red-top tube); collect serum *before* administration of antitoxin
- Collect stool, gastric aspirate, and vomitus (if available)
- Collect suspect food(s) or have family member hold suspect food(s) in refrigerator, if relevant
- Refrigerate specimens after collection while preparing to ship
- Ship specimens per Health Department instructions for toxin and *C botulinum* testing

↓

Perform other diagnostic tests as needed (eg, LP, brain imaging, edrophonium challenge)

↓

- Assess and monitor patient closely for evidence of airway obstruction, aspiration, decreased respiratory function (follow O_2 saturation, vital capacity, inspiratory force)
- Intubate if respiratory function deteriorates and concern of impending respiratory failure exists

↓

- Administer antitoxin as soon as available
- Provide ongoing patient monitoring and supportive care

Continued...

Differential Diagnosis for Botulism

- Guillain-Barre syndrome (including Miller Fisher variant)
- Myasthenia gravis
- Tick paralysis
- Lambert-Eaton syndrome
- Toxic exposures (organophosphates, depressants [including ethanol], belladonna alkaloids, carbon monoxide, aminoglycosides, paralytic shellfish poisoning)
- Stroke or central nervous system (CNS) mass lesion
- Poliomyelitis

Note: Other conditions also may be confused with botulism; examples include other infectious conditions (viral syndromes, CNS infections [particularly brainstem], streptococcal pharyngitis), diabetic neuropathy, hyperthyroidism, inflammatory myopathy, psychiatric conversion reaction

Continued...

Comparison of Electromyographic Findings in Botulism and Similar Illnesses

Disease	Characteristic EMG findings
Botulism*	• Incremental response (facilitation) to repetitive stimulation (not always present and often seen only at 50 Hz) • Short duration of MUPs; polyphasic MUPs • Decreased amplitude of CMAPs after a single nerve stimulus (most prominent in proximal muscle groups) • Normal sensory nerve function • Normal nerve conduction velocity (motor and sensory)
Guillain-Barre syndrome	Abnormal nerve conduction velocity; no facilitation with repetitive nerve stimulation
Myasthenia gravis	Decrease in muscle action potentials with repetitive nerve stimulation
Tick paralysis	Abnormal nerve conduction velocity and unresponsiveness to repetitive stimulation
Lambert-Eaton syndrome	Similar to those in botulism, but repetitive nerve stimulation shows much greater augmentation of muscle action potentials, particularly at 20-50 Hz

Abbreviations: CMAPs, compound muscle action potentials; MUPs, motor unit potentials.

*From Cherington M. Clinical spectrum of botulism. Muscle Nerve 1998:21;701-10, and Maselli RA, Bakshi N. American Association of Electrodiagnostic Medicine (AAEM) case report 16: botulism. *Muscle Nerve* 2000;23:1137-44

PLAGUE (YERSINIA PESTIS)

IMPORTANT FEATURES

- There are an average of 10 cases of naturally occurring plague in the U.S. per year, but primary plague pneumonia is rare—there have been seven cases in the past 50 years. This diagnosis strongly suggests bioterrorism.
- Clinical clues to plague pneumonia: pneumonia in previously healthy persons that is characterized by fulminent course, hemoptysis, shock, and high mortality.
- Standard antibiotic treatment is streptomycin or gentamicin; in a mass casualty setting, it may be necessary to rely on oral doxycycline and fluoroquinolones.
- Prophylaxis with doxycycline and fluoroquinolones is probably very effective and a critical part of the response plan.
- Person-to-person transmission risk—prophylaxis for being within four feet of a person who is untreated or treated <48 to 72 hours.
- There are no rapid diagnostic tests for clinical labs—all rapid tests are in public health labs

---

BACKGROUND

Yersinia pestis has ideal characteristics as a biological weapon:
- The organisms can be delivered by aerosol to cause pneumonic plague, which is a serious illness with a high fatality rate.
- Pneumonic plague is communicable, thus posing the risk of secondary cases.
- The organism has a special place in the history of medicine as a result of the 14th century pandemic, which killed one-third of the European population; thus, this organism instills special fear.
- Initial cases may not be easily recognized, since they may resemble community-acquired pneumonia.
- A WHO report estimated that a 50 kg release of *Y pestis* spores over a city of 5 million people would cause severe illness in 150,000 and 36,000 deaths. (This estimate did not consider secondary cases caused by person-to-person spread).

In the U.S., plague occurs naturally primarily in three forms:
- **Bubonic plague** usually represents transmission by a flea from a rodent source, resulting in a local skin lesion at the site of the bite (which is rarely recognized), followed by transmission via lymphatics to lymph nodes, causing the characteristic painful buboes, followed by septicemia, then DIC, shock, and death.
- **Pneumonic plague** results from inhalation, usually from droplets from infected humans or animals. The estimated inoculum size necessary to cause disease is 100 to 500 microbes. The initial clinical event is lobar pneumonia, then septicemia with DIC and death. The mortality approaches 100% in the absence of treatment.
- **Septicemic plague** results from bacteremia with the sepsis syndrome and multi-organ failure and death without an identified portal of entry.

With bioterrorism, it is suspected that the most common form would be inhalation plague as a result of aerosol delivery, and then secondary cases reflecting person-to-person spread. Since these account for only about 2% of about 10 cases per year in the U.S., any case of inhalation plague should strongly suggest bioterrorism.

The main challenges for detection of inhalation plague are suspicion of this diagnosis at a time when community-acquired pneumonia is usually treated empirically with minimal use of diagnostic testing. Once a bioterrorism event is described, the challenge is to rapidly identify exposed persons for early treatment and prophylaxis, and to prevent secondary spread through infection control precautions. In terms of the initial detection, this diagnosis should be suspected when:
- There is severe pneumonia in previously healthy persons, often with multiple cases at two to four days after exposure to a common source.
- The characteristic features of endemic plague would not apply—e.g., exposure in plague-endemic areas and the characteristic of buboes would not be found.

HOSPITAL PREPARATION

Important needs for hospital preparedness for aspects involving pneumonic plague are:

- A plan for prophylaxis for all potentially exposed persons from a common source release. This should not be in a hospital, but in a conveniently located facility that can rapidly evaluate potential exposures and expeditiously give prophylactic antibiotics. Prophylaxis is virtually 100% effective; those who present with pneumonic plague may have overwhelming septicemia and death despite appropriate antibiotics. *Prophylaxis to exposed persons is critical.*
- Special precautions to protect healthcare personnel with appropriate infection control sometimes combined with antibiotic prophylaxis.
- A plan for triage of substantial numbers of patients in the event of a large release. Efficiency here is critical because a delay of antibiotics for pneumonic plague for >24 hours is usually fatal.
- A plan to deal with large numbers of patients who require isolation by cohorting in individual rooms. Hospital personnel, especially emergency department personnel, need to be alert to the clinical and epidemiological clues that suggest pneumonic plague. The initial case will be the major diagnostic challenge. The major clinical clues: pneumonia with sepsis and hemoptysis in a previously healthy host and/or multiple cases.
- Once cases are identified, there needs to be a plan for dealing with mass numbers of cases in terms of infection control, prophylaxis, and health care worker education. This planning needs to include a high priority for specialized personnel, including emergency department personnel, infection control, pulmonary and critical care, laboratory personnel, mental health, and infectious disease.
- Established or suspected cases of plague (all forms) must be reported to public health authorities.
- Lab personnel need to be warned of possible *Y pestis* in clinical specimens.

PERSONAL PROTECTION

- Plague is transmitted primarily by fleas from a rodent source or by respiratory secretions. In a bioterrorism event, the transmission would probably be by aerosol, causing pneumonic plague or secondary cases of pneumonic plague through exposure to contaminated secretions. The health care provider dealing with cases is at risk from droplets nuclei of respiratory secretions at a distance of approximately 3.7 feet. Thus, anyone within four feet of a person with pneumonic plague and antibiotic treatment <48 to 72 hours is considered exposed and should receive prophylactic doxycycline or ciprofloxacin.
- Prevention of exposure is achieved with standard precautions including hand washing, gloves for handling any secretions, a surgical mask, eye protection or face shield, and gowns.
- All health care workers should wear a surgical mask when working within three to four feet of a patient treated <48 hours.

DECONTAMINATION

Survival outside the host is short. Following an aerosol release, *Y pestis* is considered potentially infectious for a maximum of only about one hour. Consequently, environmental decontamination has generally not been recommended.

QUARANTINE PROCEDURES

- Plague can be transmitted from person to person, although transmission can generally be prevented with infection control, with or without prophylactic antibiotics.
- Quarantine with a substantial number of exposures is a possible consideration, and the President has the authority to invoke quarantine, but this seem unlikely, given the effectiveness of antibiotic prophylaxis.

CLINICAL PRESENTATION

- Epidemiology is important in any case of plague, since this will represent an important

Table 1. Types of Plague

Type	% of Cases Endemic in U.S.	Clinical Features	Mortality with No Rx	Mortality with Antibiotics
Bubonic	85%	Regional adenopathy (buboes)	50%	<5%
Septicemic	13%	No pulmonary Involvement or buboes	100%	30-50%
Pneumonic	2%	Dyspnea, cough and infiltrate	100%	5-15%

clue to possible bioterrorism. The "hot spots" for plague in the world are Madagascar, Eastern and Southern Africa, Southeast Asia (especially Vietnam and Myanmar), parts of South America, the western U.S., Mongolia, Northern China, and parts of Russia. Cases in the U.S. are primarily in California, New Mexico, Arizona, and Colorado.

- Naturally acquired disease may occur as a result of living in or visiting an endemic area. The incubation period for bubonic plague is one to seven days; for pneumonic plague it is usually two to four days. Persons who are outside an endemic area or other potential source will not get plague.

BUBONIC PLAGUE

This is the most common clinical form and accounts for about 85% endemic cases in the U.S. The usual presentation is sudden onset of fever (mean 39.4°C) and chills, followed within one day by tender adnopathy involving the cervical, axillary, or inguinal nodes, which are enlarged and extremely tender. Nodes are usually confined to the site draining the bite site. Laboratory features show a leukocytosis (average 21,000/mm³). The course is characterized by secondary pneumonia in 5% to 15% of patients and septicemia that may result in shock and multi-organ failure. The mortality rate is approximately 50% without antibiotics and less than 5% with antibiotics.

SEPTICEMIC PLAGUE

This accounts for 13% of plague cases in the U.S. It is defined as septicemia without primary pneumonia or buboes. Presenting findings include fever, gastrointestinal symptoms, and leukocytosis. The course is rapid, with DIC, shock and multi-organ

failure. The mortality is about 100% without antibiotics and 30% to 50% with antibiotics.

PNEUMONIC PLAGUE

This is the inhalation form that would be seen with an aerosol source (bioterrorism) or from person-to-person transmission with pneumonic plague. The incubation period is one to seven days, usually one to four days. Characteristic clinical features include fever, dyspnea, cough productive of bloody sputum, and tachypnea. Laboratory studies show alveolar infiltrates in all patients and pleural effusions in about 50%. Occasional patients develop a cavity, but this is a late complication. Most commonly, the chest x-ray shows a consolidated pneumonia.

These cases are rapidly progressive with bacteremia, sepsis, DIC, and multi-organ failure. Death usually occurs with two to five days after the onset of illness. In the absence of antibiotics, mortality approaches 100% within 24 hours of the onset of symptoms.

DIAGNOSIS

CLINICAL FEATURES

- Important clinical clues to plague pneumonia are: 1) the fulminant clinical course progressing to death in two to five days after onset of symptoms, and 2) pneumonia associated with hemoptysis.
- Differential diagnosis with an epidemic of fatal pneumonia include: legionella (patients >45 yrs, positive urinary antigen in 80%), influenza (seasonal and serious disease only in elderly, unless there is a uniquely virulent strain such as avian flu), histoplasmosis (rarely fatal and endemic), inhalation anthrax

Table 2. Treatment Recommendations Based on the Consensus Statement of the Working Group on Civilian Biodefense*

Adults

Preferred	Alternative
Streptomycin[†§] 1gm IM bid x 10 days	**Doxycycline** 100 mg IV bid or 200 mg IV qd x 10 days
or	*or*
Gentamicin[†] 5 mg/kg qd IM	**Ciprofloxacin**[††] 400 mg IV bid x 10 days
or	*or*
2 mg/kg loading dose, then 1.7 mg/kg tid IM or IV x 10 days	**Chloramphenicol** 25 mg/kg IV qid x 10 days

Pregnant Women

Preferred	Contraindicated
Gentamicin[†] the dose above	**Streptomycin**

Children

Preferred	Alternative
Gentamicin[†] 2.5 mg/kg IM or IV tid x 10 days	**Doxycycline** >45 kg: adult dose
Streptomycin[†§] 15 mg/kg IM tid x 10 days	<45 kg: 2.2 mg/kg IV bid x 10 days
	or
	Ciprofloxacin[††] 15 mg/kg IV bid x 10 days
	or
	Chloramphenicol 25 mg/kg IV qid for 10 days

*Inglesby T, et al. *JAMA*. 2000;283:2281; [†]Renal dosage adjustment needed; [§]Avoid in pregnant women; [††]Fluoroquinolones other than ciprofloxacin are probably equally effective

(characteristic wide mediastinum and bloody pleural effusions), and pneumonic tularemia (far less serious, with mortality rate of 7% in pre-penicillin era).

CDC DIAGNOSTIC CRITERIA

- Confirmed diagnosis: Clinically compatible case *plus*:
  1) Isolation of *Y pestis* from a clinical source
  2) A four-fold or greater increase in serum antibody to *Y pestis* F1 antigen (F1 antigen is found in all strains that are pathogenic to humans)
- Presumptive diagnosis: Clinically compatible case *plus*:

1) Antibody titer 2 F1 antigen without prior vaccination (without the four-fold increase)
2) Detection of F1 antigen by fluorescent assay in a clinical specimen

STANDARD DIAGNOSTIC TESTS

GRAM STAIN

The organism appears as a small, plump GNB in clinical specimens, including sputum and blood. It may appear bipolar ("safety pin" appearance), but this is more easily demonstrated by Giemsa stain than by gram stain, and other organisms have this appearance.

Table 3. Prophylaxis Recommendations based on the Consensus Statement from the Working Group on Civilian Defense*

Adults	
Preferred	**Alternative**
Doxycycline 100 mg bid x 7 days *or* **Ciprofloxacin** 500 mg PO bid x 7 days	**Chloramphenicol** 25 mg/kg PO qid x 7 days
Pregnant Women	
Recommended	
Doxycycline 100 mg bid x 7 days *or* **Ciprofloxacin** 500 mg PO bid x 7 days	
Children	
Preferred	**Alternative**
Doxycycline 45 kg: adult dose <45 kg: 2.2 mg/kg PO bid x 7 days *or* **Ciprofloxacin** 20 mg/kg PO bid x 7 days	**Chloramphenicol** 25 mg/kg PO qid x 7 days

*Inglesby T, et al. *JAMA*. 2000;283:2281.

CULTURE

If plague is suspected, use standard agar plates, which should be taped shut and incubated at 28° C as well as the usual 35° C to 37° C.

DIRECT FLUORESCENT ANTIBODY STAIN (DFA)

A presumptive identification can be made on direct smears of clinical specimens or of organisms in cultures; this antigen detection system can be used only for cultures grown at 35° C to 37° C.

SEROLOGY

Paried sera collected at four to six weeks apart can be used for a retrospective diagnosis if there is a fourfold increase in titer or a single titer greater than 1:128 in an unvaccinated person.

ELISA AND PCR

Other diagnostic tests are ELISA for detection of F1 antigen in clinical specimens and PCR for the detection of *Y pestis*.

TREATMENT

- Antibiotic recommendations noted above are based on drugs that have been approved by the FDA for treatment of plague, in vitro activity, clinical experience, and activity in experimental animals.
- However, the clinical experience is modest and a strain with resistance to streptomycin and tetracyclines has been reported from Madagascar. With a bioterrorism event, there is likely to be a single strain, and antibiotic recommendations for treatment and prophylaxis would need to utilize data from in vitro sensitivity tests of that strain.

- In the event of antibiotic shortages, it should be noted that gatifloxacin and moxifloxacin appear to be as effective as ciprofloxacin.
- Amikacin and tobramycin appear to be as active as streptomycin.
- Most strains are sensitive in vitro to minocycline, trimethoprin-sulfamethoxzole, and cephalosporins (cefixime, ceftazidime, and ceftriaxone).
- Resistance has been noted to imipenem and macrolides.

PREVENTION

ANTIBIOTIC PROPHYLAXIS

This is highly effective in two settings:
1. Exposure from a common source such as an aerosol with a bioterrorism attack
2. Exposure by proximity of <3.6 feet to a patient treated for less than 48 hours and absence of adequate infection control

INFECTION CONTROL

Standard precautions for pneumonic plague include the following:
1. Hand washing following contact with body fluids or contaminated materials, even if gloves have been worn
2. Gloves for hand contact with body fluids or contaminated items
3. A gown, mask (could be a surgical mask), and eye protection or face shield
4. Patients should be in a private room for cohorting
5. The "four-foot rule": Visitors, other patients, and health care workers should maintain a distance of at least four feet to avoid exposure to respiratory droplets (not droplet nuclei). A surgical mask should be worn if there is closer contact
6. There is no necessity for a negative pressure room, special air handling methods, or a necessity to close the room door
7. *Y pestis* is not transmitted after treatment for 48 hours

Clinical Pathway: Pneumonic Plague

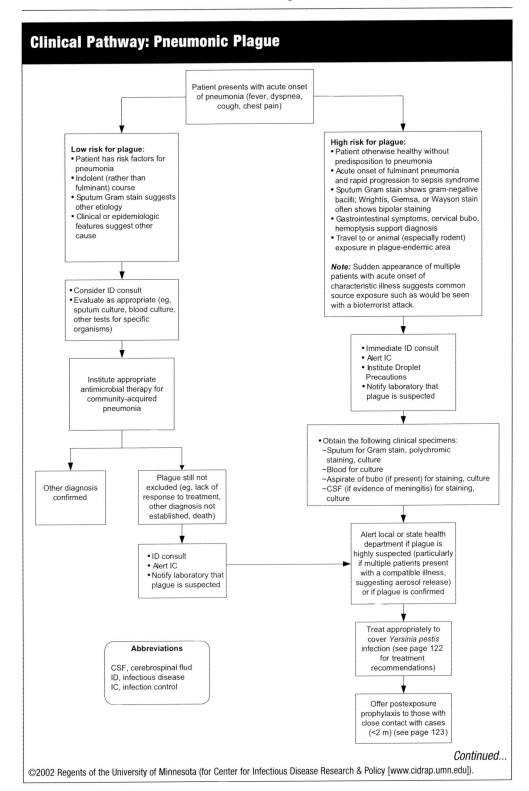

Patient presents with acute onset of pneumonia (fever, dyspnea, cough, chest pain)

Low risk for plague:
- Patient has risk factors for pneumonia
- Indolent (rather than fulminant) course
- Sputum Gram stain suggests other etiology
- Clinical or epidemiologic features suggest other cause

- Consider ID consult
- Evaluate as appropriate (eg, sputum culture, blood culture, other tests for specific organisms)

Institute appropriate antimicrobial therapy for community-acquired pneumonia

Other diagnosis confirmed

Plague still not excluded (eg, lack of response to treatment, other diagnosis not established, death)

- ID consult
- Alert IC
- Notify laboratory that plague is suspected

Abbreviations

CSF, cerebrospinal fluid
ID, infectious disease
IC, infection control

High risk for plague:
- Patient otherwise healthy without predisposition to pneumonia
- Acute onset of fulminant pneumonia and rapid progression to sepsis syndrome
- Sputum Gram stain shows gram-negative bacilli; Wrightis, Giemsa, or Wayson stain often shows bipolar staining
- Gastrointestinal symptoms, cervical bubo, hemoptysis support diagnosis
- Travel to or animal (especially rodent) exposure in plague-endemic area

Note: Sudden appearance of multiple patients with acute onset of characteristic illness suggests common source exposure such as would be seen with a bioterrorist attack.

- Immediate ID consult
- Alert IC
- Institute Droplet Precautions
- Notify laboratory that plague is suspected

- Obtain the following clinical specimens:
  ~Sputum for Gram stain, polychromic staining, culture
  ~Blood for culture
  ~Aspirate of bubo (if present) for staining, culture
  ~CSF (if evidence of meningitis) for staining, culture

Alert local or state health department if plague is highly suspected (particularly if multiple patients present with a compatible illness, suggesting aerosol release) or if plague is confirmed

Treat appropriately to cover *Yersinia pestis* infection (see page 122 for treatment recommendations)

Offer postexposure prophylaxis to those with close contact with cases (<2 m) (see page 123)

Continued...

Recommendations from the Working Group on Civilian Biodefense for Treatment of Pneumonic Plague During a Bioterrorism Event

Choices by Patient Category	Therapy Recommendations*
Adults: Preferred choices	Streptomycin, 1 gm IM twice daily for 10 days† *or* Gentamicin, 5 mg/kg IM or IV once daily or 2 mg/kg loading dose followed by 1.7 mg/kg IM or IV 3 times daily for 10 days‡§
Adults: Alternative choices**	Doxycycline, 100 mg IV twice daily or 200 mg IV once daily for 10 days§ *or* Ciprofloxacin, 400 mg IV twice daily for 10 days§†† *or* Chloramphenicol, 25 mg/kg IV 4 times daily for 10 days‡‡
Children: Preferred choices	Streptomycin, 15 mg/kg IM twice daily (maximum daily dose, 2 gm) *or* Gentamicin 2.5 mg/kg IM or IV 3 times daily for 10 days‡
Children: Alternative choices**	Doxycycline: ≥45 kg, give adult dosage <45 kg, give 2.2 mg/kg IV twice daily for 10 days (maximum, 200 mg/day) *or* Ciprofloxacin, 15 mg/kg IV twice daily for 10 days (maximum daily dose, 1 gm)†† *or* Chloramphenicol, 25 mg/kg IV 4 times daily for 10 days (maximum daily dose, 4 gm)‡‡§§

Abbreviations: IM, intramuscularly; IV, intravenously.

* These recommendations are most appropriate for the contained casualty setting where resources are adequate to treat all patients with intravenous antibiotics. In the mass casualty setting where the medical care delivery system is not able to meet the demands for patient care, oral antibiotics may need to be substituted for intravenous antibiotics for treatment of patients with plague. In such a situation, the recommendations in the table on postexposure prophylaxis should be followed for treatment, except that treatment should be continued for 10 days instead of 7 days.

† Streptomycin is not acceptable for use in pregnant women because irreversible deafness in children exposed in utero has been reported.

‡ Aminoglycosides must be adjusted according to renal function.

§ Acceptable for pregnant women. Although fetal toxicity may occur with doxycycline use, the Working Group recommended doxycycline or ciprofloxacin if gentamicin is not available or if oral antibiotics must be used.

** Trimethoprim-sulfamethoxazole has been used successfully to treat plague; however, the Working Group considers this agent as a second-tier choice.

††Other fluoroquinolones may be substituted at dosages appropriate for age.

‡‡Concentration should be maintained between 5 and 20 μg/mL; concentrations >25 μg/mL can cause reversible bone marrow suppression. The oral formulation is available only outside the United States. Some experts have recommended that chloramphenicol be used to treat patients with plague meningitis, since chloramphenicol penetrates the blood-brain barrier (AAP. Plague. In: Pickering LK, ed. 2000 Red Book: report of the Committee on Infectious Diseases. Ed 25. Elk Grove Village, Ill: American Academy of Pediatrics, 2000:450-2; Butler T. Plague. In: Strickland GT, ed. Tropical medicine. Philadelphia, Pa: WB Saunders, 1991:408-16; Dennis D, Meier F. Plague. In: Horsburgh CR, Nelson AM, eds. Pathology of emerging infections. Washington, DC: ASM Press, 1997:21-47). However, controlled trials to verify improvement in outcome have not been performed.

§§According to the Working Group, children younger than 2 years of age should not receive chloramphenicol. However, the American Academy of Pediatrics (AAP) has recommended chloramphenicol as the drug of choice for treating plague meningitis in children. The AAP *Red Book* (see reference above) does not indicate that chloramphenicol should not be given to children with serious infections who are beyond the newborn period but younger than 2 years of age.

Adapted from Inglesby TV, et al. Plague as a biological weapon: medical and public health management. JAMA 2000;283(17):2281-90 [http://jama.ama-assn.org/issues/v283n17/ffull/jst90013.html].

Continued...

Recommendations for the Working Group on Civilian Biodefense for Antibiotic Postexposure Prophylaxis During an Outbreak of Pneumonic Plague Following a Bioterrorism Event

Choices by Patient Category	Therapy Recommendations*
Adults: Preferred choices	Doxycycline, 100 mg PO twice daily for 7 days†‡ *or* Ciprofloxacin, 500 mg PO twice daily for 7 days‡§
Adults: Alternative choice**	Chloramphenicol, 25 mg/kg PO 4 times daily for 7 days††
Children: Preferred choices	Doxycycline: if ≥45 kg, give adult dosage; if <45 kg, give 2.2 mg/kg PO twice daily for 7 days† *or* Ciprofloxacin, 20 mg/kg PO twice daily for 7 days (maximum daily dose, 1 gm)§
Children: Alternative choice**	Chloramphenicol, 25 mg/kg PO 4 times daily for 7 days (maximum daily dose, 4 gm)††‡‡

Abbreviation: PO, orally.

* Recommendations were reached by consensus of the Working Group on Civilian Biodefense and may not necessarily be approved by the Food and Drug Administration. Although these recommendations are intended for postexposure prophylaxis, they also can be used for treatment of plague cases in the mass casualty setting where the number of patients is too great for all patients to receive intravenous antibiotics and oral antibiotics must be substituted (except that treatment should be continued for 10 days instead of 7 days as for prophylaxis).

† Tetracycline can be substituted for doxycycline at a dose of 10-25 mg/kg/day divided into 2-4 doses.

‡ Acceptable for pregnant women. Although fetal toxicity may occur with doxycycline use and toxic effects on the liver in pregnancy have been noted with the tetracycline class, the Working Group recommended doxycycline or ciprofloxacin for postexposure prophylaxis of pregnant women or for treatment of infection in the mass casualty setting.

§ Other fluoroquinolones may be substituted at dosages appropriate for age.

** Trimethoprim-sulfamethoxazole (40 mg sulfa/kg/day administered orally in 2 divided doses for 7 days) has been recommended for postexposure prophylaxis in children younger than 8 years old and pregnant women (AAP. Plague. In: Pickering LK, ed. 2000 Red book: report of the Committee on Infectious Diseases. Ed 25. Elk Grove Village, Ill: American Academy of Pediatrics, 2000:450-2; McGovern. Plague. In: Zajtchuk R, Bellamy RF, eds. Textbook of military medicine: medical aspects of chemical and biological warfare. Washington, DC: Office of the Surgeon General, Borden Institute, Walter Reed Army Medical Center, 1997 [http://www.nbc-med.org/SiteContent/HomePage/WhatsNew/MedAspects/contents.html].

†† Concentration should be maintained between 5 and 20 µg/mL; concentrations >25 µg/mL can cause reversible bone marrow suppression. The oral formulation is available only outside the United States.

‡‡ According to the Working Group, children younger than 2 years of age should not receive chloramphenicol.

Adapted from Inglesby TV, et al. Plague as a biological weapon: medical and public health management. JAMA 2000;283(17):2281-90 [http://jama.ama-assn.org/issues/v283n17/ffull/jst90013.html].

SMALLPOX (VARIOLA MAJOR)

IMPORTANT POINTS

- As a naturally occurring disease, smallpox was eliminated from globe in 1977, the mortality rate is 30%, and nearly all people are susceptible.
- Any announcement of smallpox would cause global panic. Announcements should only be made by designated facility representatives, usually through public health authorities.
- State and local public health authorities must immediately know about any likely or possible case (see the definitions below).
- Any case of smallpox means bioterrorism, a criminal investigation should be anticipated, and relevant evidence should be preserved.
- A smallpox vaccination within four days of exposure is protective or partially protective.
- The diagnosis of smallpox is suspected locally and established only in designated public health labs.
- Risk of transmission is defined by lack of immunity—plus being within 6.5 feet of a case during the rash stage. Contacts are defined as household members of a case or persons with face-to-face contact of a case during the rash. They should be vaccinated and monitored for temps.
- Vaccination policies: 1) preemptive (no smallpox risk) includes essential medical personnel, but excludes those with risks or family members with risks; 2) smallpox exposure—usually vaccinate everyone within the 6.5 foot ring and/or contacts of a case, as well as persons with a common source exposure from the bioterrorism event.
- Established and suspected cases should be isolated in negative-pressure rooms with airborne and contact precautions.

BACKGROUND

Smallpox is generally considered the most feared potential bioweapon on the basis of multiple factors:

- The disease occupies a prominent place in medical history as one of the most feared contagious diseases in terms of the potential for epidemic spread and high mortality.
- The mortality for *Variola major* is recorded at 15% to 45%, with an average of 30%.
- The disease is highly transmissible. The average case is historically the source of 3.6 to six additional cases as a result of contact within 6.5 feet.
- Routine smallpox examination was abandoned in the U.S. in 1972, and in most of the world by 1980. Most of those born in the U.S. after 1973 are immunologically naïve, and most of those vaccinated before that time are considered vulnerable as well, but possibly less so.
- There is no effective treatment for smallpox.
- Epidemics of smallpox in susceptible populations show waves of ten- to twentyfold increases in cases at intervals of 12 to 14 days—the incubation period. Thus, a small number of cases could rapidly become a major global epidemic.

The major limitation to the potential bioterrorist is the availability of the agent, *Variola major*. WHO declared smallpox eradicated in December 1979, and then recommended destruction of all existing supplies of *Variola* virus, except for stores maintained by the CDC in Atlanta and the Russian State Center for Research on Virology and Biotechnology in Russia. There is concern that there may be additional supplies of the virus, but specific locations are not known.

Smallpox vaccination is highly effective for preventing smallpox, as demonstrated by the global eradication program. In view of the potential threat of bioterrorism, President George W. Bush announced on December 13, 2002, a plan for vaccinating 500,000 public health staff and health care workers who would represent the first responders in the event of a bioterrorism attack with smallpox. However, only 39,000 health care workers were vaccinated due to concerns about adverse events, workmen's compensation issues, and liability.

Current recommendations for smallpox vaccination fall into in two categories: 1) smallpox response teams and health care worker teams who need to be ready for a smallpox attack (e.g., in 2003, the Department of Defense gave smallpox vaccinations to more than 450,000 U.S. military forces, as well as to certain emergency-essential civilians and contractors), and 2) a completely different recommendation that would apply to the use of the vaccination in the event of an attack.

HOSPITAL PREPARATION

A hospital response to a smallpox outbreak needs to include the following components:
- There needs to be education regarding recognition of smallpox. Any single case is, by definition, an act of bioterrorism that needs the immediate involvement of a medical response, a public health response, and an FBI response.
- Medical care facilities need to know the method for managing a potential case in terms of collecting specimens and use of the appropriate resource laboratories.
- There needs to be substantial attention to infection control, including patient isolation in negative-pressure rooms.
- In the event of a smallpox case in a facility in a city or in a region, there needs to be a planned response for management with vaccine strategies in two categories:
    ✔ Essential medical personnel with priority over those with prior smallpox vaccination to achieve an accelerated response
    ✔ Persons exposed to smallpox with the "ring vaccination plan" (described below)

- In the event of an outbreak, critical health care workers would be a high priority for immediate vaccination, as would be an aggressive education program regarding the reality of the risk to both healthcare workers and their families.
- Hospital planning needs to identify health care workers who are essential: emergency medicine, critical care, infectious disease, infection control, dermatology, pathology, and respiratory therapy. High priority should be given to persons who are protected by previous vaccination (first, recent vaccinees with a "take;" then, remote vaccine recipients).

- Regional planning would be critical. In prior times, it was common to divert smallpox cases to a single hospital; no hospital wants to be the "smallpox hospital," so this plan becomes feasible only in the event that there is an available facility that is not in use.

PERSONAL PROTECTION

- Smallpox is transmitted person-to-person by droplet nuclei in respiratory secretions. The risk of transmission begins with the onset of the rash and lasts until the scabs have fallen off. The proximity to a case that defines risk is being within 6.5 feet.
- Smallpox vaccination with a "take" indicates immunity, but the duration of protection is not well defined. The reason is that humoral response decreases with time, but cell-mediated immunity may persist much longer.
- A "take" is defined as a vesicular response at the site of vaccination or a scar at a prior vaccination site. Persons with recent vaccination and a "take" are protected. Those who had a vaccination more than five to 10 years ago should be revaccinated, although they are likely to have partial protection without the vaccine and will have an accelerated response with revaccination. For this reason, persons born before 1973 are often the highest priority for the initial care plan for vaccination.
- Patients with smallpox should have airborne and contact precautions in addition to standard precautions.

DECONTAMINATION

Variola is usually inactivated within one hour in the environment. Hypochlorite and quaternary ammonium compounds are adequate to clean surfaces. Laundry should be placed in a biohazard container and autoclaved before being laundered. An alternative is to launder in water to which bleach has been added. The virus may survive long periods, possibly months or years, in scabs or in cool environmental temperatures, but these are not thought to be important sources of cases.

Table 1. Comparison of Smallpox and Chickenpox

Prodromal Stage	Smallpox	Chickenpox
Duration	2-4 days	1 day
Severity	High fever	Mild
Rash Stage		
Initial	Oral mucosa	Trunk
Location	Most—face and distal extremities	Trunk
Stage	Lesions evolve together	Lesions are at different stages
Pain	Painful	Not painful
Depth	Deep dermis	Superficial
Other Considerations		
Duration	14-21 days	4-7 days
Age	All ages	Children
Severity	Toxic	Not toxic
Mortality	30%	Nil

QUARANTINE PROCEDURES

- Quarantine has been implemented in prior outbreaks of smallpox, including an outbreak in the former Yugoslavia which appeared to contribute to containment.
- The President of the United States has the authority to invoke quarantine in an effort to control smallpox and other major health hazards, including SARS and avian influenza.
- Despite precedent and presidential authority for quarantine, it is anticipated that ring vaccination and education will be satisfactory to deal with an outbreak of smallpox.

CLINICAL PRESENTATION

- The incubation period is usually 12 days, with a range of seven to 16 days.
- *Prodrome:* Characteristic features that precede the rash include fever in all patients, usually with headache and backache, and usually sufficiently severe to send the patient to bed. Thus, most transmissions occur in the hospital or in the home.
- The rash begins on the oral mucosa, then the face. Then there is centrifugal spread to the trunk and proximal extremities, and then to distal extremities. The most extensive involvement is on the face and distal extremities.
- The lesions evolve simultaneously, starting with macules (day one), then papules (day two), then vesicles (days three to five), then pustules (days seven to 14), and then scabs (days 14 to 20). These lesions are deeply imbedded in the dermis; they form firm nodules and leave scars.
- Patients with smallpox are severely ill, may appear toxic, and have a mortality rate of about 30%.
- Other forms of smallpox include:
  Variola minor—This is caused by a distinct strain of variola virus; it was the predominant form of smallpox in the U.S. and Great Britain, and it is a much milder form. The epidemiology, vaccine protection, and management issues are all the same, but the mortality rate is <1%. It seems unlikely that a bioterrorist would use this strain if there was any option.
  Hemorrhagic smallpox—This is an especially severe form of smallpox associated with bleeding from mucosal surfaces (hence the name), DIC, and thrombocytopenia. The mortality rate is about 95%.
  Flat-type smallpox—Another relatively rare form of smallpox, it is associated with lesions that evolve slowly, remain flat, and do not progress to the pustular stage (hence the name).

This is associated with severe toxicity and a mortality rate of about 95%.

- Differential diagnoses
    - ✔ **Chickenpox** (see **Table 1**)
    - ✔ **Monkeypox**
      Seventy-one cases in the U.S. in 2003. No further cases reported after 2003.
    - ✔ **Disseminated herpes zoster**
      Disease of the compromised host with a diagnosis by Tzanck prep, PCR, DFA stain, and/or culture.
    - ✔ **Disseminated herpes simplex**
      Disseminated disease occurs in the compromised host. The diagnoses are established with Tzanck prep; PCR, DFA stain and/or culture.
    - ✔ **Coxsackie virus**
      Hand, foot, and mouth disease, usually in children and often limited to hands and feet.
    - ✔ ***Molluscum contagiosum***
      Usually occurs in healthy children or HIV-infected adults. Lesions are painless. This disease is usually chronic rather than acute.
    - ✔ **Drug eruptions**
      Association with a drug—usually not severe, and the rash is usually not pustular.
    - ✔ **Secondary syphilis**
      VDRL or RPR—always positive.

DISEASE FEATURES

- The diagnostic challenge will be the first case. After that, patients with typical exposure history and symptoms will be managed presumptively.
- The CDC has identified the following three criteria for determining the probability of smallpox in a patient with a generalized vescicular or pustular rash.

CDC CRITERIA FOR DETERMINING THE PROBABILITY THAT A PATIENT HAS SMALLPOX

HIGH PROBABILITY

All three of the following:
- Fever for one to four days before the onset of

the rash and measuring $\geq 102°$ F, plus at least one of the following: prostration, headache, backache, chills, vomiting, or severe abdominal pain
- Classic smallpox lesions that are deep in the dermis, firm, round, often umbilicated, and may be discreet or confluent
- Lesions at the same stage of development

MODERATE PROBABILITY

- Febrile prodrome plus at least one of the smallpox criteria listed above

or

- Febrile prodrome and four of the following minor criteria: lesions primarily on face and distal extremities, initial lesions on oral mucosa or face, patient appears toxic or moribund, slow evolution of lesions over several days, and/or lesions on palms and soles

LOW PROBABILITY

- Lack of a febrile prodrome or febrile prodrome and fewer than four of the five minor criteria.

LABORATORY DIAGNOSES

CASE CLASSIFICATION

CONFIRMED CASE

Smallpox that is laboratory-confirmed or a patient that meets the case definition that is epidemiologically linked to a laboratory confirmed case

PROBABLE CASE

Case that meets the case definition or one that does not meet the case definition but is clinically consistent with smallpox and is epidemiologically linked to a confirmed case

SUSPECTED CASE

Febrile—a rash illness with fever preceding the rash by one to four days

COLLECTION OF SPECIMENS

- ✔ If probable case (defined above): The state or local health department should be contacted immediately for instructions on collecting specimens
- ✔ Dermatologic specimens should be obtained with barrier precautions, preferably by a person with smallpox vaccination within three years. If done by an unvaccinated person, it should be done by someone with no contraindication to vaccination in the event smallpox is confirmed, and the specimen collector should use barrier precautions plus a N95 respirator.
- ✔ The usual samples are a scraping of the base of a vesicle or pustule or a 3.5 mm to 4 mm dermal punch biopsy
- ✔ Specimens should be shipped to the CDC according to their specified conditions

VIRAL DETECTION (REQUIRES BSL-4 LAB)

- ✔ EM: The exam shows the very characteristic brick-shaped viron measuring about 200 nm in diameter. This is detected in about 95% of specimens from patients with *variola*
- ✔ Growth on egg chorioallantoic membrane (requires a BSL-4 isolation laboratory)
- ✔ PCR: This will permit detection of *variola*, vaccinia, and monkeypox

TREATMENT

- Treatment is supportive, with appropriate attention to infection control.
- There are no antiviral agents with established efficacy. Some agents with possible in vitro activity versus orthopox viruses (including variola) are cidofovir, adofovir, and rivavirin.

PREVENTION

CONTACT

A contact is a household member with face-to-face contact with an infected person during the period of rash. Contacts should be vaccinated and monitored for fever; they probably do not need to be isolated.

WHO SHOULD GET A SMALLPOX VACCINATION?

HEALTH CARE WORKERS

Health care workers considered essential for initial response as defined above should receive a smallpox vaccination. Contraindications to the vaccine include the presence of one of the following conditions in the potential vaccine recipient or in their household (family) members:

- History of eczema or atopic dermatitis
- Presence of an acute or chronic exfoliative skin condition
- Immunosuppressive condition, including HIV infection or high-dose steroids
- Physician-diagnosed heart disease, including risk for heart disease, defined as three or more of the following:
  - ✔ Hypertension
  - ✔ Diabetes
  - ✔ Increased cholesterol
  - ✔ Heart disease at age 50 in a first degree relative
  - ✔ Smoking
  - ✔ Women who are pregnant or are likely to become pregnant in the next four weeks

POSTEXPOSURE PROPHYLAXIS

- Immunity to variola virus develops within eight to 11 days after vaccination, and the incubation period for smallpox averages 10 to 13 days.
- Consequently, vaccination within four days of exposure reduces the rate of infection and also reduces the severity of the disease.
- This strategy would be expected to be particularly effective in persons who have previously been vaccinated, since revaccination could prompt an anamnestic immune response.
- The benefit of vaccine administration after four days following smallpox contact is not known.

VACCINATION IN A SMALLPOX EMERGENCY

The strategy currently favored is "ring vaccination,"

Table 2. Adverse Reactions to Smallpox Vaccination (Rate/1 Million)

Type of Reaction	1968 Survey*		2003 Experience**
	Primary	Revaccination	71% primary
Generalized Vaccinia	242	9	82
Eczema Vaccinatum	39	3	0
Progressive Vaccinia	1.5	3	0
Postvaccination Encephalitis	12	2	2
Myopericarditis	ND	ND	82

* Ten-state survey, 1968
** U.S. military experience with 450,293 vaccine recipients, 2003

which means vaccination to persons identified as "at risk" by any of the following:

- Face-to-face contact with, a household member of, or proximity contact of up to 6.5 feet of a person with confirmed or suspected smallpox, plus contact that takes place after the onset of fever and prior to dislodging of scabs
- Persons who are exposed to any defined release
- Medical personnel with priority to persons involved in the medical care of cases or public health evaluation of cases, and laboratory personnel who are responsible for collecting and transporting specimens

VACCINE SUPPLY

There is now sufficient smallpox vaccine in the U.S. to supply the entire population. The CDC is the exclusive vaccine distributor.

DURATION OF IMMUNITY

This has not been adequately defined. Standard teaching is a duration of five to 10 years. Neutralizing antibodies can be found for up to 30 years after three doses, and some studies have found evidence of cell-mediated immune response even longer. The assumption is that those who were vaccinated prior to 1973 are vulnerable to infection, but may have some protection against serious disease; persons who were not vaccinated within five years—and those vaccinated within five years and did not have a take—should be revaccinated.

RESPONSE TO VACCINATION

With primary vaccination (no prior vaccination), the usual sequence is: a red papule at three to five days, a vesicle at five to eight days, and then a pustule at eight to 10 days. The pustule then separates a dark crust and heals at 14 to 21 days. A pitted scar remains. Persons who develop a vesicle or pustule, or who have a pitted scar, are defined as having a "take," which indicates an immune response.

ADVERSE REACTIONS

- **Table 2** summarizes the serious and life-threatening reactions experienced with smallpox vaccinations during two periods of study—the first a 10-state 1968 report, the second the 2003 military experience.
- It is noted that the more recent experience was nearly devoid of any of the three potentially life threatening complications, including eczema vaccinatum, progressive vaccinia, and postvaccination encephalitis.
- The 2003 experience with smallpox vaccinations showed 37 cases of acute myopericarditis among 450,000 military vaccines, a complication that was not a recognized problem with the vaccine in the earlier period of study. All of these patients subsequently recovered, and all were primary vaccines.

VACCINA IMMUNE GLOBULIN (VIG)

This hyperimmune globulin is advocated for severe adverse reactions to smallpox vaccination that are caused by uncontrolled replication of vaccinia—

progressive vaccinia, eczema vaccinatum, generalized vaccine, and periorbital edema.

PATIENT CARE

All patients with suspected or established smallpox
should be isolated in a single room with negative
pressure and closed door, as well as on airborne
and contact precautions.

See next page for Clinical Pathways.

Clinical Pathway: Vesicular or Pustular Rash Illness

Patient with acute pustular or vesicular rash illness

↓

- Institute Airborne and Contact Precautions
- Alert IC on admission

Illness suggestive of smallpox

High-risk (meets all three *major criteria*):
- Febrile prodrome lasting 1-4 days with at least 1 of the following: prostration, headache, backache, chills, vomiting, severe abdominal pain *and*
- Classic smallpox lesions (deep-seated, firm, well-circumscribed, round, may be umbilicated) *and*
- Lesions in same stage of development

Moderate risk:
- Febrile prodrome *and*
- At least one other major criteria (see above)

  OR
- Febrile prodrome and ≥4 *minor criteria*:
  −Centrifugal distribution (greater concentraion of lesions on face, distal extremities)
  −First lesions on oral mucosa/ palate, face, forearms
  −Patient appears toxic or moribund
  −Slow pregression of lesions from macules to papules to pustules over days
  −Lesions on palms and soles

Note: Sudden appearance of multiple patients with acute onset of characteristic illness suggests common source exposure such as would be seen with a bioterrorist attack.

↓

- Immediate ID and derm consults
- Alert IC

↓

Contact local or state health department immediately

↓

Response team advises on management and specimen collection

↓

Testing at CDC

Illness suggestive of chickenpox

- No or minimal prodrome
- Lesions occur in crops (ie, are at different stages on any one area of body)
- Lesions are superficial (ie, "dew drop on rose petal" appearance)
- Lesions are usually not present on palms and soles
- Rash pattern is centripetal (ie, greater concentration on trunk)
- Lesions may be pruritic and usually are not painful
- Lesions progress quickly (>24 hr) from macules to papules, then to crusted lesions
- Patient does not appear toxic

↓

Test for VZV if diagnosis is in question

Abbreviations

CDC, Centers for Disease Control and Prevention
IC, infection control
ID, infectious disease
VZV, varicella-zoster virus

History and PE suggest diagnosis other than smallpox or chickenpox

- Disseminated herpes zoster
- Impetigo
- Drug eruption
- Contact dermatitis
- Erythema multiforme
- Disseminated herpes simplex
- Hand, foot, and mouth disease
- Molluscum contagiosum
- Secondary syphilis
- Scabies
- Insect bites
- Bullous pemphigoid

↓

ID and/or derm consults

↓

Evaluate as appropriate

↓

Other diagnosis confirmed

Re-evaluate patient if no diagnosis confirmed

↓

Contact local or state health department if smallpox is still under consideration

TULAREMIA (FRANCISELLA TULARENSIS)

IMPORTANT POINTS

- Following aerosol delivery, there would be multiple presentations based on the site of aerosol exposure, most commonly pneumonic tularemia, but also less common forms— ulceroglandular (from contaminated wounds), ocular, oropharyngeal, and typhoidal (sepsis).
- Clues to tularemic pneumonia are early prostration, delayed infiltrate, x-ray showing hilar adenopathy, a pulse-temperature disassociation, and low mortality.
- Antibiotic recommendation is streptomycin or gentamicin, with standard treatment of CAP. Fluoroquinolones may work. The experience with betalactams and macrolides is limited, failures are reported, and these are not recommended.
- In mass casualty setting, it may be necessary to rely on oral treatment with doxycycline, fluoroquinolone, or other agent selected by in vitro sensitivity test of the epidemic strain.
- There is no person-to-person spread, but warn the microbiologist.
- Microbiological identification is slow.

BACKGROUND

- Tularemia is a serious disease with multiple forms that is found in the U.S., primarily from two mechanisms of transmission: bites of infected insects and contact with rabbits and other small mammals.
- There are about 170 cases per year, with most in Arkansas, Oklahoma, Missouri, Kansas, South Dakota, and Montana.
- The highest rates are in persons ages five to nine years and 75 to 84 years.
- Most cases occur in the summer, and most are in rural areas; tularemia is rarely found in urban areas.
- There are periodic outbreaks. The last in the

U.S. was at Martha's Vineyard in 2000, when there were 15 cases; most had pneumonic disease, one patient died, and the epidemiologic risk was lawn mowing about two weeks before the onset of disease.

- Outside the U.S., the highest number of cases are in Russia and Scandinavian countries.
- Tularemia can present with several clinical syndromes. The most common with naturally occurring disease is ulceroglandular (cutaneous ulcer with regional adenopathy) and glandular tularemia (regional adenopathy with no ulcer). These two forms account for 50% to 90% of naturally occurring cases in the U.S.
- The forms of tularemia that would be expected in a bioterrorism event would be pneumonic tularemia (a primary pulmonary disease), which now accounts for less than 5% of naturally occurring disease, and occasional other forms, including oculoglandular tularemia (conjunctivitis and preauricular adenopathy).

Some of the issues regarding bioterrorism with tularemia are the following:

- Both the United States and the former Soviet Union developed, stockpiled, and weaponized *F tularensis* as a component of their bioterrorism programs in the 1950s and 1960s. The program in the Soviet Union included the development of weaponized strains of F *tularensis* that were resistant to antibiotics and vaccines.
- WHO estimated that an aerosol dispersal of 50 kg of *F tularensis* over a metropolitan area of 5 million people would result in 250,000 cases of tularemia and 19,000 deaths.
- In the event of bioterrorism, the following atypical features should specifically suggest a bioterrorism source rather than a naturally occurring disease:
  - Most patients would have primary pneumonic tularemia
  - The incubation period would be expected at three to five days for those with a heavy exposure, but up to 14 days for those who have a smaller inoculum size
  - The disease might occur in an urban area, which is unusual for tularemia, and it would involve patients who do not have the usual

risk factors in terms of age, exposure to insects or rabbits, or location in states with high numbers of those creatures

– Strains with antibiotic resistance would specifically suggest a bioterrorism source

HOSPITAL PREPARATION

- Hospitals need to be alert to the possibility of tularemia if there is an outbreak of pneumonia, especially community-acquired pneumonia with the characteristics summarized above.
- Other potential sources of an epidemic of pneumonia include Legionnaires' disease, influenza, and occasionally histoplasmosis or other endemic fungus.
- Other considerations within the context of bioterrorism include plague and inhalation anthrax.
- In sharp contrast to inhalation anthrax and pneumonic plague, patients with pneumonic tularemia have a less serious disease, usually respond to antibiotics within 24 to 48 hours, and have a case fatality rate of <2%.
- There is no patient-to-patient transmission of *F tularensis,* so infection control is not an important issue.
- There is some risk to the laboratory technicians who process the specimens containing *F tularensis.* The laboratory needs to be warned of this possibility.
- Patients exposed to a bioweapon attack should receive prophylaxis. Patients who are exposed and develop fever within 14 days should be treated presumptively.
- In a large-scale exposure, a plan is needed for mass application of prophylaxis and treatment.

PERSONAL PROTECTION

With tularemia in all its forms, standard precautions are appropriate, since there is no person-to-person transmission.

DECONTAMINATION

- Surfaces and medical devices can be cleaned with bleach (a 1:10 dilution of household bleach) and/or 70% alcohol. Body surfaces and clothing can be washed with soap and water.
- With aerosolized delivery and widespread surface contamination, no special environmental decontamination procedures are generally recommended.
- There is no person-to-person transmission of this pathogen.
- Standard chlorination should protect water supplies.
- With adequate public education, the risk of exposed animals or insects is regarded as low.

QUARANTINE PROCEDURES

Due to the absence of person-to-person transmission, quarantine is unnecessary.

CLINICAL PRESENTATION
PNEUMONIC TULAREMIA

- The incubation period is usually three to five days after an aerosol exposure.
- Clinical features are those of community-acquired pneumonia with the acute onset of fever, dry cough and dyspnea.
- A characteristic feature is rapid and profound prostration, mental impairment and, in 40% of cases, a pulse-temperature disassociation.
- Chest x-ray shows patchy infiltrates, often accompanied by hilar adenopathy and pleural effusions, but the x-ray changes are usually not apparent in early-stage disease.
- The course without therapy is highly variable—sometimes rapid but more often slowly progressive. In the pre-chemotherapeutic era, the mortality rate of pneumonic tularemia was only 7%.

ULCEROGLANDULAR AND GLANDULAR TULAREMIA

- In ulceroglandular tularemia, the organisms enter by an insect bite, there is an ulcerating lesion at the bite site, and the organism then spreads to regional lymph nodes, where it causes a necrotizing lymphadenitis.

Table 1. Treatment Recommendations for All Forms of Tularemia

Adults

Preferred	Alternative
Streptomycin[†] 1 gm IM bid x 10 days *or* **Gentamicin**[†] 5 mg/kg IM or IV qd x 10 days *or*	**Doxycycline** 100 mg IV bid x 14-21 days *or* **Chloramphenicol** 15 mg/kg qd x 14-21 days **Ciprofloxacin** 400 mg IV bid x 10 days

Pregnant Women

Recommended	
Gentamicin[†] 5 mg/kg IM or IV qd x 10 days *or* **Ciprofloxacin** 400 mg IV bid x 10 days	

Children

Preferred	Alternative
Streptomycin[†] 15 mg/kg IM (max 1 gm) bid x 10 days *or* **Gentamicin**[†] 2.5 mg/kg IM or IV tid x 10 days	**Doxycycline** >45 kg – adult doses 14-21 days <45 kg 2.2 mg/kg IV bid x 14-21 days *or* **Ciprofloxacin** 15 mg/kg IV bid x 10 days (maximum dose 1 gm) *or* **Chloramphenicol** 15 mg/kg IV qid x 14-21 days

[†] Renal dosage adjustment needed

- Clinical features include an incubation period of three to five days followed by fever, skin ulcer, and regional adenopathy (primarily axillary and epitrochlear adenopathy); about 30% of patients develop secondary pneumonia.
- Glandular tularemia has the same presentation as ulteroglandular tularemia, but without the recognition of the cutaneous lesion.
- The ulceroglandular and glandular forms of tularemia account for the majority of naturally occurring cases of tularemia and might account for a small percentage of cases in a bioterrorism attack by aerosol, due to contamination of pre-existing cutaneous lesions.

MISCELLANEOUS FORMS

OCULOGLANDULAR TULAREMIA

Oculoglandular tularemia is a result of ocular exposure, which may occur from an aerosol delivery. The presentation is conjunctivitis and preauricular adenopathy. This is associated with fever, periorbital edema, and an ocular exam that shows yellow conjunctival nodules, ulcers, and/or chemosis.

ORAL PHARYNGEAL TULAREMIA

Oral pharyngeal tularemia is a result of aerosol contamination of the oral pharynx. The presentation

Table 2. Antibiotic Recommendation for Patients with Aerosol Exposure to *F tularensis*
Adults
Doxycycline   100 mg PO bid x 14 days   *or*   **Ciprofloxacin**   500 mg PO bid x 14 days
Pregnant Women
Doxycycline   100 mg PO bid x 14 days   *or*   **Ciprofloxacin**   500 mg PO bid x 14 days
Children
Doxycycline   > 45 kg – 100 mg PO bid x 14 days   < 45 kg – 2.2 mg/kg PO bid x 14 days   *or*   **Ciprofloxacin**   15 mg/kg bid x 14 days

is pharyngitis, which may show an exudate or diphtheritic membrane, often with cervical adenopathy and fever. There may also be pneumonic tularemia.

TYPHOIDAL TULAREMIA

Typhoidal tularemia is characterized as a febrile illness without localizing signs or symptoms, and may be an important category with an aerosol delivery. Characteristic features include fever, prostration, gastrointestinal symptoms, leukocytosis, and bacteremia; the course may be rapid, with sepsis, coma, shock, and death. It should be noted that this is a relatively rare form of naturally occurring tularemia, accounting for less than 5% of cases. But it would be expected to be more common with an aerosol delivery, and it represents the form of tularemia with the highest mortality rates.

DIAGNOSIS

CDC CASE DEFINITION

CONFIRMED CASE

- Recovery of *F tularensis* in a clinical specimen
- A fourfold rise in antibody titer to *F tularensis*

PROBABLE CASE

A clinically consistent case with laboratory tests showing a presumptive diagnosis based on a single elevated antibody titer (in the absence of vaccination) or detection of *F tularensis* in a clinical specimen by fluorescent assay.

CULTURE

- The organism grows on conventional bacterial culture media, but poses a risk to laboratory personnel if there is aerosolization or skin contact at sites of open sores. Thus, warning the microbiologist is important so that microbial manipulations can be done in a biologic safety hood with gloves.
- The organism grows on blood agar, and plates should be taped shut. Growth is slow in broth and agar media, usually requiring two to five days in agar and a minimum of 10 days in broth.
- Level A laboratories can make a presumptive identification, but complete characterization should be done by a reference laboratory due to the risk associated with microbial manipulations.

STAINS

F tularensis is a tiny, faint-staining plemorphic GNB which is difficult to detect on direct gram stains of clinical specimens such as sputum. There are a variety of additional tests that are available at BSL3 labs to facilitate stain detection using DFA, PCR, and immunohistochemistry.

SEROLOGY

Commercially available serologic tests show an increased titer at about two weeks and peak titer at four to seven weeks.

TREATMENT

- The greatest experience is with aminoglycosides, primarily streptomycin and gentamycin, which appear to be equally effective.

- Ciprofloxacin and other fluorquinolones have been used successfully, but the experience is less extensive.
- Tetracycline and chloramphenacol can be used to treat tularemia, but experience is limited here as well, and there have been relapses, so these antibiotics are advocated for use primarily in combination with aminoglycosides.
- Supportive care is important, including fluid management.
- Exposed persons who develop fever within 14 days of exposure should be treated expectantly.
- In the event of mass attack, it may be necessary to rapidly treat large numbers of patients using oral regimens of doxycycline (100 mg twice a day) or ciprofloxacin (750 mg twice a day).

PREVENTION

ANTIBIOTIC PROPHYLAXIS

VACCINE

A live attenuated vaccine has been developed in the U.S. However, serologic response requires two weeks, and the incubation period for tularemia following exposure is generally three to five days.

INFECTION CONTROL

- There has been no documented person-to-person transmission of *F tulararensis*. Standard precautions are advocated.
- Contacts of cases should not be given prophylaxis.

See following pages for Clinical Pathways.

Clinical Pathway: Pneumonic Tularemia

Patient presents with acute onset of pneumonia (fever, dyspnea, cough, chest pain)

Low risk for tularemia:
- Patient has risk factors for pneumonia
- Sputum Gram stain suggests other etiology
- Clinical or epidemiologic features suggest other cause

- Consider ID consult
- Evaluate as appropriate (eg, sputum culture, blood culture, other tests for specific organisms)

Institute appropriate antimicrobial therapy for community-acquired pneumonia

Other diagnosis confirmed

Tularemia still not excluded (eg, lack of response to treatment, other diagnosis not established)

- ID consult
- Alert IC
- Notify laboratory that tularemia is suspected

High risk for tularemia:
- Rapid progression to severe, life-threatening pneumonia in relatively high proportion of cases
- Characteristic CXR findings: peribronchial infiltrates leading to bronchopneumonia in 1 or more lobes; hilar adenopathy and pleural effusions relatively common; nodular parenchymal pattern may be seen
- Sputum Gram stain generally not helpful, since organisms are difficult to visualize
- Concomitant presentation of cases with other clinical manifestations of tularemia (ie, ocular, oropharyngeal, ulceroglandular, glandular, or typhoidal tularemia)
- Less severe respiratory illnesses than those expected to be caused by anthrax or plague (anthrax cases would likely have characteristic mediastinal widening on CXR or chest CT; plague cases would likely have higher rates of hemoptysis and rapid progression to shock)

Note: Sudden appearance of multiple patients with acute onset of characteristic illness suggests common source exposure such as would be seen with a bioterrorist attack.

- Alert IC
- Immediate ID consult
- Notify laboratory that tularemia is suspected

Obtain the following clinical specimens:
- Sputum for Gram stain, culture, DFA testing through the LRN
- Blood for culture, serologic testing
- Aspirate of pleural fluid (if present) for staining, culture, DFA testing
- Biopsy specimen, scraping, swab, or aspirate of cutaneous ulcer (if present) for staining, culture, DFA testing

Alert local or state health department if tularemia is highly suspected (particularly if multiple patients present with a compatible illness, suggesting aerosol release) or if tularemia is confirmed

Treat appropriately to cover *F tularensis* infection (see page 139)

Follow public health recommendations for postexposure prophylaxis of potentially exposed persons, if indicated (see page 140)

Abbreviations

CT, computed tomography
CXR, chest x-ray
DFA, direct fluorescent antibody
ID, infectious disease
IC, infection control
LRN, laboratory response network

Clinical Pathway: Pneumonic Tularemia

Recommendations for Treatment of Tularemia During a Bioterrorism Event

Choices by Patient Category	Therapy Recommendations*†
Adults: Preferred choices	Streptomycin, 1 gm IM twice daily for 10 days‡§** *or* Gentamicin, 5 mg/kg IM o r IV once daily for 10 days‡**
Adults: Alternative choices	Doxycycline, 100 mg IV twice daily for 14-21 days‡ *or* Chloramphenicol, 15 mg/kg IV 4 times daily for 14-21 days†† *or* Ciprofloxacin, 400 mg IV twice daily for 10 days‡
Children: Preferred choices	Streptomycin, 15 mg/kg IM twice daily (maximum daily dose, 2 gm) for 10 days** *or* Gentamicin, 2.5 mg/kg IM or IV 3 times daily for 10 days**
Children: Alternative choices	Doxycycline ≥45 kg: give adult dosage for 14-21 days <45 kg: give 2.2 mg/kg IV twice daily for 14-21 days *or* Ciprofloxacin, 15 mg/kg IV twice daily for 10 days (maximum daily dose, 1 gm) *or* Chloramphenicol, 15 mg/kg IV 4 times daily for 14-21 days (maximum daily dose, 4 gm)††

Abbreviations: IM, intramuscularly; IV, intravenously.

*In the mass casualty setting where the medical care delivery system is not able to meet the demands for patient care, oral antibiotics may need to be substituted for intravenous antibiotics for treatment of patients with tularemia. In such a situation, the recommendations in the table above on postexposure prophylaxis should be followed for treatment.
†These treatment recommendations reflect those of the Working Group on Civilian Biodefense and may not necessarily be approved by the Food and Drug Administration.
‡Acceptable for pregnant women.
§Streptomycin is not as acceptable as gentamicin for use in pregnant women because irreversible deafness in children exposed in utero has been reported with streptomycin use.
**Aminoglycosides must be adjusted according to renal function.
††Concentration should be maintained between 5 and 20 µg/mL; concentrations >25 µg/mL can cause reversible bone marrow suppression.

Adapted from Dennis DT, Inglesby TV, Henderson DA, et al, for the Working Group on Civilian Biodefense. Tularemia as a biological weapon: medical and public health management. JAMA 2001;285:2763-73.

Continued...

Clinical Pathway: Pneumonic Tularemia

Recommendations for Antibiotic Postexposure Prophylaxis During an Outbreak of Tularemia Following a Bioterrorism Event*

Patient Category	Therapy Recommendations†
Adults (including pregnant women)	Doxycycline, 100 mg PO twice daily for 14 days‡ *or* Ciprofloxacin, 500 mg PO twice daily for 14 days‡
Children	Doxycycline ≥45 kg: give adult dosage <45 kg: give 2.2 mg/kg PO twice daily for 14 days *or* Ciprofloxacin, 15 mg/kg PO twice daily for 14 days (maximum daily dose, 1 gm)

Abbreviation: PO, orally.

*In the mass casualty setting where the medical care delivery system is not able to meet the demands for patient care, oral antibiotics may need to be substituted for intravenous antibiotics for treatment of patients with tularemia. In such a situation, the recommendations in this table should be followed for treatment as well as for prophylaxis.
†Recommendations were reached by consensus of the Working Group on Civilian Biodefense and may not necessarily be approved by the Food and Drug Administration.
‡Although fetal toxicity may occur with doxycycline use, the Working Group recommended doxycycline or ciprofloxacin for postexposure prophylaxis of pregnant women or for treatment of infection of pregnant women in the mass casualty setting.

Adapted from Dennis DT, Inglesby TV, Henderson DA, et al, for the Working Group on Civilian Biodefense. Tularemia as a biological weapon: medical and public health management. JAMA 2001;285:2763-73.

VIRAL HEMORRHAGIC FEVER (VHF)

IMPORTANT POINTS

- The characteristic features are fever and hemorrhage from any site; the hemorrhage is usually due to thrombocytopenia, and the frequency with different VHF viruses is highly variable.
- None of these viruses is found in the U.S. Detection in a U.S. patient without travel to an endemic area within 21 days prior to the onset of symptoms means bioterrorism.
- Contagion begins with fever.
- These viruses are transmitted person-to-person primarily by contact with blood and body fluids; airborne transmission is also possible.
- The primary concern for transmission is nosocomial and household spread. The infection control recommendation would require complex changes in standard practice in dealing with patients, lab specimens and corpses.
- Containment will require placement of patients in isolation or by cohorting in a negative-pressure room with access restricted to essential personnel.
- Management, risks, and mortality show substantial differences for the various agents within the class of VHF viruses.

BACKGROUND

The hemorrhagic fever viruses are a diverse group of viruses found primarily in Africa and Asia that cause hemorrhagic conditions. They are attractive for bioterrorism due to the following properties:
- The minimum infection dose is as low as 10 virions.
- They can be distributed and cause disease through aerosols.
- The mortality and morbidity rate is usually high.
- They cause great fear.

- There are no effective vaccines and antiviral agents are limited or nil.
- Some agents in this category are apparently transmitted person to person.

The former Soviet Union maintained stocks of viral hemorrhagic fever viruses (Marburg, Ebola, Lassa, Junin, and Machupo) in their bioterrorism arsenal. To our knowledge, there has not been attempted bioterrorism with these agents.

The organisms included in this category that are considered the best candidates for bioterrorism are the following:
- Ebola virus
- Marburg virus
- Lassa virus
- New World arenaviruses
  - Machupo (Bolivian hemorrhagic fever)
  - Junin (Argentine hemorrhagic fever)
  - Guanarito (Venezuelan hemorrhagic fever)
  - Sabia (Brazilian hemorrhagic fever)
- Rift Valley fever virus
- Yellow fever virus
- Kyasanur forest disease virus
- Omsk hemorrhagic fever virus

The properties these viruses have in common are: 1) all are single-stranded RNA viruses; 2) all possess a lipid envelope; 3) none has ever been found in the U.S. or Europe, so their presence indicates either importation or bioterrorism; and 4) they cause fever and thrombocytopenia and/or platelet dysfunction, resulting in bleeding.

HOSPITAL PREPARATION

This is a diverse group of viruses that share some properties, although risk of transmission is somewhat variable (see **Table 1**). The following represent the general issues for the hemorrhagic fever viruses in terms of hospital response:
- All of the viruses in this class may be delivered by an aerosol attack, which is regarded as the most likely mechanism with bioterrorism. Hospitals consequently need to be prepared for evaluating large numbers of cases, including some patients who are critically ill or who will become critically ill.

Table 1. Clinical Features of Hemorrhagic Fever Viruses

Virus(es)	Clinical	Person-to-person transmission	Incubation period	Mortality	Antiviral agent with in vitro activity
Ebola	High fever, severe prostration, DIC M-P rash, DIC	Yes	2-21 days	50%-90%	None
Marburg arenavirus	High fever, M-P rash, DIC	Yes	2-14 days	23%-80%	None
Lassa fever	Fever, severe pharyngitis, conjunctivitis, GI sx	Yes	5-16 days	15%-20%	Ribavirin
New World	Fever, myalgias, GI sx, conjunctivitis, general adenopathy ± CNS sx	Yes	7-14 days	15%-30%	Ribavirin
Rift Valley fever	Fever, headache, jaundice, photophobia	No	2-6 days	<1%	Ribavirin
Yellow fever	Fever, conjunctivitis, flushing, remission—then + fever, renal failure, jaundice	No	3-6 days	20%	None
Omsk hemorrhagic fever	Fever, conjunctivitis, red face and trunk, general adenopathy, pneumonia, CNS, biphasic	No	2-9 days	.05% to 10%	None
Kyasanur	Like Omsk hemorrhagic fever—biphasic with CNS sx	No	2-9 days	3%-10%	None

- There will be large numbers of "worried well."
- The response in terms of treatment or vaccine is virus-dependent.
- Hospital laboratory personnel are at great risk. This risk applies to microbiologists who may manipulate cultures and technicians working with other specimens as well.
  - In general, laboratory testing should be held to a minimum, pneumonic transmission of specimens should not be done.
  - Technicians who handle the specimens should be limited to those with special training.
  - Serum samples need to be pretreated with Triton X-100 or samples should be heated to 60° C for one hour.
  - Laboratory workers need to wear protective equipment and processing should usually be done in a BSL-3 facility.
  - It is emphasized that these restrictions apply to all specimens, not just microbiology specimens. The reason is that these viruses are transmitted primarily by blood or body fluids.

- Large numbers of patients may require large stocks of ribavirin for viral hemorrhagic fever of unknown cause or if the identified cause or virus specifically is arenavirus or bunyavirus.
- For large numbers of patients with extensive bleeding there will need to be substantial supplies of platelets, fresh frozen plasma, and clotting factor concentrates.
- Nosocomial transmission usually results from contact with infected blood or body fluids, making contact precautions the highest priority. Person-to-person airborne transmission appears to be rare. Nevertheless, the combination of airborne and contact precautions is usually advised.
- With admission of multiple patients, the recommendation is for cohorting to reduce exposure of other patients and to reduce the contact with health care workers.
- Any case of suspected or established VHF infection must be reported immediately to infection control and public health authorities.

PERSONAL PROTECTION

- Risk for non-laboratory health care workers is largely defined by contact with mucous membranes or body fluids of patients with viral hemorrhagic fever after the onset of fever. Airborne transmission appears to be plausible, but rare; airborne precautions are appropriate, but not nearly as important as blood and body fluid precautions.
  - The specifics of the recommendations for protecting healthcare workers are described on the next page under "Prevention."

- Persons (patients and health care workers) who have high risk (contact with mucous membranes or percutaneous injury involving exposure to secretions) or close contact (live with, shake hands with, provide medical care, or process laboratory specimens from a patient with viral hemorrhagic fever) are at risk.
- Ribavirin prophylaxis is not generally advocated, but should be considered for high-risk exposures.
- Exposed persons should have careful temperature monitoring for 21 days; with fever they should be referred to an appropriate provider for monitoring of temperature and symptoms.

DECONTAMINATION

- The hemorrhagic fever viruses have lipid envelopes, which mean that they are not stable in the environment for more than one hour. Consequently, decontamination of the environment is generally not necessary, but this decision should be made by an expert based on the type of contamination.
- For environmental surfaces and contaminated objects, disinfection with EPA-registered hospital disinfectants or a 1:100 dissolution of household bleach should be adequate.
- Excreta should be disinfected with 0.6% sodium hydrochlorite.
- Bedding and clothes should be incinerated, autoclaved, or placed in double bags and washed without sorting with a normal hot water cycle and bleach.

QUARANTINE PROCEDURES

It is possible that quarantine would be considered appropriate.

CLINICAL PRESENTATION

- The common features in all patients are fever, usually accompanied by myalgia, and prostration.
- A variable finding is hemorrhages, which may be from mucous membranes, hemoptysis, hematemsis, bloody diarrhea, petechiae, and ecchymosis. With many of the agents in this group, hemorrhage is actually quite rare.
- Characteristics of the individual conditions are summarized in **Table 1**.

DISEASE FEATURES

- All patients are febrile, and this defines the beginning of potential transmission.
- The hemorrhage can be a purpuric rash, hematemesis, hemoptysis, and/or melena.
- There is variable severity and great differences in the number of patients who actually have hemorrhage with different viral agents. The usual cause of hemorrhage is thrombocytopenia, which is a characteristic laboratory finding when hemorrhage is found.

DIAGNOSIS

- Laboratory personnel should be warned, and only designated technicians should be assigned to processing specimens. This applies to all specimens, not just microbiology specimens.
- Hazards include respiratory exposure to aerosols, mucous membrane exposures, or accidental parenteral inoculation.

Specimens from patients with suspected VHF should be referred for diagnostic testing to the CDC or the U.S. Army Research Institute of Infectious Diseases (USAMRIID) at Fort Detrick, MD (USAMRIID's emergency response line is: 888-872-7443; the duty officer will provide

Table 2. Treatment Recommendations for Viral Hermorrhagic Fever of Unknown Cause or Known to be Caused by Arenavirus of Bunyavirus

Contained-Casualty Setting	Mass-Casualty Setting
Adults	
Ribavirin*	Ribavirin*
32 mg/kg (Max: 2 gm) x 1 IV	2 gm PO x 1
then	*then*
16 mg/kg (Max: 1 gm) q 6h IV x 4 days	600 mg bid (weight >75 kg)
then	*or*
8 mg/kg (Max: 500 mg) q 8h x 6 days	1,000 mg/day in 2 doses (weight ≤75mg) x 10 days
Pregnant Women	
Category X	Category X
Children	
Ribavirin*	Ribavirin*
32 mg/kg (Max: 2 gm) x 1 IV	30 mg/kg PO or IV
then	*then*
16 mg/kg (Max: 1 gm) q 6h IV x 4 days	30 mg/kg PO or IV
then	*then*
8 mg/kg (Max: 500 mg) q 8h x 6 days	15 mg/kg/day in 2 doses x 10 days

* Ribavirin is not FDA approved for VHF. It must be used under an investigational new drug protocol.

direction). These are the only level D labs in the U.S. that can do viral isolation of the VHF.

- The preferred diagnostic method for most of these agents is with antigen detection using ELISA on serum or RT-PCR, 1 gm serology, and viral isolation. The CDC requires one day for a preliminary analysis.

TREATMENT

- Ribavirin has in vitro activity against Lassa fever, New World arenaviruses, and bunyaviruses.
- The ribavirin regimen recommended is summarized in **Table 2**. This provides recommendations for a contained-casualty setting and a mass-casualty setting. The former would apply to a limited number of cases where there would be the ability to rapidly administer IV treatment; the mass casualty setting assumes the need for oral treatment.
- Supportive care will include management of any bleeding complications with clotting factors, platelets, and fresh frozen plasma.

- Other forms of supportive care include mechanical ventilation, dialysis, and antibiotic treatment for secondary infections.
- Steroids have no influence on the course of the disease.

PREVENTION

The major concern is nosocomial and household transmission by contact with blood and body fluids. The second category of concern is close contact by people living with, shaking hands with, or processing laboratory specimens from a patient with VHF. Exposed persons by this definition should be on temperature surveillance, usually for two to three weeks, depending on the incubation period of the virus (see **Table 1**).

BARRIER PRECAUTIONS

- Healthcare personnel should use N-95 respirators or PAPR, double gloves, impermeable gowns, goggles or face shields, and leg and shoe coverings.

- Patients should be placed in a private room with negative pressure and six to 12 air exchanges per hour.
- The rooms with patients should be restricted from nonessential staff, visitors, and health care personnel. Cohorting may be an efficient way to reduce exposures.
- Rooms should contain dedicated medical equipment in such as stethoscopes, point-of-care analyzer—if available for laboratory testing, etc.

VACCINATION

- The only currently available vaccine for hemorrhagic fever viruses is yellow fever vaccine, a live-virus vaccine.
- However, this vaccine is in limited supply, has substantial side effects, and is thought to be relatively useless in a yellow fever bioterrorism attack. That is because the incubation period for the disease is three to six days, and the immune response requires 10 days.

MANAGING CORPSES

- Disposition of the dead is particularly important, because this has been noted as a source of transmission and sometimes a substantial contribution to outbreaks.
- Contact with corpses should be limited to trained personnel and only those who are considered essential.
- Autopsies should be limited in frequency and require the full contact and airborne precautions described above. These include eye protection, full body protection, and the N-95 respirator or PAPRs.

ENVIRONMENTAL SURFACES AND CONTAMINATED OBJECTS

Environmental surfaces and contaminated objects should be cleaned with an Environmental Protection Agency-registered hospital disinfectant or a 1:100 dissolution of household bleach. Cloth items should be incinerated, autoclaved, or placed in a double bag.

BODY FLUIDS

Body fluids, including stool, should be decontaminated when possible by autoclave, chemical toilet, or application of household bleach.

See following pages for Clinical Pathways and additional charts.

Clinical Pathway: Viral Hemorrhagic Fever

Patient presents with:
- Fever $\geq$101°F (38.3°C) of <3 wk duration
- At least two of the following:
  --Hemorrhagic or purple rash
  --Epistaxis
  --Hematemesis
  --Hemoptysis
  --Blood in stools
  --Petechiae in nondependent areas
- No predisposing factors for hemorrhage and no established alternative diagnoses

Note: Sudden appearance of multiple patients with acute onset of characteristic illness suggests common source exposure such as would be seen with a bioterrorist attack.

↓

Report immediately to local and/or state health department

↓

- Initiate appropriate infection control practices (see page 147)
- Send clinical specimens for VHF testing directly to CDC
- Initiate ribavirin therapy (see page 148)

←

- If arenavirus or bunyavirus infection confirmed, administer ribavirin therapy for 10 days
- If VHF ruled out, or if flavivirus or filovirus infection confirmed, discontinue ribavirin

↓

Identify close and high-risk contacts (see page 149) and place them under medical surveillance

↓

If VHF ruled out for index patient, disconitinue surveillance

If contacts have no fever or symptoms suggestive of VHF for 21 days after last exposure, discontinue surveillance

If fever $\geq$101°F (38.3°C) or other symptoms suggestive of VHF develop in contacts, initiate treatment, evaluation, and infection control practices as appropriate

Abbreviations

CDC, Centers for Disease Control and Prevention
VHF, viral hemorrhagic fever

Continued...

Isolation Precautions for Patients with Suspected Viral Hemorrhagic Fever

Type of Precaution	Procedures
Airborne Precautions	Place the patient in a private room with: • Negative air pressure • 6 to 12 air changes per hour • Restricted access of nonessential staff and visitors
VHF-specific personal protective equipment*	Provide the following PPE for healthcare providers: • N-95 respirator or powered air-purifying respirator • Double gloves • Impermeable gowns • Face shields • Goggles for eye protection • Leg and shoe coverings
Hand hygiene	All healthcare providers should adhere to the following practices: • Clean hands prior to donning PPE for patient contact • After patient care, remove gloves, gown, and leg and shoe coverings, and immediately clean hands • Clean hands prior to the removal of facial protective equipment to minimize exposure of mucous membranes with potentially contaminated hands • Clean hands again after all PPE is removed
Handling of medical equipment	Dedicate medical equipment such as: • Stethoscopes • Blood pressure cuffs • Glucose monitors • Point-of-care analyzers (if available)
Environmental decontamination	• Environmental surfaces, inanimate contaminated objects, or contaminated equipment should be disinfected with an EPA-registered hospital disinfectant or a 1:100 dilution of household bleach using standard procedures • Contaminated linens should be incinerated, autoclaved, or placed in double (ie, leak-proof bags) bags at the site of use and washed without sorting in a normal hot water cycle with bleach • Hospital housekeeping staff and linen handlers should wear appropriate PPE when handling or cleaning potential contaminated material or surfaces
Patient cohorting	If multiple patients with suspected VHF are admitted to one healthcare facility: • Cohort them in the same part of the hospital to minimize exposure to other patients and healthcare workers • Dedicate staff trained in appropriate infection control practices to care for them • If large number of patients must be cared for in 1 facility, then recommendations to place all patients under Airborne Precautions (see above) may need to be modified

Abbreviations: EPA, Environmental Protection Agency; PPE, personal protective equipment; VHF, viral hemorrhagic fever.

*The most common forms of exposure involve accidental parenteral inoculation; therefore, particular attention should be paid to handling of needles and sharp instruments.

Continued...

Ribavirin Therapy Recommendations for Patients with Viral Hemorrhagic Fever of Unknown Cause or Known to Be Caused by an Arenavirus or Bunyavirus*

Patient Group	Contained-Casualty Setting	Mass-Casualty Setting†
Adults (including pregnant women)‡	—Loading dose of 30 mg/kg IV once (maximum dose, 2 gm) —Then 16 mg/kg IV every 6 hr for 4 days (maximum dose, 1 gm) —Then 8 mg/kg IV every 8 hr for 6 days (maximum dose, 500 mg)	—Loading dose of 2,000 mg PO once —*Weight >75 kg:* 1,200 mg/day PO in 2 divided doses for 10 days§ —*Weight ≤75 kg:* 1,000 mg/day PO in divided doses (400 mg in AM and 600 mg in PM) for 10 days§
Children	—Loading dose: 30 mg/kg IV once (maximum dose, 2 gm) —Then 16 mg/kg IV every 6 hr for 4 days (maximum dose, 1 gm) —Then 8 mg/kg IV every 8 hr for 6 days (maximum dose, 500 mg)	—Loading dose of 30 mg/kg PO once —Then 15 mg/kg/day PO in 2 divided doses for 10 days

Abbreviations: IV, intravenously; PO, orally.

*Recommendations are from the Working Group on Civilian Biodefense; ribavirin is not approved by the US Food and Drug Administration for treatment of viral hemorrhagic fever and must be used under an Investigational New Drug (IND) protocol, although in a mass-casualty setting these requirements may need to be modified.

†The decision to use oral rather than parenteral medication will depend on available resources.

‡Generally, ribavirin is contraindicated in pregnant women; however, the Working Group indicated that the benefits appear to outweigh the fetal risk of ribavirin therapy. Also, the mortality of viral hemorrhagic fever appears to be higher in pregnancy.

§A 1,000-mg/day dosage given in 3 divided doses has been used to treat patients with Lassa fever; however, this regimen cannot be used in the United States because the current available formulation of ribavirin is 200-mg capsules, which cannot be broken open.

Adapted from Borio L, Inglesby T, Peters CJ, et al. Hemorrhagic fever viruses as biological weapons: medical and public health management. JAMA 2002 May 8;287:2391-405 (http://jama.ama-assn.org/issues/v287n18/ffull/jst20006.html).

Continued...

Medical Surveillance for Contacts of Patients with Suspected Viral Hemorrhagic Fever

Initial medical surveillance:
Place all persons (including medical and laboratory personnel) who have had close or high-risk contact with patient within 21 days following onset of the patient's symptoms (and before onset of appropriate barrier precautions) under medical surveillance.

> High risk is defined as:
> —Mucous membrane contact
> —Percutaneous injury involving contact with secretions, excretions, or blood
>
> Close contact is defined as:
> —Living with, shaking hands with, or hugging patient
> —Processing laboratory specimens from patient

If filovirus or arenavirus infection is confirmed:
Continue medical surveillance for all contacts for 21 days

If Rift Valley fever or a flavivirus infection is confirmed:
Only those who process laboratory specimens from an infected patient prior to initiation of appropriate precautions need to be continued on medical surveillance (since these conditions are transmitted in the laboratory setting but not via person-to-person transmission)

CDC CATEGORY B BIOLOGICAL TERRORISM AGENTS

BRUCELLOSIS

BACKGROUND

- Brucellosis is a disease of animals that is transmittable to humans and can cause a diverse array of symptoms.
- The disease is worldwide, but occurs especially in the Mediterranean, India, Mexico and parts of Central and South America.
- Brucellosis is nearly eliminated from the U.S., where most cases occur from ingestion of unpasteurized goat milk products from Mexico.
- For bioterrorism, the organism could be introduced through animals, as food-borne (milk or cheese) or aerosolized.
- Brucellosis is highly infectious, with only 10 to 100 aerosolized organisms required to cause disease.
- With brucellosis, there is no person-to-person spread. If recognized, the disease is easily treated.

HOSPITAL PREPARATION

- The major challenge is diagnosis for a disease that has such incredibly protean clinical features manifested by bacteria that take ≥ four weeks to grow.
- Infection control is not an issue since there is no person-to-person spread.
- In a large outbreak, access to large supplies of tetracyclines and rifampin will be needed.
- Providers need awareness of the extraordinary array of drug interactions with rifampin.
- Patients with serious illness may need ICU and respiratory support.

PERSONAL PROTECTION

No precautions are necessary.

DECONTAMINATION

- Environmental sources are not a concern. The disease is transmitted by ingestion of contaminated food or by aerosol delivery to the lungs.
- The inoculum size necessary to cause infection is 10 to 100 organisms by inhalation.

QUARANTINE PROCEDURES

Quarantine is not necessary.

CLINICAL PRESENTATION

- It is said of brucellosis that there are no diseases other than syphilis and tuberculosis that have more variation in clinical expression.
- The incubation period is five to 60 days.
- The usual initial complaints are a flu-like illness with fever, sweats, malaise, anorexia, back pain, and headache.
- This is a systemic infection that may involve any organ causing acute ileitis, hepatitis, sacroiliitis, acute or chronic meningitis, endocarditis, bronchopneumonia, nephritis, orchitis, salpingitis, marrow suppression, uveitis, etc.
- Symptoms may be acute or chronic. A physical exam may show fever, adenopathy and/or hepatomegaly or splenomegaly.
- Airborne transmission may result from bioterrorism or occur naturally in slaughterhouses.
- In addition to flu-like symptoms, the presentation usually includes a chest x-ray that may be normal or show pneumonia, nodules, miliary lesions, hilar adenopathy, or pleural effusions.

DIAGNOSIS

- Blood cultures are positive in 15% to 70% of cases. The yield is higher with cultures of bone marrow.

- The lab needs to be warned, as this is a biohazard BSL-3 pathogen, and because cultures need to be held a minimum of four weeks.
- Serology may support this diagnosis. No single titer is considered diagnostic, but titers over 1:160 are supportive.
- With bioterrorism, the challenge will be detection of the initial cases, since the organism takes a long time to grow and identify, and serologic response is slow and often nonspecific.
- In the event of a large-scale attack, the diagnosis will usually be made presumptively on the basis of characteristic symptoms and exposure.

TREATMENT

- Antibiotic treatment relieves symptoms and prevents late sequelae.
- Standard treatment recommended by WHO is doxycycline (200 mg/day) combined with rifampin (600 mg/day to 900 mg/day), both given orally for six weeks.
- With single-drug therapy, the rate of relapse is high.
- More recent studies also support the use of doxycycline plus streptomycin or possibly gentamicin (which is more active in vitro and less toxic compared with streptomycin).

PREVENTION

- Control of naturally occurring brucellosis depends on elimination of the animal source.
- There are no vaccines for human use. There are also no data dealing with prophylactic antibiotics, although exposed persons might be treated with doxycycline 100 mg bid plus rifampin 600 mg qd x 3 weeks.

CHOLERA

BACKGROUND

- Cholera has been responsible for devastating epidemics, with seven pandemics in the last two centuries.

- The organism typically causes epidemics but has the potential to cause pandemics and to remain endemic once introduced.
- The organism exists in water and is introduced to humans from water sources or contaminated food.
- *Vibro cholerae* is found in the U.S., but clinical cases are extremely rare, presumably due to sanitation standards.
- With exposure in nonimmune populations, such as are found in the U.S., the disease is clinically severe, and rates of secondary spread are high.

HOSPITAL PREPARATION

- A newly developed vaccine is highly effective and might be considered for health care workers who have risk of repeated exposure.
- Another option would by doxycycline or ciprofloxacin prophylaxis.
- Nevertheless, person-to-person transmission is rare; the major risk to patients is transmission through water or food, and rates of household transmission by these routes have been high.
- There is no risk of airborne transmission.
- The major challenge to hospitals with any large-scale outbreak would be to provide supportive care for patients who have devastating diarrhea.
- The preferred mechanism of rehydration is the oral route, although some will require IV support.
- As such, hospital preparation should include methods to obtain massive supplies of oral rehydration solutions (which can be easily prepared in the pharmacy) for rapid administration to a large number of patients, with a much smaller number of patients to receive IV Lactated Ringers solution.
- An adequate supply of simple antibiotics, primarily doxycycline or fluoroquinolones, would be needed as well.

PERSONAL PROTECTION

There are four components:
- Contact precautions, including careful hand hygiene

- The potential use of the new cholera vaccine
- Prophylactic antibiotics
- Careful avoidance of contaminated food and water

DECONTAMINATION

Waterborne sources of *V cholerae* can be easily eliminated by boiling or chlorination. Acidic beverages and carbonated water are also safe.

QUARANTINE PROCEDURES

Quarantine is not necessary.

CLINICAL PRESENTATION

- The hallmark of cholera is watery diarrhea that is devastating, particularly in immunologically naïve population.
- Disease onset is abrupt, it is sometimes associated with vomiting, fever is noted in less than 5% of cases, and the diarrhea is typically "small bowel" with "rice-water stools" and without cramps, white cells, blood, or tenesmus.
- Laboratory tests show hemoconcentration, prerenal azotemia, metabolic acidosis, and hypokalemia.

DIAGNOSIS

- The initial cases may prove challenging simply because cholera is so rare in nonendemic areas.
- Once an outbreak is recognized, most cases can be managed empirically while cultures are pending.
- The organism is generally easy to recover from stool cultures, but laboratories need to be warned, as these stool cultures require specialized media.

TREATMENT

- Antibiotic treatment is relatively easy with doxycycline (300 mg as a single dose),

ciprofloxacin (250 mg/day for three days), other fluoroquinolones, or trimethoprim-sulfamethoxazole (1 DS bid times 3 days).
- Most important will be rapid fluid support, preferably with oral rehydration solutions given at a rate of 500 mL/hour to 1,000 mL/hour, usually for two to four hours.
- The "maintenance phase" consists of replacing losses. Indications for IV rehydration are inability to tolerate the oral route, severe diarrhea with purging of more than 10 mL/kg/hour to 20 mL/kg/hour, and patients with severe dehydration as indicated by hypotension, mental status changes, and fluid losses estimated as exceeding 10%.
- Treatment guidelines suggest oral rehydration solution in the maintenance phase of 800 mL/hour to 1,000 mL/hour matching ongoing losses.
- Recommendations for discharge are: oral tolerance of at least one liter/hour by mouth, urine volume exceeding 40 mL/hour, and stool volume at less than 400 mL/hour. These recommendations are particularly important in the context of maintaining optimal capacity in an epidemic.

PREVENTION

- The new cholera vaccine would be particularly useful if there is a risk of ongoing new cases. Hand hygiene would be particularly important as a preventive strategy in the health care setting, but also for patients managed at home.
- As noted, household transmission has been well established in prior outbreaks. Fecal contamination is the major source. Water can be made safe by boiling or chlorination.

CRYPTOSPORIDUM

BACKGROUND

- Cryptosporidum is the only protozoan parasite included as a category A, B, or C bioterrorism agent.

- Cryptosporidum was considered a relatively rare form of enteric infection until the infamous 1993 epidemic of 400,000 cases in Milwaukee, WI, which gave new respect to its epidemic potential.
- The usual source is waterborne disease from contaminated swimming pools or municipal supplies, but contaminated beverages have also been sources of outbreaks.
- Person-to-person transmission may occur.
- The disease is characterized by large-volume diarrhea that may last weeks, may be particularly devastating in immunosuppressed hosts, and has no specific treatment.

HOSPITAL PREPARATION

- The hospital should be prepared to manage large numbers of patients, most of whom will not require hospitalization. They will, however, require education about symptomatic treatment and methods to prevent person-to-person transmission.
- Some patients will have relatively devastating diarrhea, particularly those with compromised cell-mediated immunity, such as those with HIV advanced infection.
- Of special concern are children and the elderly.

PERSONAL PROTECTION

Most important for personal protection would be standard contact precautions and hand hygiene. There is no airborne transmission

DECONTAMINATION

Nearly all cases are food-borne or water-borne and reflect inadequate treatment (filtration or chlorination) or distribution. Decontamination may occur with implementation of these strategies. Also effective are point-of-use filters.

QUARANTINE PROCEDURES

Quarantine is not necessary.

CLINICAL PRESENTATION

- The initial presentation of an outbreak may be subtle. With the Milwaukee outbreak traced to the municipal water supply, the initial clue was that drug stores in the city were completely depleted of antidiarrheal agents.
- The incubation period is two to 10 days, and the clinical expression is with watery diarrhea that may be mild and persistent or large volume, with up to 12 liters/day to 17 liters/day.
- Symptoms often wax and wane, lasting up to one month in the healthy host.
- The major concerns are the age extremes and patients who are immunosuppressed. These patients are most likely to have life-threatening diarrhea and most likely to require hospitalization.
- The great majority of cryptosporidiosis cases can be managed as outpatients.

DIAGNOSIS

The diagnosis is relatively easy, with a modified acid-fast stain of stool.

TREATMENT

- The disease is generally self-limited, except in the immunosuppressed host.
- Multiple trials for effective drugs have shown unimpressive results. Nitazoxanide (500 mg PO q6-12h times 3 days) has been FDA-approved for children with cryptosporidiosis.
- Most important is supportive care with oral replacement and antidiarrheal agents.

EASTERN EQUINE ENCEPHALITIS

(also see "Venezuelan equine encephalitis" and "Western equine encephalitis" in this section)

BACKGROUND

- Eastern equine encephalitis (EEE) is found in the

eastern U.S. and Gulf Coast.

- Like the other alphaviruses (Venezuelan equine encephalitis and western equine encephalitis), this agent causes encephalitis in horses and people, and it is mosquito borne.
- The usual presentation is headache, high fever, nausea, chills, and vomiting.
- There are a few human cases each year in the U.S. Outbreaks are easy to detect because the mortality rate is 50% to 70%.
- Any bioterrorism event would probably result from aerosolization, and would be expected to present with deaths in both horses and people.

HOSPITAL PREPARATION

- In a bioterrorism event, hospitals should be prepared to deal with a large number of seriously ill patients with encephalitis and a high mortality rate.
- In this context, it will be particularly important to:
  - Establish the mechanism and area
  - Assure health care workers that there is no person-to-person transmission
  - Be prepared to provide supportive medical care for patients with exposure plus typical symptoms.

PERSONAL PROTECTION

- There is no person-to-person transmission.
- Risk would be defined by people with a common exposure, presumably to aerosol delivery.

DECONTAMINATION

EEE is a mosquito-borne disease, so decontamination would not be a high priority.

QUARANTINE PROCEDURES

Quarantine is not necessary.

CLINICAL PRESENTATION

- The incubation period is one to six days, and this is followed by the onset of headache, high fever, nausea, chills, and vomiting.
- Many patients develop progressive disease, with nuchal rigidity, seizures, and coma.
- A CSF exam typically shows a mononuclear pleocytosis with 600/mm^3 to 2,000/mm^3 and an elevated protein.
- The mortality rate is 50% to 70%—probably higher in an aerosol attack.

DIAGNOSIS

- CSF changes are noted above.
- An MRI usually shows changes in the basal ganglia and thalamus, and this focal distribution may be helpful in distinguishing this infection from herpetic encephalitis.
- The virus can often be isolated from serum during the prodrome stage, which may be helpful in the event of multiple cases.
- However, the usual method to establish the diagnosis is with acute and convalescent serology and IgM.
- In the event of a common source outbreak due to an aerosol terrorism attack, a presumptive diagnosis could be made of EEE in any patient who presents with suspected exposure and acute febrile illness, especially if accompanied by the characteristic clinical and CSF findings and symptoms of encephalitis.

TREATMENT

Treatment is supportive. No known antiviral agents are thought to be effective.

PREVENTION

There is no vaccine or other preventive intervention—except for mosquito control—to prevent mosquito-borne disease.

EPSILON TOXIN

BACKGROUND

- Epsilon toxin is produced by *Clostridium perfringens* types B and D. It is responsible for a fetal intestinal disease in several animal species presumably by producing large membrane pores that permit an influx of ions and other molecules, resulting in cell death.
- There are no data on epsilon toxin for disease in humans. It is presumed that use of this toxin as an agent of bioterrorism would be by aerosolization and that patients would present with shock and multiorgan failure based on multiple studies in animals.
- There is no antitoxin or vaccine, and antibiotics directed against *C perfringens* would be useless.
- The presumed presentation with bioterrorism would be multiple critically ill patients, as well as animals.
- There is no person-to-person or animal-to-person transmission.

HOSPITAL PREPARATION

- With a large attack, hospitals would need to be prepared for managing large numbers of critically ill patients who require substantial supportive care for shock, renal failure, and pulmonary edema.
- Concern about patient-to-patient transmission of epsilon toxin is not necessary.

PERSONAL PROTECTION

No precautions are necessary.

QUARANTINE PROCEDURES

Quarantine is not necessary.

CLINICAL PRESENTATION

There are no data for humans with this toxin, but the presumed presentation based on animal studies would be inhalation followed by pulmonary edema, renal failure, and shock.

DIAGNOSIS

- Multiple assays are available for detection of epsilon toxin in intestinal contents and other body fluids of animals. It is presumed that these techniques would be used in humans.
- The assays include polyclonal capture ELISA, monoclonal capture ELISA, mouse neutralization test, and counterimmunoelectrophoresis.
- All these techniques appear to be highly specific, although they vary in sensitivity, and there seems to be some inconsistency between the tests.
- As such, in a bioterrorism attack, it is likely that testing would be done in reference public health laboratories using specimens submitted from hospitals.
- Once the bioterrorism agent is identified, however, most patients would be treated presumptively.

TREATMENT

- There is no antitoxin.
- The presumed mechanism of bioterrorism would be with toxin rather than in vivo production of toxin. As such, there is no rationale for treating *C perfringens* unless that agent is used for toxin delivery. In that case, clindamycin or penicillin would presumably be the preferred agents.

PREVENTION

- There is no vaccine and no preventive strategy.
- Delivery in the food or water supply would require identification of the source through public health studies.
- The obvious admonition would be to avoid this source, which would need to be removed from the food chain as quickly as possible.

ESCHERICHIA COLI 0157:H7 (E COLI)

BACKGROUND

- *E coli* has multiple mechanisms to cause diarrhea, but the one that is most likely as a bioterrorism agent is *E coli* that produces Shiga toxin, the toxin responsible for dysentery with shigellosis; it is also implicated in the hemolytic-uremic syndrome (HUS).
- The usual strain is *E coli* 0157:H7, but other serotypes have also been implicated.
- *E coli* was first described as an enteric pathogen in 1982 as a result of a food-borne outbreak that caused serious disease, including HUS.
- Most serious cases and deaths from *E coli* infection occur in children.

HOSPITAL PREPARATION

- The putative agent may be transmitted from person-to-person by the fecal-oral route.
- Naturally occurring disease and the presumed mechanisms that would be used with a bioterrorism attack are contaminated food or water, especially ground beef, salami, lettuce, sprouts, unpasteurized milk, juice, underchlorinated drinking water, and swimming pools and other bodies of water.
- Hospitals need to be alert to the clinical features that specifically suggest this diagnosis (bloody, nonfebrile diarrhea), as well as to the possibility of a terrorism attack when there is more than one case, promptly reporting an outbreak or even a single confirmed case to appropriate health officials.
- Hygiene is important for protection of health care workers and other patients.

PERSONAL PROTECTION

Most important are contact precautions and hand hygiene to prevent fecal-oral contamination.

DECONTAMINATION

It is conceivable that surfaces could be a potential source for transmission of these organisms, but this has not been an important source of cases.

QUARANTINE PROCEDURES

Quarantine is not necessary.

CLINICAL PRESENTATION

The incubation period is three to eight days. The usual presentation is watery diarrhea followed by bloody diarrhea without fever.
- About 2% to 5% of cases are complicated by HUS.
- The mortality rate in outbreaks is 0% to 2%.

DIAGNOSIS

Obtain a stool culture, but the lab must be alerted of suspicion of *E coli* 0157, since this requires special media and testing to distinguish this *E coli* from bacteria.

TREATMENT

- Treatment consists of supportive care, including dialysis for patients who have renal failure from HUS.
- Antibiotics are thought to be unwarranted; they may, in fact, be contraindicated due to concern that this might prompt toxin release, with an increased risk of HUS.

PREVENTION

There is no vaccine for *E coli*. Prophylactic antibiotics are not recommended.

GLANDERS

BACKGROUND

- *Burkholderia mallei* (formerly *Pseudomonas mallei*) is traditionally considered a veterinary pathogen.
- One hundred years ago, glanders was an important cause of death in horses, and there were often secondary fatal infections in humans.
- Subsequent aggressive veterinary control measures have essentially eliminated glanders from the West; there has been only one human case in the U.S. in the past 50 years. This was in a lab technician working with *B mallei*.
- The disease in humans was characterized by necrosis of the tracheobronchial tree, pustular skin lesions, pneumonia, and sepsis.
- If the source of exposure was by skin, there were usually multiple abscesses reflecting that portal of entry; if it was inhaled, the presentation was predominantly pneumonia.

HOSPITAL PREPARATION

- There is no person-to-person spread by aerosol, but *B mallei* might be transmitted by cutaneous contact with lesions, so contact precautions are important.
- It is presumed that any bioterrorism event would present by an aerosol delivery, with presentation of multiple patients with severe pneumonia and sepsis.
- These patients would require respiratory support and antibiotics—probably ceftazidime, imipenem, piperacillin, and/or tetracyclines—based on sensitivity of the strain used.

PERSONAL PROTECTION

More important than preemptive personal protection would be contact precautions after the fact.

QUARANTINE PROCEDURES

Quarantine was an important method to control this disease in horses and presumably would be used again in the event of a bioterrorism attack in which sick horses were a by-product. However, the necessity of quarantine of patients would be unlikely.

CLINICAL PRESENTATION

- The incubation period is 10 to 14 days.
- With aerosol delivery, the anticipated presentation would be pneumonia with severe sepsis.
- Other features include fever, generalized erythroderma, hepatosplenomegaly with hepatic abscesses, and possibly pustular skin lesions that may suggest smallpox.

DIAGNOSIS

- *B mallei* is a gram-negative bacillus with a safety-pin shape. It is usually recovered from blood cultures, but they may be positive only in relatively late stage disease.
- Most laboratories will not be able to readily distinguish this organism from *Pseudomonas fluorescens* or *P putida*.
- *B mallei* requires precautions by microbiologists and is usually referred to a BSL-3 lab.
- Serologic tests include a compliment fixation test and an ELISA.
- A concern is that most laboratories would have difficulty distinguishing this organism from others that would not be agents of bioterrorism, as the resources available in most microbiology labs do not permit these distinctions. As such, suspected isolates must be referred to reference labs for sophisticated techniques, such as cellular analysis of fatty acid and 16S ribosomal RNA gene sequencing.

TREATMENT

- Treatment would be with systemic antibiotics that would depend to a large extent on the sensitivity profile of the bioterrorism strain. Most are susceptible to ceftazidime, imipenem, piperacillin, and doxycycline.
- Treatment is usually lengthy, with initial treatment

by IV, followed by a prolonged course of oral agents.

PREVENTION

- There is no vaccine for *B mallei*, and no drug has been tested for prophylaxis.
- The control of glanders in horses was accomplished primarily by identifying infected animals and then quarantining them.
- Antibiotics might be useful, including trimethoprim-sulfamethoxazole, doxycycline, or amoxicillin-clavulanate.

MELIOIDOSIS

BACKGROUND

- Melioidosis is a severe disease caused by *Burkholderia pseudomallei*, which is endemic in southeast Asia and northern Australia.
- Disease presentations are variable, including severe sepsis and acute or chronic pneumonia. There may also be skin lesions, including pustules, which may suggest smallpox.
- There is no rapid diagnostic test available to most hospitals, and the diagnosis is unlikely to be made efficiently with initial cases.
- Melioidosis is not normally seen in the U.S.; as such, initial cases presumably would be suspected of tuberculosis or an epidemic of disease manifested by severe pneumonia, as in *Legionella pneumophila*, histoplasmosis, or influenza.

HOSPITAL PREPARATION

- In the event of bioterrorism or a multiple-case outbreak, hospitals must be prepared for managing large numbers of patients with a severe illness who require prolonged therapy.
- There is no person-to-person spread by air, but there may be transmission by contact with skin lesions.

PERSONAL PROTECTION

- The most important personal protection is not preemptive, but contact precautions after the fact.
- It is possible that prophylaxis with trimethroprim-sulfamethoxazole, doxycycline, or a fluoroquinolone may confer additional protection.

QUARANTINE PROCEDURES

Quarantine is not necessary.

CLINICAL PRESENTATION

- Melioidosis may be acute or chronic.
- The acute form is characterized by a fulminant pneumonia with fever, sputum, and a pulmonary infiltrate that usually shows a diffuse patchy alveolar infiltrate with multiple nodular lesions.
- The chronic form may resemble tuberculosis with cavity formation and upper-lobe involvement.
- Many patients, about 30% in most series, have septicemia with liver or splenic abscesses.
- The mortality rate is about 20%, usually due to sepsis or pulmonary failure.

DIAGNOSIS

- *B pseudomallei* may be grown from blood or respiratory secretions or skin lesions, but it represents a risk to laboratory technicians and consequently is preferably cultured in a BSL-3 laboratory.
- An immunofluorescent test has been developed that will quickly identify this organism; this test has good specificity and a 60% to 65% sensitivity.
- There is also a complement fixation test in which a titer exceeding 1:160 is supportive of this diagnosis.

TREATMENT

- Antibiotics that have been used most extensively are ceftazidime, trimethoprim-sulfamethoxazole, or both.

- Doxycycline is also effective.
- Fluoroquinolones are active against most strains in vitro but have not done well in experimental animal studies.
- Most patients require treatment for prolonged periods, and much of this can be done with oral trimethroprim-sulfamethoxazole.

PREVENTION

- There is no vaccine for B pseudomallei, but one is currently in development.
- It is possible that trimethroprim-sulfamethoxazole would be effective in preventing disease in those who are exposed.

PSITTACOSIS

BACKGROUND

- Psittacosis is a systemic infection acquired by inhalation with bird exposure.
- Psittacosis has protean manifestations, but the most characteristic is pneumonia.
- With a bioterrorism attack, the assumption is that it would be from an aerosol. Infection of birds might also be attempted, but 5% to 8% of most bird populations are already infected.
- The prognosis with antibiotic therapy is good; mortality rates of 20% are decreased to 1% with tetracycline.

HOSPITAL PREPARATION

- Human-human transmission is possible but very rare. Health care workers and the general population need to know this.
- Tetracyclines, including doxycycline, are the favored drugs, so any large terrorism attack would require a substantial supply that would presumably be used for treatment and probably prevention.

PERSONAL PROTECTION

Human-to-human transmission is presumably possible but rare.

DECONTAMINATION

Aerosolization from bird droppings has been an important mechanism of transmission; widespread environmental contamination could presumably be an indirect source.
- Chlamydophila psittaci can be eliminated from environmental sources with standard detergents using hypochlorite or a 1:10 dilution of household bleach.

QUARANTINE PROCEDURES

Quarantine is not necessary.

CLINICAL PRESENTATION

- The incubation period is five to 15 days, followed by what is usually described as a "non-specific viral-like illness."
- At this stage, the findings are fever, pharyngitis, cough that is usually nonproductive, hepatosplenomegaly, and adenopathy.
- Common clinical syndromes include atypical pneumonia with nonproductive cough.
- Chest x-rays often show changes that are quite variable, including an interstitial infiltrate, patchy reticulum radiating from the hilus, lobar, or segmental consolidation, and hilar adenopathy.
- Other findings may include mental status changes, pericarditis, hepatitis, cranial nerve palsies, encephalitis, and/or a blanching, maculopapular rash.
- Laboratory tests include a pulmonary infiltrate in about 75% of cases, as well as abnormal liver function tests suggesting cholestasis in 50% of cases.

DIAGNOSIS

- C psittaci is not seen on gram stain and not

grown with routine cultures.

- There are serologic tests for detection of psittacosis; the expected response with CF or MIF is a titer of at least 1:64.
- The organism can be cultured from blood, but this is dangerous due to the risk to laboratory workers. Preferred newer tests include detection by DFA stain, EIA, and PCR.
- Serologic tests are genera specific, but do not distinguish *C psittaci* from *Chlamydophila trachomatis* or *Chlamydophila pneumoniae.*
- It is anticipated that the greatest challenge would be the detection of the initial cases, and that, with any sizable outbreak, the diagnosis would be made presumptively on the basis of typical clinical findings and exposure.

TREATMENT

- The preferred treatment is tetracycline (500 mg qid) or doxycycline (100 mg PO bid), each for 10 to 21 days.
- The potential role of macrolides and fluoroquinolones is simply unknown.
- With tetracycline, the response is impressive, usually with improved clinical status within one day.
- The mortality rate with untreated disease is 20%; with tetracycline treatment, it is 1%.

PREVENTION

There is no vaccine for *C psittaci.* Prophylactic antibiotics are not generally recommended.

Q FEVER

BACKGROUND:

- Q Fever is a zoonotic disease caused by *Coxiella burnetii,* which is distributed throughout the world.
- The primary reservoirs are cattle, sheep, and goats, but infection may involve many animal species, including cats.

- The organisms are excreted in the milk, urine, and stool of infected animals and reach concentrations of 109/gm of placental tissue in sheep.
- Infection occurs by inhalation from airborne sources.
- The organisms are highly resistant to heat, drying, and common disinfectants, and environmental contamination becomes a particularly important source of infection in the context of bioterrorism.
- As little as one to five inhaled organisms may cause disease.
- Diagnosis is difficult due to *C burnetii's* protean clinical features, the infrequency of this disease in the U.S. and the unlikelihood of physicians considering it, as well as the fact that it is not seen on gram strain or grown with conventional cultures.
- A potentially important clue in the context of bioterrorism is simultaneous disease in animals and people.

HOSPITAL PREPARATION

- Hospitals need to be alert to the possibility of Q fever when there are multiple patients with an illness characterized by fever, pneumonia (in 30% to 50% of cases), and abnormal liver function tests.
- Infection control includes bagging, autoclaving, and washing of contaminated clothes.
- There may be a role for prophylactic antibiotics in health care workers and others who are exposed.

DECONTAMINATION

- *C burnetii* is resistant to heat and drying, and therefore can persist in the environment for long periods. Environmental longevity becomes an important potential source of disease, as the inoculum size necessary to cause infection is as low as one microbe.
- Environmental cleaning may be achieved with hypochloride or a 1:10 dilution of household bleach. Clothing should be subject to standard wash protocol.

QUARANTINE PROCEDURES

Quarantine might be an issue for infected or exposed animals.

CLINICAL PRESENTATION

- About half of patients who are exposed develop a clinical illness.
- Acute Q fever is associated with incubation period of two to three weeks, followed by sudden onset of a flu-like illness with fever—often of 104° F to 105° F, headache, malaise, myalgias, confusion, chills, sweats, nonproductive cough, sore throat, vomiting, diarrhea, abdominal pain, and chest pain.
- Thirty percent to 50% of patients develop pneumonia characterized by patchy infiltrates or rounded opacities with or without hilar adenopathy on chest x-ray.
- Most patients would have abnormal transaminase levels.
- Most patients fully recover even without therapy; the mortality rate is only 1% to 2%.
- A small number of patients develop chronic disease that includes Q fever endocarditis; it may last up to 20 years. These are primarily patients with prosthetic heart valves, especially aortic heart valves.
- Compromised hosts also are at risk for chronic Q fever.

DIAGNOSIS

- Laboratory clues to the diagnosis include the abnormal liver function tests, the characteristic findings on chest x-ray, and thrombocytopenia.
- A confirmed diagnosis requires positive serology, preferably with the indirect immunofluorescence assay (IFA).
- *C burnetii* may be detected in tissue with immunohistochemical staining and DNA detection.

TREATMENT

- The standard treatment is doxycycline 100 mg twice daily for two to three weeks.

- Fluoroquinolones are active in vitro, but clinical experience is limited.

PREVENTION

- There are no FDA-licensed vaccines for treating Q fever, but there are investigational vaccines.
- Prophylactic antibiotics with doxycycline or tetracycline may be effective, but experience is limited and prophylaxis given too early in the course of the disease may simply delay onset.
- Particularly important in controlling the disease is attention to animal sources with education of the public, testing of animals with possible quarantine and treatment.

RICIN

BACKGROUND

- Ricin is a widely available and an easily ingested, inhaled, or injected phytotoxin.
- The toxin is produced from the residue from processing castor beans.
- Ricin is a 66 kD protein with an A and B chain. The B chain binds to surface glycoproteins to permit entry of A chains, which interfere with protein synthesis at the 60S ribosomal subunit, leading to cell death.
- The structure of ricin is similar to cholera toxin, diphtheria toxin, tetanus toxin, and insulin.
- Ricin was reportedly found in al-Qaeda caves in Afghanistan. It was also discovered in mailroom of the Dirksen Senate Office Building in Washington, DC, in 2004, as well as in the possession of extremists.
- The lethal dose is 500 mg (about 3 mcg/kg) with onset of symptoms in about 12 hours and death in 36 to 72 hours, depending on the exposure dose.
- These data sound alarming, but to cause a mortality rate comparable to 1 kg of aerosolized anthrax spores would require four metric tons of ricin.
- Of particular concern is the potential use of ricin in contaminating food and water, as

large-scale production is so simple. Patients are unlikely to detect exposure and would present with acute symptoms that relate to the portal of entry.

- There is no effective therapy for ricin poisoning other than supportive care.

HOSPITAL PREPARATION

- The main challenge with isolated cases is recognition of ricin toxicity as an explanation of a patient with an acute febrile illness, usually expressed by rapid progression to ARDS or acute gastroenteritis, with GI bleeding and death within 36 to 72 hours.
- Multiple cases with such symptoms would be extraordinary and strongly suggestive of a terrorism attack.

PERSONAL PROTECTION

- There is no person-to-person transmission.
- Cutaneous exposure from contaminated clothing of patients or other sources is a minimal risk, because ricin is not absorbed cutaneously.
- Cutaneous exposure should nevertheless be avoided by removal of patient clothing with gloves, and patient cleansing using 0.1% Na hypochlorite or soap and water.
- Irrigation of the eyes is also recommended.

DECONTAMINATION

- When a diagnosis of ricin toxicity is suspected, health care workers should decontaminate exposed patients by removing their clothing using gloves to avoid contact. Patients should also be cleaned with soap and water.
- Clothing should be double-bagged using plastic bags.
- Once bagged, clothing is forensic evidence and should not be discarded.

QUARANTINE PROCEDURES

Quarantine is not necessary.

CLINICAL PRESENTATION

Morbidity and mortality is dose dependent. The presenting symptoms are dictated by the type of exposure:

INGESTION

- The LD50 is 30 mcg/kg or tenfold less than with aerosol exposure due to poor absorption.
- With sufficient exposure there is severe gastroenteritis, GI hemorrhage, shock, and death.
- The onset of symptoms occurs approximately 12 hours after exposure, and death ensues at one to three days; patients who survive longer than five days usually live.

AEROSOL EXPOSURE

- The LD50 is 3 mcg/kg.
- Symptoms of aerosol exposure to ricin include weakness, fever and cough within 12 to 18 hours, and a chest x-ray showing infiltrates.
- Aerosol ricin toxicity progresses to respiratory failure with ARDS and then death at 36 to 72 hours.

INJECTION

- The LD50 is 3 mcg/mL.
- Ricin toxicity as a result of injection can cause muscle necrosis and lymph adenopathy, followed by death.
- Bulgarian dissident Georgi Markov was killed when he was jabbed in the leg with an umbrella tipped by a ricin-filled dart in London in 1978. He developed severe gastroenteritis and died three days later.

DIAGNOSIS

- There is no diagnostic laboratory test for ricin toxicity.
- In isolated events, the patient is unlikely to be aware of exposure via inhalation or ingestion; injection will initially show symptoms related only to pain at the site of injection.

TREATMENT

- Treatment is supportive. Antibiotics are useless; there is no definite antidote to ricin toxicity.
- Possible antidotes under investigation are pteroic acid, neopterin, and guanine tautomer.
- There should be decontamination of gastric contents by superactivated charcoal. Dose is 25 g to 100 g given as a suspension in water.
- With inhalation, there should be early intubation.
- With injection, resect the injection site, when possible.
- For supportive care, use dopamine 2 mcg/min to 4 mcg/min IV, increased by 2 mcg/min to 4 mcg/minute q 5-10 minutes.

PREVENTION

There is no effective prevention strategy. The best that can be done is to:
- Avoid exposure
- Remove ricin surface contamination using irrigation on mucous membranes and sodium hypochlorite (0.1%) or soap and water on skin.

SALMONELLA

BACKGROUND

- Salmonella bacteria are the most common identifiable form of food-borne disease in the U.S.
- A wide range of food has been implicated in salmonella poisoning; precedent as a bioweapon was set in Oregon, where the organism was intentionally used to contaminate salad bars in restaurants.
- The organisms may also cause waterborne disease.
- Salmonella are enteric pathogens that may cause serious disease, but they are easily diagnosed and easily treated.
- Typhoid fever is a form of salmonellosis that often presents with constipation and vomiting.

HOSPITAL PREPAREDNESS

- Most important is recognition of the role of person-to-person transmission, which can be prevented with contact precautions and hand hygiene.
- There is no person-to-person spread by aerosol.
- This is a reportable disease. Health authorities will be responsible for identifying the source in the outbreak setting.

PERSONAL PROTECTION

- Contact precautions with careful hand hygiene are considered the keys to preventing disease spread by person-to-person transmission.
- Spread is by direct contact or by contaminated food or water. There is no person-to-person airborne transmission.

DECONTAMINATION

- Environmental contamination is an unlikely source for disease acquisition.
- Surfaces are easily cleansed of salmonella with standard disinfectants, including hypochlorite and 1:10 household bleach.

QUARANTINE PROCEDURES

Quarantine is not necessary.

CLINICAL PRESENTATION

- The incubation period for salmonella is eight to 46 hours.
- The most common form infection is gastroenteritis with diarrhea and fever.
- However, some patients develop enteric fever or focal infections, such as an endovascular infection, osteomyelitis, or septic arthritis.
- Some patients become chronic carriers of the disease.
- Particularly vulnerable to severe disease are infants, people over 50 years, and patients with

prostheses, artificial heart valves, severe ather-osclerosis, cancer, uremia, AIDS, and other reasons for immunosuppression. In a mass attack, such people who should be given treatment priority.

DIAGNOSIS

The diagnosis is usually easily established with culture of blood and stool. Serology plays no important role here.

TREATMENT

- Presuming a single epidemic strain, to some extent treatment guidelines would be dictated by in vitro sensitivity tests and the clinical symptoms.
- Most cases of uncomplicated gastroenteritis should not be treated with antibiotics, as this may prolong the carrier state.
- However, treatment is recommended for patients who have severe disease, including all patients with typhoid fever and those with non-typhoid salmonellosis, patients who are over 50 years, and those who have a prosthesis (joint or heart valve), severe atherosclerosis, cancer, uremia, or immunosuppression.
- The usual treatment is trimethoprim-sulfa-methoxazole 1 DS bid, ciprofloxacin 500 mg bid, or ceftriaxone 2 gm IV/day for five to seven days.
- Treatment for patients who are immunosup-pressed would be longer.
- Patients with complicated diseases—osteomyelitis, septic arthritis, endocarditis, etc.—would also be treated for prolonged periods.

PREVENTION

- This is an easily transmitted pathogen that can be efficiently delivered to a large population by contaminating food, water, or beverages.
- Keys to controlling the epidemic include:
  - Identification of the common source
  - Implementation of appropriate hygiene
  - Appropriate preparation of food derived from

animals if these are determined to be the source of the epidemic (ie, adequate cooking of meat, poultry, and eggs)
- Possible use of prophylactic antibiotics.

SHIGELLA

BACKGROUND

- Shigella is the most efficiently transmitted enteric bacterial pathogen, as an inoculum as little as 10 microbes is sufficient to cause severe disease.
- The usual presentation is acute diarrhea that is often bloody.
- Contaminated water is the usual source of outbreaks.

HOSPITAL PREPARATION

- Hospitals need to be prepared for a large number of patients with relatively severe dysentery caused by a very efficiently transmitted enteric pathogen.
- All patients with this diagnosis should be treated. In an outbreak setting this would be done empirically.
- The disease is easily treated with simple antibiotics.

PERSONAL PROTECTION

- Most important will be great care in enforcing to contact precautions, including hand hygiene.
- Spread is by hand contact and contaminated food or water.
- There is no airborne spread.

DECONTAMINATION

Contaminated surfaces may be cleaned with hypochlorite or 1:10 dilution of household bleach. Soiled bedding and clothes can be cleaned with standard washing with detergent.

QUARANTINE PROCEDURES

Quarantine is not necessary.

CLINICAL PRESENTATION

- Shigella is a toxin-mediated enteric pathogen characterized by invasion.
- Shigella manifests with symptoms of colitis, including cramps, fever, and bloody diarrhea.
- Nevertheless, the initial symptom is watery diarrhea.
- At greatest risk are children ages one to four years.
- Hemolytic-uremic syndrome is a potential complication.
- Adults often acquire the disease from their children.

DIAGNOSIS

- The organism is easily recovered with routine stool cultures.
- With outbreaks, patients with typical symptoms will be treated empirically using standard antibiotics, possibly modified only if there are unique sensitivity test results.

TREATMENT

- This is an enteric infection in which all patients are treated. The rationale is based on the severity of the illness in most cases, but also on the high rates of transmission.
- Standard treatment is trimethoprim-sulfamethoxazole (160 mg to 800 mg PO q12h for three to five days) or a fluoroquinolone such as ciprofloxacin (500 mg bid PO for three to five days).
- Other quinolones that appear to be equally effective are norfloxacin, ofloxacin, or nalidixic acid; in fact, probably all fluoroquinolones are acceptable if supplies are short.
- Patients may also require rehydration for severe fluid losses.

PREVENTION

- Particularly important is hygiene, including identification of the source, effective treatment of contaminated water (such as with chlorination), fastidious adherence to contact precautions, and hand hygiene.
- Based on multiple studies showing intrafamily transmissions, patients managed on an outpatient basis need appropriate warning to adhere to these principles in the home environment.
- Prophylactic antibiotics are an attractive option for patients who have been exposed to a common source.
- There is no vaccine for shigella.

STAPHYLOCOCCUS ENTEROTOXIN B

BACKGROUND

- The staphylococcal enterotoxins are polypeptides in the bacterial superantigen protein family.
- The clinical expression will depend on the route of exposure.
  - Ingestion—the most common naturally occurring route is via contaminated food—causes "food poisoning," with vomiting and cramps with or without diarrhea. Symptoms appear one to six hours after ingestion and last one to two days.
  - Inhalation, as a result of which there may be fever, pulmonary symptoms, and GI symptoms.
- Use of staphylococcal enterotoxins for bioterrorism presumably would either be by aerosol if pulmonary symptoms are evident or by contamination of food or fluids in the event of GI symptoms.

HOSPITAL PREPARATION

- Hospitals should be prepared for large numbers of patients with gastroenteritis or with the pneumonic form of the toxin, which can be serious and even lethal.

- It will be difficult to establish a diagnosis of staphylococcus enterotoxin B. The toxin exists in many body fluids, but methods for detection are limited.
- Initial cases may present as an epidemic of gastroenteritis, suggesting common form of food poisoning, or as an epidemic of afebrile illness associated with pulmonary edema, suggesting severe pneumonia such as *Legionella*.
- There is no person-to-person spread, but avoiding a common source of food or fluids is necessary.

PERSONAL PROTECTION

There is no risk in terms of patient contact, but there needs to be caution in avoiding any common source of food or fluids.

DECONTAMINATION

Decontamination is not necessary.

QUARANTINE PROCEDURES

Quarantine is not necessary.

CLINICAL PRESENTATION

- Inhalation is associated with an incubation period of three to 12 hours and then is characterized by a flulike condition with fever, cough, chest pain, and dyspnea.
- The patient may go on to have respiratory failure.
- Chest x-rays may show pulmonary edema.
- With the aerosol delivery, there may also be conjunctivitis and cutaneous swelling at one to six hours after exposure.
- With ingestion, the incubation period is one to 12 hours and then is associated with vomiting and abdominal pain with or without diarrhea. This is self-limited to 24 to 48 hours.

DIAGNOSIS

The diagnosis is based on detection of enterotoxin B in body fluids by PCR. Toxin may also be found in food or ingested fluids.

TREATMENT

The only treatment is supportive.

PREVENTION

The main method of prevention is to avoid a common source (eg, contaminated food or an area of aerosol delivery).

TYPHUS

BACKGROUND

- Louse-borne typhus is a rickettsial disease caused by *Rickettsia prowazekii*. It is transmitted from person to person by lice and consequently requires close personal to clothing contact.
- The mechanism of action is: The louse takes a blood meal and then defecates, which causes irritation; the host then scratches the bite site, giving entry to *R prowazekii*.
- Medical history shows 30 million cases of typhus in the former Soviet Union and Eastern Europe from 1918 to 1922, resulting in 3 million deaths.

HOSPITAL PREPARATION

- Particularly important would be recognition of the condition, which is very rare in the U.S. Once identified, public education and public health would be important methods to control this disease.
- Detection would likely be delayed because the organism cannot be seen on gram stain nor recovered in standard cultures.

- The disease, however, is easily treated; a single dose of doxycycline 100 mg is curative.

PERSONAL PROTECTION

- Scrub areas harboring rodents with mites living on them are risk areas to transmit the disease. Humans are infected by the bites of infected mites. When walking through such areas, use insect repellent and wear a protective long-sleeve shirt and trousers.
- Maintaining good personal hygiene can also be effective in the prevention of spread of louse-borne typhus.

QUARANTINE PROCEDURES

Quarantine is not necessary.

CLINICAL PRESENTATION

- The incubation period is about one week, followed by an abrupt, flulike illness with fever, headache, chills, and myalgia.
- The particularly characteristic feature is a rash, which is first noted in the axillary folds and the upper trunk at about Day 5 of the illness.
- The rash then spreads centrifugally and consists of nonconfluent, pink macules that blanch with pressure.
- The rash then becomes maculopapular, confluent, darker, and petechial. It covers the body but spares the face, palms of the hands, and soles of the feet.
- Without treatment, the fever usually resolves after two weeks, but the mortality may be relatively high—as high as 40%, with most deaths occurring in people over 65 years.

DIAGNOSIS

- Most important are the clinical features, particularly the rash with involvement of axillary folds.
- The differential diagnosis includes meningococcemia, measles, secondary syphilis, leptospirosis, Rocky Mountain spotted fever, rubella, mononucleosis, and relapsing fever.
- The Weil Felix reaction is often positive but non-specific.
- Preferred newer assays for detection of typhus include PCR or rickettsia culture, which would require specialized laboratories.

TREATMENT

Standard treatment has generally been doxycycline 100 mg bid until two to three days after fever resolution. Most patients become afebrile within 24 to 48 hours.

PREVENTION

No vaccine is FDA-approved. However, a vaccine may be available and advocated for medical personnel exposed to these cases, as well as for laboratory personnel who work with the putative agent.

VENEZUELAN EQUINE ENCEPHALITIS

(also see "Eastern equine encephalitis" and "Western equine encephalitis" in this section)

BACKGROUND

- Venezuelan equine encephalitis (VEE) is an alphavirus found primarily in South America and Central America, where it is responsible for thousands of encephalitis cases in horses and humans.
- VEE is transmitted by mosquitoes. Epidemics usually start with horses and progress to people one to two weeks later. Severe disease is most common in children.

HOSPITAL PREPARATION

- There is no person-to-person transmission and no treatment.

- The role of the hospital is patient/public education, reassurance of safety of health care workers in caring for these patients, supportive care, and notification of the public health authorities.

PERSONAL PROTECTION

VEE has been recovered from throat washings, but there has not been confirmed transmission from person to person.

DECONTAMINATION

Transmission occurs by the mosquito vector. Protection from mosquito bites is therefore important. Visitors to endemic areas should take appropriate precautions, including wearing long-sleeve shirts and trousers, using insect repellant, and using mosquito nets.

QUARANTINE PROCEDURES

Quarantine is not necessary.

CLINICAL PRESENTATION

- The presentation in patients is an incubation period of one to six days followed by a febrile illness—usually a severe illness characterized by chills, myalgia, and headache.
- There may also be photophobia, conjunctivitis, seizures, confusion, hyperesthesia, and vomiting.
- About 1% of adults and 4% of children go on to develop severe encephalitis; this rate would be expected to be higher in an aerosol attack due to direct entry of the virus into brain via the olfactory nerve instead of indirectly via mosquito exposure.
- CSF shows the typical mononuclear pleocytosis.
- The overall case mortality rate is less than 1%, but in patients who develop encephalitis, it is 20%.

DIAGNOSIS

- VEE can be recovered from blood when obtained within 48 hours of onset of symptoms, but can't usually be found after there is fully developed encephalitis.
- The CSF typically shows mononuclear cells; an elevated protein VEE-specific IgM can be found in sera and CSF by EIA.

TREATMENT

There is no specific treatment other than supportive care.

PREVENTION

- There is a highly effective VEE vaccine for horses but none for people.
- Preventive care in people consists of avoiding mosquitoes.
- There is no horse-to-person or person-to-person transmission.

WESTERN EQUINE ENCEPHALITIS

(also see "Eastern equine encephalitis" and "Venezuelan equine encephalitis" in this section)

BACKGROUND

- Western equine encephalitis (WEE) is found primarily in the Americas and primarily west of the Mississippi, hence the name.
- WEE is similar to other alphaviruses that cause encephalitis: eastern equine encephalitis (EEE) and Venezuelan equine encephalitis (VEE).
- The disease is transmitted by the mosquito vector, and disease may be epidemic in horses and humans.
- Serologic studies show that less than 1:1,000 older adults have clinical expression, but the ratio in infants is 1:1.
- Encephalitis is consequently most common in

children less than one year, and it is most frequently severe and fatal in the elderly.
- The overall case fatality rate is 3% to 4%, but it would probably be higher in an aerosol attack.

HOSPITAL PREPARATION

The main role of the hospital would be education of the public, reassurance to health care workers concerning the safety of care (since there is no person-to-person transmission), and supportive care of patients who present with encephalitis.

PERSONAL PROTECTION

- There is no person-to-person transmission.
- It is likely that this virus, like other alphaviruses, would be delivered by aerosol in a bioterrorism attack.
- Health care workers who become cases should be warned that illness would more likely represent exposure to a common source than person-to-person transmission.

DECONTAMINATION

This is a mosquito-borne disease, so decontamination should not be necessary.

QUARANTINE PROCEDURES

Quarantine is not necessary.

CLINICAL PRESENTATION

- A minority of exposed persons develop symptoms.
- Patients who do develop symptoms present with high fever, headache, chills, nausea, and vomiting.
- Also common are vertigo, pharyngitis, and respiratory symptoms.
- There are often mental status changes, which may progress to coma, seizures, and death.
- CSF usually shows a monocytic pleocytosis of $50/mm^3$ to $500/mm^3$ and elevated protein.
- Neurologic sequelae are common, but less common with WEE compared with EEE.

DIAGNOSIS

- Diagnosis is usually established with serology, including IgM.
- Unlike the VEE virus, the WEE virus cannot easily be detected in blood in the early viremic stage.

As with VEE and EEE, the CSF shows mononuclear cells and elevated protein.

TREATMENT

Treatment is supportive care.

PREVENTION

- The major mechanism of controlling naturally occurring disease is mosquito control.
- There is no WEE vaccine.

NOTES

PART FIVE

CHEMICAL TERRORISM AGENTS IN DEPTH

By:
Michael I. Greenberg, MD, MPH
Professor of Emergency Medicine
Drexel University College of Medicine
Professor of Public Health
Drexel University School of Public Health
Philadelphia, PA

With contributions from:
Matthew Salzman, MD
John Curtis, MD
Kimber Bogush, MD
Sobia Ansari, MD
Department of Emergency Medicine
Drexel University College of Medicine
Philadelphia, PA

Continued...

NOTE: In each monograph in this section, under "Synonyms and Trade Names," is the agent's "CAS number." The Chemical Abstract Service Registry, a division of the American Chemical Society, is the largest, most current database of chemical substance information, with more than 26 million entries. To learn more about a given chemical terrorism agent on the Internet, enter into a search engine the letters CAS, followed by that agent's registry number.

NOTE: In each monograph in this section, under "Synonyms and Trade Names," is the agent's "CAS number." The Chemical Abstract Service Registry, a division of the American Chemical Society, is the largest, most current database of chemical substance information, with more than 26 million entries. To learn more about a given chemical terrorism agent on the Internet, enter into a search engine the letters CAS, followed by that agent's registry number.

ACIDS

HYDROCHLORIC ACID (HCl)

SYNONYMS AND TRADE NAMES

Chlorohydric acid, hydrogen chloride, marine acid, muriatic acid, soldering acid, spirit of salt, and spirits of salts.
(CAS No. 7647-01-0)

BACKGROUND

Hydrochloric acid is usually found as a colorless liquid with a pungent, "acid-like" odor. However, it may exist as a colorless to slightly yellow gas often shipped in the form of a liquefied compressed gas.

ROUTINE USE

- HCl is used in a wide variety of manufacturing processes, including in the manufacture of phosphoric acid, ammonium chloride, fertilizers, dyes, artificial silk, and pigments for paints. It is used in refinement and production of tin and tantalum, as a lab reagent, to clean boilers and heat-exchange equipment, clean membranes in desalination plants, and clean the surface of various metals in preparation for the application of various coatings.
- HCl may be used to neutralize industrial waste streams in the recovery of zinc from scrap, as well as in the production of chloride chemicals, vinyl chloride, manufacture of sodium glutamate and gelatin, sugar refining, electroplating, soap refining, and leather tanning.
- HCl also has applications in the photographic, textile, brewing, and rubber industries.
- HCl is the primary product of combustion emanating when polyvinyl chloride burns at high temperatures.

POTENTIAL TERRORIST USE

- Given the wide presence of this chemical in bulk, it is possible that terrorists may attempt to release HCl as an aerosolized mist in locales where large numbers of people may gather, such as theaters, sports venues, or shopping malls.
- In addition, terrorists may mix hydrochloric acid with common oxidizing chemicals, such as bleach (NaOCl) or potassium permanganate ($KMnO_4$), in order to liberate chlorine gas.
- HCl may be contemplated for use as an unconventional weapon by terrorists. For example, in 1993, two members of the radical Japanese Aum Shinrikyo group were arrested for carrying dangerous chemicals aboard an aircraft after customs officials found two black plastic containers of hydrochloric acid labeled "hand soap" in their luggage.
- Chlorine gas combines with water in the respiratory tree, as well as mucous membranes, to form HCl. Thus, HCl is, in part, responsible for the pathophysiological damage induced by the inhalation of chlorine gas.

MECHANISM OF ACTION

HCl is readily soluble in water and, as such, tends to rapidly dissolve in mucous-membrane and upper-airway water. This may alter the local pH of the tissues in question, causing local irritation at low concentrations and tissue damage at higher concentrations.

POTENTIAL ROUTES FOR EXPOSURE

Dermal, inhalational, ingestion, and ocular.

TARGET ORGANS/SYSTEMS

Skin, upper respiratory tract, pulmonary tree, and GI tract (if ingested).

CLINICAL FEATURES

- Inhalation of HCl mists or vapors may cause coughing, hoarseness, choking, and inflammation, and ulceration of the nose, throat, and upper respiratory tract.
- In severe cases, inhalation of HCl mists or

vapors may cause noncardiogenic pulmonary edema, circulatory failure, and death.
- If ingested, HCl may cause immediate pain and burns of the mouth, throat, esophagus, and gastrointestinal tract, as well as nausea, vomiting, and diarrhea.
- Ingestion of HCl may be fatal.
- Dermal contact with HCl may cause redness, pain, and variable degrees of skin injury.
- HCl-containing mists or vapors tend to be irritating and may cause ocular damage. High concentrations may cause severe ocular burns and permanent eye damage.
- Long-term exposure to concentrated HCl vapors may cause dental erosions.

DIAGNOSIS

The diagnosis of HCl exposure depends upon situational recognition and reports from prehospital personnel, who may be aware of the release of HCl at a given incident site.

LABORATORY TESTING AND IMAGING

- There is no specific laboratory assay available to confirm or exclude exposure to HCl, and HCl blood levels or chloride levels are of no clinical value.
- Patients should have meticulous supportive care with special attention to respiratory status.
- If substantial inhalation is suspected, baseline chest x-rays should be obtained and oxygen saturation monitored.

TREATMENT AND DISPOSITION

- There is no specific antidote for HCl exposure.
- Supportive care—with special attention to airway, hemodynamic, and cardiac monitoring—is paramount.
- Prehospital treatment begins with the removal of victims from exposure.
- Next, decontaminate with copious amounts of water and, if available, soap.
- Identify and treat hypotension with fluids and direct pressors, if needed.
- Administer humidified oxygen, if needed.
- If the patient begins to seize, administer benzodiazepines.

- If treatment with benzodiazepines fails, administer barbiturates or propofol and consider chemical paralysis, endotracheal intubation, and continuous EEG monitoring.
- Identify and treat electrolyte abnormalities.
- Treat bronchospasm with inhaled beta agonists, such as albuterol, and parenteral or oral steroids.
- Treat arrhythmias when identified.
- In an ocular exposure, irrigate the eyes with copious amounts of water or saline. The use of a Morgan lens may facilitate this process.

REFERENCES

International Agency for Research on Cancer. Hydrochloric acid. In: *IARC Monographs on the Evaluation of Carcinogenic Risks to Humans.* Lyons, France: International Agency for Research on Cancer; 1992, v. 54:189-211.

Technology Transfer Network Air Toxics Website, U.S. Environmental Protection Agency. *Hydrochloric acid (Hydrogen chloride);* Washington, DC: Technology Transfer Network Air Toxics Website, U.S. Environmental Protection Agency; 2000. Available at: http://www.epa.gov/ttn/atw/hlthef/hydrochl.html. Accessed September 26, 2005.

HYDROFLUORIC ACID

SYNONYMS AND TRADE NAMES

Antisal 2B, HF, fluorhydric acid, and fluoric acid. (CAS No. 7664-39-3)

BACKGROUND

- Hydrofluoric acid (HF) is a colorless gas or, below 67° F, a fuming liquid.
- HF has a strong, irritating odor.
- Anhydrous HF is a strong protonic acid.
- In the aqueous form, however, HF is a weak acid.
- The minimum lethal dose is considered to be 1 mg/kg of fluoride ion.
- Exposure to HF generally occurs via inhalation; however, dermal and ocular exposure are also of great concern.

ROUTINE USE

- HF is used to produce high-octane fuel, aerosols, plastics, and refrigerants.
- HF is also used in the electronics industry and in chemical manufacturing.
- HF is used to clean stone, marble, bricks, and

metal. It has been used in glass etching since the 17th century.

POTENTIAL TERRORIST USE

If used as a terrorist weapon, HF would be expected to be released into the air as a gas in a densely populated area, potentially causing massive numbers of exposed victims. This release could be accomplished by targeting an industrial storage facility or a transport vehicle, such as a truck or rail car.

MECHANISM OF ACTION

- Contact with HF may result in local irritation and burns.
- Of greater concern, however, is HF's ability to dissociate and penetrate deep into subcutaneous tissues. The fluoride ion is able to cross lipid membranes and, once in deep tissues, binds intracellular calcium and magnesium, resulting in cellular dysfunction, liquefactive necrosis, and cell death.
- HF also binds to calcium, making it systemically unavailable, thereby predisposing the victim to hypocalcemia-related arrhythmias.
- The pain associated with HF exposure is often described as a deep burning pain, believed to be caused by calcium immobilization, resulting in potassium shifts and nerve stimulation.

POTENTIAL ROUTES FOR EXPOSURE

Dermal contact, inhalation, ocular exposure, and ingestion.

TARGET ORGANS/SYSTEMS

Cardiovascular, dermal, musculoskeletal, ocular, and pulmonary.

CLINICAL FEATURES

- Ocular exposure to HF may result in rapid onset of eye irritation and pain. Conjunctival injection, corneal abrasion or ulcer, corneal vascularization and stromal scarring, and corneal opacification may then appear. Visual deficits may be permanent.

- Dermal exposure may result in local irritation and chemical burns. However, HF notoriously penetrates into deeper tissues, including muscle and bone. This results in severe pain, with tissue destruction and necrosis. If the victim survives the incident, permanent scarring and disfiguration are likely.
- Inhalation of HF causes airway irritation and burning. Additionally, laryngospasm, laryngeal edema, bronchospasm, hemoptysis, tracheobrochitis, and ARDS may occur. Pulmonary edema may be delayed up to 72 hours after the exposure.
- Arrhythmias after exposure to HF, such as ventricular tachycardia and fibrillation, are not uncommon. These are generally a result of hypocalcemia, hypomagnesemia, and hyperkalemia. Profound hypotension may also be present. While there are reports of patients surviving these events, death is more commonly the outcome.

DIAGNOSIS

The diagnosis is based on the history of exposure in conjunction with the clinical findings.

LABORATORY TESTING AND IMAGING

- Most patients with inhalation exposure will require continuous pulse oximetry and cardiac monitoring.
- Routine labs and studies, such as electrolyte panels and chest x-rays, are often warranted following an acute exposure.
- Of particular importance are serum calcium, potassium, and magnesium levels, as these patients are predisposed to electrolyte abnormalities and associated arrhythmias.
- Electrocardiograms should also be performed on these patients. Serum electrolyte levels and ECGs may need to be repeated frequently.
- Fluoride levels are not clinically useful in the acute management of HF-exposed victims, as they are not readily available and are probably not as important as calcium, magnesium, and potassium levels.

TREATMENT AND DISPOSITION

- There are many treatment options for patients exposed to HF.
- Supportive care is critical, with close attention to the patient's airway.
- Hypotension should be treated with intravenous fluids.
- Pulse oximetry and continuous cardiac monitoring are essential.
- Prehospital treatment starts with removal from exposure and decontamination, with removal of clothing and washing with copious amounts of water, if available.
- Bronchospasm should be treated with inhaled beta agonists and oral or parenteral steroids. Some authors also recommend nebulized 2.5% calcium gluconate.
- Dermal exposure should be treated with calcium gluconate or calcium carbonate gel in 2.5% to 3.3% concentration. Topical treatment with a quaternary ammonium compound, such as Hyamine® 0.2% or Zephiran® 0.13% (benzalkonium chloride), may be useful in a superficial exposure.
- Some authors recommend local infiltration with 0.5 mL of 10% calcium gluconate per cm² of exposed tissue.
- Of note, calcium chloride should never be used, as it is also irritating to tissues.
- Other authors recommend intravenous infusion of calcium gluconate using the Bier block technique.
- Another possibility is intra-arterial infusion of calcium gluconate. This may be particularly useful after hand exposure to HF. Such infusion should be performed after consultation with a burn specialist and an interventional radiologist.
- Some authors recommend early excision of the wound, as well as blisters and necrotic tissue.
- Hypocalcemia should be treated with intravenous calcium gluconate or calcium chloride.
- Arrhythmias should be treated according to ACLS protocol, with additional treatment with intravenous calcium and magnesium.
- Ocular exposure should be treated with anesthetic drops and copious irrigation. A Morgan lens may facilitate this process. Some authors suggest a 1% calcium gluconate eye drop applied every two to three hours. Others recommend irrigation with a solution of 50 mL of 10% calcium gluconate with 500 mL of normal saline.
- Ophthalmology should be consulted immediately. There may be a role for cycloplegics and steroids in treatment in order to inhibit fibroblast proliferation. This should be determined in consultation with the ophthalmologist.
- Patients who are symptomatic after an inhalation exposure may need to be admitted for symptomatic care and monitoring for arrhythmias and pulmonary edema.
- Once stabilized, patients who sustain a significant dermal exposure may need to be transferred to a local burn center.

REFERENCES

Horton DK, Berkowitz Z, Kaye WE. Hydrofluoric acid releases in 17 states and the acute health effects associated, 1993-2001. *J Occup Environ Med.* 2004; 46(5):501-508.

Wing JS, Brender JD, Sanderson LM, et al. Acute health effects in a community after a release of hydrofluoric acid. *Arch Environ Health.* 1991;46(3):155-160.

BLOOD AGENTS

ARSINE (AsH₃)

SYNONYMS AND TRADE NAMES

Arsenic hydrid, arsenic hydride, arsenic trihydride, arseniuretted hydrogen, arsenous hydride, arsenowodor, and hydrogen arsenide. (CAS No. 7784-42-1)

BACKGROUND

- Arsine is a colorless, flammable gas formed when arsenic comes into contact with a reducing agent.
- Arsine is heavier than air and consequently tends to collect along the ground surface and in areas below grade.
- Arsine is reported to have a garlic-like odor.

ROUTINE USE

Arsine is used as a dopant in the semiconductor industry and in the manufacture of light emitting diodes (LEDs).

POTENTIAL TERRORIST USE

- Arsine is an attractive terrorism agent because it has minimal warning properties.
- Arsine is generally nonirritating and does not cause potential victims to evacuate the scene.
- Severe health effects related to arsine are usually delayed, thereby causing further difficulty in pinpointing the site and time of release.

MECHANISM OF ACTION

- Following inhalation, arsine is absorbed from the lungs and binds to sulfhydryl groups within red blood cells, inhibiting enzymes and depleting the cell of reduced glutathione.
- Varying degrees of intravascular hemolysis may result, and that, in turn, may lead to acute tubular necrosis and renal failure.

POTENTIAL ROUTES FOR EXPOSURE

Inhalational and mucous membranes.

TARGET ORGANS/SYSTEMS

Pulmonary, hematological, and CNS.

CLINICAL FEATURES

- After a latent period of up to one day, exposed persons may develop massive intravascular hemolysis.
- Early symptoms are nonspecific and may include frontal headache, vomiting, and malaise.
- Colicky abdominal and flank pain as well as jaundice may also be present.
- Hemaglobinuria causes discoloration of the urine and may lead to oliguric renal failure within as few as one to three days.
- Severe exposures may result in death within a matter of hours.

DIAGNOSIS

- While elevations of blood and urine arsenic levels would be expected following arsine exposure, these tests are rarely available in time to aid in acute diagnosis.
- The diagnosis is therefore primarily a clinical one, relying on a high level of suspicion and a patient presenting with acute, massive hemolysis and its complications, as well as situational analysis.

LABORATORY TESTING AND IMAGING

- A hemoglobin level that declines for approximately 36 hours, often accompanied by a moderate leukocytosis, may be apparent in blood counts.
- Peripheral smears may show "ghost cells" depleted of hemoglobin.

- Blood chemistries may show an elevated bilirubin level and declining renal function.
- Urinalysis shows hemoglobinuria.

TREATMENT AND DISPOSITION

- Decontaminate the patient. This involves removal of clothing of those exposed to the gas to prevent contamination of the treatment area and exposure of health care providers.
- Consider early exchange transfusion for significant or symptomatic exposures.
- Dimercaprol may be beneficial if administered within 24 hours.
- Other dithiol-containing agents, such as DMSA, may help prevent hemolysis if administered early.
- Mannitol may promote an osmotic diuresis and protect the kidneys from pigment-induced renal tubular necrosis.
- Hemodialysis may be required in the event of renal failure resulting from acute tubular necrosis.

REFERENCES

Klimecki WT, Carter DE. Arsine toxicity: Chemical and mechanistic implications. *J Toxicol Environ Health*. 1995;46(4):399-409.

Rael LT, Ayala-Fierro F. The effects of sulfur, thiol, and thiol inhibitor compounds on arsine-induced toxicity in the human erythrocyte membrane. *Toxicol Sci.* 2000;55(2):468-477.

CYANIDE (CN)

SYNONYMS AND TRADE NAMES

Carbon hydride nitride, cyanure, hydrocyanic acid, hydrogen cyanide, and prussic acid.
(CAS No. 57-12-5)

BACKGROUND

- Cyanide is a fast-acting, potentially lethal chemical that can exist in various forms, including hydrogen cyanide (HCN) and cyanogen chloride (CNCl), as well as salts such as sodium cyanide (NaCN) and potassium cyanide (KCN).
- Cyanide may, in some instances, have a faint "bitter almond" smell, but some people lack a genetic ability to detect this odor.
- Cyanide compounds are also known by the military designations AC (hydrogen cyanide) and CK (cyanogen chloride).

ROUTINE USE

- Cyanide and related compounds are found in a variety of industries, including electroplating, metallurgy, organic chemical production, photo developing, plastic manufacturing, fumigation, and mining industries.
- Cyanide is also a product of combustion in structure fires.

POTENTIAL TERRORIST USE

- Terrorists may try to disseminate cyanide as a gas or in conjunction with various explosive devices.
- A terrorist attack using cyanide may involve dispersion of gas or vapor containing cyanide or tainting of consumer products or food using cyanide.
- Logistical problems make the contamination of reservoir water supplies with cyanide an unlikely mechanism for terrorist attack.

MECHANISM OF ACTION

- Cyanide acts as a cellular asphixiant by binding to cytochrome oxidase to interfere with the utilization of oxygen and production of ATP.
- Exposure to cyanide gas, even at very low levels, may be fatal. However, if patients arrive at the hospital with intact vital signs, the potential for survival is favorable.

POTENTIAL ROUTES FOR EXPOSURE

Inhalation is the primary route of exposure; however, it is possible to ingest cyanide in contaminated food or water.

TARGET ORGANS/SYSTEMS

Respiratory tree and cellular oxygen-utilization systems.

CLINICAL FEATURES

- Cyanide poisoning should be considered in any cyanotic patient with hypoxia.
- The smell of bitter almonds on the breath or in vomitus may be a useful clinical clue to CN exposure.
- Symptoms of mild poisoning include headache, dizziness, drowsiness, nausea and vomiting, and mucosal irritation.
- Severe effects may include dyspnea, altered level of consciousness, tachydysrhythmias and bradydysrhythmias, hypotension, cardiovascular collapse, coma, seizures, and death.
- Death can occur rapidly (within minutes) following inhalational exposure.
- Metabolic acidosis is related to lactic acid accumulation.
- A decrease in the arterial-venous difference in PO_2 is usually evident.

DIAGNOSIS

The diagnosis of cyanide poisoning is based primarily on the exposure history in conjunction with rapid progression of clinical symptoms and the findings listed above.

LABORATORY TESTING AND IMAGING

- Elevated serum lactate levels and lactic acidosis are hallmarks of cyanide poisoning.
- Specific blood/body fluid cyanide levels are not usually helpful since the clinical syndrome progresses very quickly and lab results are usually not available in time to alter treatment decisions.

TREATMENT AND DISPOSITION

- Except for trivial exposures, all patients should receive the contents of a commercially available cyanide antidote kit.
- In Europe, dicobalt edetate and hydroxocobalamin are commonly used antidotes, but they are not yet available in the U.S.
- Supportive treatment measures include prompt removal from exposure, high-concentration oxygen, correction of acidosis, treatment of seizures, and cardiovascular support.

- Cyanide is lighter than air, so its volatility limits its toxicity in the open air.
- Most survivors are without sequelae, although anoxic encephalopathy has resulted in some long-term neurological effects.
- IV sodium thiosulfate provides sulfur substrate to facilitate the formation of thiocyanate by rhodanese.
- Inhaled amyl nitrate initiates the formation of methemoglobin, the ferric ion of which has a greater affinity for cyanide than hemoglobin. The cyanide is then slowly released from the methemoglobin and detoxified by the body. Intravenous sodium nitrate continues this process and may have additional beneficial cardiovascular effects.
- Extreme caution is required, since methemoglobin induction may adversely affect patients with underlying cardiac or pulmonary disease or those suffering from smoke inhalation.

REFERENCES

Bismuth C, Borron SW, Baud FJ, et al. Chemical weapons: Documented use and compounds on the horizon. *Toxicol Lett.* 2004;149(1-3):11-18.

SODIUM MONOFLUOROACETATE ($C_2H_3FO_2Na$)

SYNONYMS AND TRADE NAMES

1080, compound 1080, fratol, furatol, ratbane 1080, SMFA, sodium fluoacetate, and TL 869. (CAS No. 62-74-8)

BACKGROUND

- Sodium monofluoroacetate (commonly referred to as "SMFA") occurs naturally in certain plants found in South America, South Africa, and Australia. When synthesized, it is usually an odorless, white powder that is readily water-soluble.
- Exposure to SMFA generally occurs via ingestion; however, ocular, dermal, and inhalational exposures are also of concern.

- SMFA primarily affects the central nervous system and the cardiovascular system. Following nonfatal cases, patients may have permanent neurologic sequelae, but may otherwise make a complete recovery.
- Most case reports in the literature are of acute, intentional ingestion, or accidental, chronic poisoning as a result of occupational hazard.

ROUTINE USE

SMFA is used as a rodenticide as well as a poison for livestock predator elimination (e.g., coyotes).

POTENTIAL TERRORIST USE

If used as a terrorist weapon, SMFA might be expected to be released into community drinking water supplies. While the dilutional effects of releasing this material into reservoirs may be protective, contamination of sources close to end-users is potentially lethal. Such contamination of drinking water has the potential to result in large numbers of casualties.

MECHANISM OF ACTION

- SMFA is metabolized to fluorocitrate, which inhibits aconitase, an enzyme in the Krebs cycle.
- Aconitase inhibition results in increased intracellular levels of citric acid, and effectively ceases oxidative energy metabolism. A lethal dose may be as low as 2 mg/kg to 10 mg/kg.

POTENTIAL ROUTES FOR EXPOSURE

- Ingestion is the primary route of exposure. However, there is one case report of a near-fatal inhalational exposure to SMFA.
- SMFA is not well absorbed through the skin, absent skin lesions and/or loss of skin integrity.
- SMFA is also known to act as an eye irritant.

TARGET ORGANS/SYSTEMS

CNS, cardiovascular, renal, hepatic, endocrine, and ocular.

CLINICAL FEATURES

- Symptoms follow shortly after exposure and may include auditory hallucinations, vomiting, and hypotension.
- Facial paresthesias, muscle twitching, pulsus alternans, tachycardia, pulmonary edema, nystagmus, liver failure, and thyroid dysfunction have all been reported.
- Shock, acute renal failure, hypokalemia, and hypocalcemia have also been reported.
- Further, the electrocardiogram may demonstrate a prolonged QTc interval and increased T–wave amplitude followed by S-T segment elevation, followed by ventricular tachycardia and ventricular fibrillation, and, ultimately, asystole.
- Patients may also experience seizures and coma, both ominous signs that may portend death.
- Symptoms usually manifest within 30 to 150 minutes. However, there is at least one case report of an individual manifesting symptoms 36 hours after exposure.

DIAGNOSIS

The diagnosis is based on the history of exposure in conjunction with the specific clinical findings and agent/contaminant identification.

LABORATORY TESTING AND IMAGING

- There is no specific laboratory assay available to confirm or exclude exposure to SMFA, and blood levels of the compound are of no clinical value.
- After an acute exposure, patients should have frequent electrolyte monitoring, with careful attention to potassium, magnesium, and calcium levels.
- Patients should have an electrocardiogram performed, as well as continuous cardiac monitoring.

TREATMENT AND DISPOSITION

- There is no specific antidote for SMFA poisoning.
- Glyceryl monoacetate (monoacetin) and ethanol have been studied in animals and shown to

reverse and/or prevent toxic effects. These treatments have not been determined to be safe or effective in humans. As such, they are not currently recommended.

- Supportive care—with special attention to airway, hemodynamic, and cardiac monitoring—is paramount.
- In the event of aerosolized particles, prehospital treatment starts with removal from exposure.
- Decontaminate with copious amounts of water and, if available, soap.
- Identify and treat hypotension with fluids and direct pressors, if necessary.
- Administer oxygen, if necessary.
- If the patient begins to seize, administer benzodiazepines.
- If treatment with benzodiazepines is ineffective, administer barbiturates or propofol and consider chemical paralysis, endotracheal intubation, and continuous EEG monitoring.
- Identify and treat electrolyte abnormalities.
- Treat bronchospasm with inhaled beta agonists, such as albuterol, and parenteral or oral steroids.
- Treat arrhythmias, when identified. Consider having a defibrillator at the patient's bedside.
- In an ocular exposure, irrigate the eyes with copious amounts of water or saline. The use of a Morgan lens may facilitate this process.

REFERENCES

Animal Health Board. *Technical review of sodium monofluoroacetate (1080) toxicology.* Wellington, New Zealand: Animal Health Board and Landcare Research New Zealand Limited; 2002. Available at: http://www.landcareresearch.co.nz/publications/downloads/AHB_1080_review.pdf. Accessed September 15, 2005.

CHOKING/PULMONARY AGENTS

AMMONIA (NH₃)

SYNONYMS AND TRADE NAMES

Nitro-sil, spirit of hartshorn, and vaporole.
(CAS No. 7664-41-7)

BACKGROUND

- Ammonia is a colorless gas that is readily water soluble at room temperature.
- Ammonia has a strong, pungent, and easily recognized odor.
- An alkali corrosive, ammonia has the potential to be extremely irritating to any surface it contacts, and it is especially irritating to mucous membranes.
- Reports in the literature include human exposures resulting from intentional as well as unintentional ingestions. In addition, numerous occupationally based exposures, many related to accidental spills during transport, have been described.

ROUTINE USE

- One of the most commonly produced chemicals in the U.S., ammonia finds widespread use as a component of fertilizers and animal feed.
- Ammonia is also used in the manufacture of various pharmaceuticals, pesticides, textiles, leather, and plastics, as well as a refrigerant and in a wide variety of household cleaning agents.
- In addition, ammonia is a product of combustion of nylon, silk, wood, and melamine.

POTENTIAL TERRORIST USE

- If used as a terrorist agent, anhydrous ammonia would be expected to be released as a gas into open areas or closed spaces where large numbers of people may congregate, either from a transport vessel, such as truck or train, or from a large storage facility.
- Ammonia is generally expected to be used as an agent of opportunity, (i.e., diverted from normal transportation routes or disseminated from manufacturing plants and/or locales storing large amounts of ammonia on site) rather than as a chemical that would be produced by terrorists.

MECHANISM OF ACTION

When ammonia mixes with water, ammonium hydroxide forms. This corrosive alkali is capable of causing liquefaction necrosis of tissues, and is able to penetrate deeper into tissues than an equally potent acid. This creates an exothermic reaction. As a result, local thermal burns may occur, in addition to chemical injuries directly attributable to skin, eye, or mucous membrane contact with ammonia.

POTENTIAL ROUTES FOR EXPOSURE

Exposures to ammonia may occur via inhalation, skin exposure, ocular exposure, or ingestion.

TARGET ORGANS/SYSTEMS

Pulmonary, ocular, dermatologic, and gastrointestinal.

CLINICAL FEATURES

- Symptoms associated with minimal exposures to anhydrous ammonia gas may include mild eye, nose, and throat irritation. As concentrations increase, symptoms may gradually become more intense.
- At higher concentrations, immediate eye injury, such as corneal ulcers or conjunctivitis, may occur, as well as caustic airway injury, leading to laryngospasm, wheezing, cough, shortness of breath, and stridor.
- At even higher concentrations, airway mucosal sloughing, chest pain, noncardiogenic pulmonary edema, and bronchospasm may occur. Seizures and coma have been reported as well.
- Large exposures may result in death.

- Ingestion of an ammonia-containing liquid may result in esophageal burns, with possible subsequent perforation. Mediastinitis is a feared consequence of esophageal rupture and may be fatal.

DIAGNOSIS

The diagnosis is based on the history of exposure in conjunction with the specific clinical findings described above.

LABORATORY TESTING AND IMAGING

- There is no laboratory test to specifically confirm or exclude an exposure to ammonia.
- Blood ammonia levels are of no clinical value.
- Symptomatic patients will require pulse oximetry and chest x-rays.
- Routine lab studies, such as CBC and electrolytes, should be considered after an acute exposure.

TREATMENT AND DISPOSITION

- There is no specific antidote for an ammonia exposure.
- After removal from the source and adequate decontamination, supportive care—with special attention to the patient's airway—is the mainstay of treatment for patients after an inhalation exposure to ammonia.
- Symptomatic patients should have continuous pulse oximetry monitoring.
- Some authors suggest treatment with inhaled bronchodilators, such as albuterol. Others suggest treatment with parenteral steroids; however, there is some evidence that treatment with steroids may actually result in higher morbidity.
- Treatment with parenteral antibiotics has never been shown to improve outcomes.
- Supplemental (moist, humidified) oxygen should be administered to symptomatic or hypoxemic patients.
- The decision to admit patients following ammonia exposure rests on the clinical judgment of the evaluating physician; however, admission should be standard for those at the extremes of age or with underlying cardiopulmonary disease.

- Patients who have suffered a dermal exposure should be decontaminated with copious amounts of tap water.
- Patients with ocular symptoms should be decontaminated and irrigated with large volumes of saline, preferably using a Morgan lens, if available. These patients should also have a slit-lamp examination with fluoroscein staining to evaluate for corneal abrasion or ulcer.
- Early ophthalmologic consultation should be considered for persons with significant corneal ulcers.
- Patients who have ingested ammonia-containing liquids should be admitted for observation and endoscopy within 12 to 24 hours after the exposure, even if initially asymptomatic.
- Treatment with steroids should only be initiated after an endoscopy and consultation with a medical toxicologist.

REFERENCES

Agency for Toxic Substances and Disease Registry, U.S. Department of Health and Human Services, Public Health Service. *Toxicological Profile for Ammonia.* Atlanta, GA: Agency for Toxic Substances and Disease Registry, U.S. Department of Health and Human Services, Public Health Service; 2004. Available at: http://www.atsdr.cdc.gov/toxprofiles/tp126.html. Accessed September 9, 2005.

Brautbar N, Wu MP, Richter ED. Chronic ammonia inhalation and interstitial pulmonary fibrosis: A case report and review of the literature. *Arch Environ Health.* 2003;58(9):592-596.

Centers for Disease Control and Prevention, U.S. Department of Health and Human Services. *Chemical Emergencies: Ammonia.* Washington, DC: Centers for Disease Control and Prevention, U.S. Department of Health and Human Services; 2005. Available at: http://www.bt.cdc.gov/agent/ammonia. Accessed September 9, 2005.

BROMINE (Br$_2$)

SYNONYMS AND TRADE NAMES

Brom, Brom-A-Gard®, brome, bromo, broom, dibromine, and UN 1744. (CAS No. 7726-95-6)

BACKGROUND

- Bromine is a naturally occurring, reddish-brown volatile element found in the earth's crust, seawater, and, to a lesser extent, well water.
- Bromine emits an odor reminiscent of bleach. It dissolves in water and exists as a liquid at room temperature.

- Bromine is denser than air and thus may be expected to concentrate in low-lying areas.
- Bromine and related compounds have come to serve as alternatives to chlorine for pool and hot tub sanitation as they are cheaper to use and have greater efficacy against *Pseudomonas* spp.
- Several bromine-containing compounds were historically used as sedatives, but they have since been removed from the U.S. market.

ROUTINE USE

- Much like chlorine, bromine has powerful oxidizing characteristics that make it and its related compounds very versatile in industrial and commercial processes such as petrochemical production, photographic-film production, and paper and dye manufacture.
- Bromine-containing products are also used in agriculture and sanitation, as well as fumigants and fire-suppression agents.

POTENTIAL TERRORIST USE

- If released by terrorists, bromine may be used to contaminate community food or drinking supplies.
- Terrorists may also attempt to release bromine as a gas into open or confined areas where large numbers of people may congregate (e.g., shopping malls, sports venues, theaters, etc.).
- Bromine may also be an agent of opportunity for terrorists, who may try to liberate bromine or bromine-containing chemicals from industrial sites, large storage facilities, or transport vessels (i.e., trucks or trains).

MECHANISM OF ACTION

- Bromine's cytotoxicity is thought to be secondary to its oxidizing properties.
- Bromine can react with water in tissue to produce hydrogen bromide (HBr) and hypobromous acid (HOBr), subsequently breaking down into free radicals.
- Bromamine and thiol radicals generated from the interaction between the acids and cellular protein may also contribute to the overall toxicity of bromine exposure.

- Bromine's high water solubility translates into significant tissue permeability, which may result in deeper, more extensive tissue damage.

POTENTIAL ROUTES FOR EXPOSURE

Inhalational, ingestion, and dermal.

TARGET ORGANS/SYSTEMS

Respiratory, mucous membranes, gastrointestinal, CNS, and ocular.

CLINICAL FEATURES

- Bromine exposure may be occupational due to its industrial uses, or as a result of swimming in bromine-sanitized pools.
- Eye and nose inflammation, sore throat, chest tightness, bronchospasm, blepharospasm, and dermatitis have been reported after occupational exposure.
- Other inhalational symptoms may include epistaxis, dizziness, headaches, upper airway edema, and pulmonary edema.
- Pneumomediastinum has also been reported.
- High concentrations of bromine may be corrosive to the skin. 1-Bromo-3-chloro-5,5-dimethylhydantoin, often used in swimming pools, has led to "spa-pool dermatitis," a pruritic, eczematoid rash that may be exacerbated upon repeated exposure.
- Bromine exposure may lead to long-term systemic health effects, including eye irritation, respiratory dysfunction, headaches, dizziness, fatigue, memory disturbances, abdominal pain, diarrhea, and constipation.
- Exposure to bromine gas may also cause ocular irritation or damage.
- Ingestion of liquid bromine may result in hemorrhagic gastroenteritis with secondary shock.

DIAGNOSIS

- Signs of bromine exposure may include brown discoloration of mucous membranes and the tongue.
- Prehospital personnel may report bromine exposure based on information obtained at the scene.

LABORATORY TESTING AND IMAGING

There is no specific test for bromine exposure, but elevated bromide serum levels may be an important qualitative indicator that exposure occurred.

TREATMENT AND DISPOSITION

- No specific antidote exists for bromine poisoning.
- Prehospital treatment begins with removal from exposure, followed by decontamination with soap and water.
- General supportive care—with special attention to the airway—is paramount.
- Administer oxygen, if needed.
- Patients with dermal or ocular exposure should be decontaminated with copious amounts of irrigation with tap water.
- The use of a Morgan lens may facilitate ocular decontamination.

REFERENCES

Burns MJ, Linden CH. Another hot tub hazard. Toxicity secondary to bromine and hydrobromic acid exposure. *Chest.* 1997;111(3):816-819.

Centers for Disease Control and Prevention. *Chemical Emergencies: Facts about Bromine.* Atlanta, GA: Centers for Disease Control and Prevention; 2004. Available at: http://www.bt.cdc.gov/agent/bromine/basics/facts.asp. Accessed October 10, 2005.

Woolf A, Shannon M. Reactive airways dysfunction and systemic complaints after mass exposure to bromine. *Environ Health Perspect.* 1999;107(6):507-509.

CHLORINE (Cl₂)

SYNONYMS AND TRADE NAMES

Bertholite and chlore. (CAS No. 7782-50-5)

BACKGROUND

- Chlorine is a greenish-yellow gas at room temperature with a distinct odor.
- Two and a half times heavier than air, chlorine is only modestly soluble in water.
- Clinically important exposure to chlorine usually occurs via inhalation. However, it is important to remember that exposure may also take place through ocular as well as dermal contact.
- Acute intoxication following exposure to chlorine generally affects the lungs, but skin and ocular exposure may result in burns and blisters.
- Because of its modest water solubility and low odor threshold, exposure to chlorine gas usually prompts the victim to flee the area, if able, and results in only mild upper airway irritation.
- After a nonfatal exposure, recovery is generally rapid; however, symptoms such as cough may last up to two weeks.

ROUTINE USE

- Commonly found in household cleaning products, chlorine is one of the 10 most produced industrial chemicals in the U.S. It is used in the pulp and paper industry, as well as in water purification and waste management.
- Chlorine is often shipped nationwide as a pressurized gas in tanks via rail and truck transport.

POTENTIAL TERRORIST USE

- A transport truck or train tanker car carrying pressurized chlorine gas may serve as a target for terrorists, who could release the contents either by activating release valves or by blowing up the container, essentially creating a chlorine gas bomb.
- A terrorist could also choose to target an industry in which chlorine is utilized and stored and attempt to release the chemical from the industrial site itself.
- If used as a terrorist agent, chlorine would be expected to be released as a gas either from a transport vessel, such as truck or train, or from a large storage facility, into large open areas or closed spaces where large numbers of people may congregate.
- Chlorine is generally expected to be used as an agent of opportunity (i.e., diverted from normal transportation routes or disseminated from manufacturing plants and/or locales storing large amounts of ammonia on site). It is less likely to be produced by terrorists as a chemical weapon.

MECHANISM OF ACTION

- Chlorine reacts with water to form hydrochloric acid and hypochlorous acid.

- Hydrochloric acid may cause local irritation and burns even at relatively low concentrations.
- Hypochlorous acid dissociates to form free radicals that can yield delayed injury.

POTENTIAL ROUTES FOR EXPOSURE

Inhalation is the primary route of concern; however, dermal and ocular contact may also occur. After skin exposure, systemic absorption is not a concern.

TARGET ORGANS/SYSTEMS

Pulmonary, ocular, dermatologic, and gastrointestinal.

CLINICAL FEATURES

- Within approximately one hour, exposure to chlorine gas at low concentrations results in mild mucous membrane irritation.
- As concentrations increase, exposed victims will begin to experience upper respiratory tract irritation and may develop a burning sensation in the nose and throat.
- At higher concentrations, exposed persons may experience chest pain, coughing, wheezing, and vomiting.
- Following substantial inhalational exposures, patients may develop chemical pneumonitis with or without noncardiogenic pulmonary edema.
- Massive exposures to high concentrations of chlorine are capable of causing rapid death.
- Patients who recover from acute illness secondary to chlorine may go on to develop chronic pulmonary problems.
- Skin contact with chlorine, especially in its liquid state, may produce local irritation, pain, and blisters.
- In some cases, ocular exposure to chlorine may result in irritation, conjunctivitis, and corneal abrasion.

DIAGNOSIS

The diagnosis is based on the history of exposure in conjunction with the specific clinical findings.

LABORATORY TESTING AND IMAGING

- Symptomatic patients presenting after inhalational exposures will all require pulse oximetry and a chest x-ray.
- Routine lab tests, such as CBC and electrolytes, should also be considered.
- There is no specific laboratory test available to confirm or exclude a diagnosis of chlorine injury.
- Patients with ocular complaints should have fluorescein staining performed to assess for corneal abrasion or ulcer. When possible, patients should undergo slit-lamp microscopy.

TREATMENT AND DISPOSITION

- There is no specific antidote for chlorine inhalational injury.
- Prehospital treatment starts with removal from exposure.
- General supportive care—with special attention to airway—is paramount.
- Administer oxygen if needed.
- Pulse oximetry is indicated if patient is symptomatic.
- Some authors suggest treatment with nebulized bronchodilators.
- The use of nebulized sodium bicarbonate has also been suggested and may be effective, but conclusive data are lacking.
- Some authors consider treatment with parenteral steroids to be beneficial, but data are lacking.
- Treatment with phosphodiesterase inhibitors, such as aminophylline and theophylline, is controversial and generally not recommended.
- Patients with dermal or ocular exposure should be decontaminated with copious amounts of irrigation with the most readily available neutral fluid, such as water. Eye irrigation may be facilitated by the use of a Morgan lens.

REFERENCES

Bosse GM. Nebulized sodium bicarbonate in the treatment of chlorine gas inhalation. *J Toxicol Clin Toxicol.* 1994;32(3):233-241.

HYDROCHLORIC ACID (HCl)

SYNONYMS AND TRADE NAMES

Chlorohydric acid, hydrogen chloride, marine acid, muriatic acid, soldering acid, spirit of salt, and spirits of salts. (CAS No. 7647-01-0)

BACKGROUND

Hydrochloric acid is usually found as a colorless liquid with a pungent, "acid-like" odor. However, it may exist as a colorless to slightly yellow gas often shipped in the form of a liquefied compressed gas.

ROUTINE USE

- HCl is used in a wide variety of manufacturing processes, including in the manufacture of phosphoric acid, ammonium chloride, fertilizers, dyes, artificial silk, and pigments for paints. It is used in refinement and production of tin and tantalum, as a lab reagent, to clean boilers and heat-exchange equipment, to clean membranes in desalination plants, and to clean the surface of various metals in preparation for the application of various coatings.
- HCl may be used to neutralize industrial waste streams in the recovery of zinc from scrap; in the production of chloride chemicals, vinyl chloride, sodium glutamate, and gelatin; and in sugar refining, electroplating, soap refining, and leather tanning.
- HCl also has applications in the photographic, textile, brewing, and rubber industries.
- HCl is the primary product of combustion emanating when polyvinyl chloride burns at high temperatures.

POTENTIAL TERRORIST USE

- Given the wide presence of this chemical in bulk, it is possible that terrorists may attempt to release HCl as an aerosolized mist in locales where large numbers of people may gather, such as theaters, sports venues, or shopping malls.

- In addition, terrorists may mix hydrochloric acid with common oxidizing chemicals, such as bleach (NaOCl) or potassium permanganate ($KMnO_4$), in order to liberate chlorine gas.
- HCl may be contemplated for use as an unconventional weapon by terrorists. For example, in 1993, two members of the radical Japanese Aum Shinrikyo group were arrested for carrying dangerous chemicals aboard an aircraft after customs officials found two black plastic containers of hydrochloric acid labeled "hand soap" in their luggage.
- Chlorine gas combines with water in the respiratory tree, as well as mucous membranes, to form HCl. Thus, HCl is, in part, responsible for the pathophysiological damage induced by the inhalation of chlorine gas.

MECHANISM OF ACTION

HCl is readily soluble in water and, as such, tends to rapidly dissolve in mucous-membrane and upper-airway water. This may alter the local pH of the tissues in question, causing local irritation at low concentrations and tissue damage at higher concentrations.

POTENTIAL ROUTES FOR EXPOSURE

Dermal, inhalational, ingestion, and ocular.

TARGET ORGANS/SYSTEMS

Skin, upper respiratory tract, pulmonary tree, and gastrointestinal tract (if ingested).

CLINICAL FEATURES

- Inhalation of HCl mists or vapors may cause coughing, hoarseness, choking, inflammation, and ulceration of the nose, throat, and upper respiratory tract.
- In severe cases, inhalation of HCl mists or vapors may cause noncardiogenic pulmonary edema, circulatory failure, and death.
- If ingested, HCl may cause immediate pain and burns of the mouth, throat, esophagus, and gastrointestinal tract, as well as nausea, vomiting, and diarrhea.

- Ingestion of HCl may be fatal.
- Dermal contact with HCl may cause redness, pain, and variable degrees of skin injury.
- HCl-containing mists or vapors tend to be irritating and may cause ocular damage. High concentrations may cause severe ocular burns and permanent eye damage.
- Long-term exposure to concentrated HCl vapors may cause dental erosions.

DIAGNOSIS

The diagnosis of HCl exposure depends upon situational recognition and reports from prehospital personnel, who may be aware of the release of HCl at a given incident site.

LABORATORY TESTING AND IMAGING

- There is no specific laboratory assay available to confirm or exclude exposure to HCl, and HCl blood levels or chloride levels are of no clinical value.
- Patients should have meticulous supportive care with special attention to respiratory status.
- If substantial inhalation is suspected, baseline chest x-rays should be obtained and oxygen saturation monitored.

TREATMENT AND DISPOSITION

- There is no specific antidote for HCl exposure.
- Supportive care—with special attention to airway, hemodynamic, and cardiac monitoring—is paramount.
- Prehospital treatment begins with the removal of victims from exposure.
- Next, decontaminate with copious amounts of water and, if available, soap.
- Identify and treat hypotension with fluids and direct pressors, if needed.
- Administer humidified oxygen, if needed.
- If the patient begins to seize, administer benzodiazepines.
- If treatment with benzodiazepines fails, administer barbiturates or propofol and consider chemical paralysis, endotracheal intubation, and continuous EEG monitoring.

- Identify and treat electrolyte abnormalities.
- Treat bronchospasm with inhaled beta agonists, such as albuterol, and parenteral or oral steroids.
- Treat arrhythmias when identified.
- In an ocular exposure, irrigate the eyes with copious amounts of water or saline. The use of a Morgan lens may facilitate this process.

REFERENCES

International Agency for Research on Cancer. Hydrochloric acid. In: *IARC Monographs on the Evaluation of Carcinogenic Risks to Humans.* Lyons, France: International Agency for Research on Cancer; 1992, v. 54:189-211.

Technology Transfer Network Air Toxics Website, U.S. Environmental Protection Agency. *Hydrochloric acid (Hydrogen chloride)*; Washington, DC: Technology Transfer Network Air Toxics Website, U.S. Environmental Protection Agency; 2000. Available at: http://www.epa.gov/ttn/atw/hlthef/hydrochl.html. Accessed September 26, 2005.

METHYL BROMIDE (CH_3Br)

SYNONYMS AND TRADE NAMES

Bromomethane, monobromomethane, and Terabol. (CAS No. 74-83-9)

BACKGROUND

- Methyl bromide is a halogenated hydrocarbon that is colorless and volatile.
- At room temperature, methyl bromide is a gas. At high concentrations, it may be identified by an odor reminiscent of chloroform.
- Exposure to methyl bromide generally occurs via inhalation and at times via skin exposure.
- Acute intoxication following exposure to methyl bromide usually affects the central nervous system.
- Following nonfatal cases, recovery is usually slow and neurological and/or psychiatric sequelae may occur.
- Most cases of acute intoxication reported in the literature are due to intentional or accidental poisoning following occupational exposures.

ROUTINE USE

- Methyl bromide is commonly used as a fumigant insecticide for foodstuffs and in structures.

- Methyl bromide is also used as a refrigerant, as well as a fire-extinguisher chemical.
- Heavier than air, methyl bromide tends to accumulate in low-lying areas.

POTENTIAL TERRORIST USE

- If used as a terrorist weapon, methyl bromide would be expected to be released as a gas into closed-space environments where large numbers of people congregate, such as theaters, sports venues, shopping malls, office complexes, or airport terminals.
- Methyl bromide may be a terrorist weapon of opportunity since it may exist in bulk at various locations, where terrorists may be able to cause its release into the atmosphere or environment.

MECHANISM OF ACTION

Methyl bromide acts as an alkylating agent that tends to bind with various amino and sulfhydryl groups in enzymes and other biological chemicals.

POTENTIAL ROUTES FOR EXPOSURE

- Inhalation is the primary route of concern. However, dermal and/or ocular contact may occur.
- Dermal absorption is known to occur and may cause systemic problems.

TARGET ORGANS/SYSTEMS

Pulmonary, CNS, renal, hepatic, and cardiac.

CLINICAL FEATURES

- Symptoms following exposure may include ocular, skin, respiratory tract, and mucous membrane irritation.
- Other symptoms may include muscle weakness, lack of muscular coordination, visual problems, dizziness, nausea, vomiting, headache, tremors, seizures, and problems with breathing.
- Following dermal exposure, vesiculation and/or frostbite may result.
- Some patients with severe acute exposures may suffer intractable seizures, which are an ominous finding.

- Following substantial inhalational exposure, respiratory failure and noncardiogenic pulmonary edema may occur.
- Chronic neurological problems may follow acute exposure and involve a variety of neurological and neuropsychiatric abnormalities, including psychosis, aphasia, ataxia, and peripheral neuropathies.
- All patients with any degree of acute exposure will require neurological follow-up.

DIAGNOSIS

The diagnosis is based on the history of exposure in conjunction with the specific clinical findings.

LABORATORY TESTING AND IMAGING

- Most patients with inhalational exposure will require pulse oximetry, as well as baseline arterial blood gases and chest x-rays.
- Routine lab studies (CBC, electrolytes, and serum glucose) should be considered following all acute exposures.
- Serum bromine levels are usually not clinically helpful in the acute setting, as low bromine levels will not necessarily rule out clinically important exposures.

TREATMENT AND DISPOSITION

- There are no specific antidotes available for methyl bromide. Some authors have suggested that N-acetylcysteine (NAC) may be useful, but there is no definitive scientific support for the efficacy of NAC in this context.
- Administer supportive care (airway maintenance, ventilation, cardiac monitoring).
- Administer oxygen as needed.
- Prehospital treatment starts with removal from exposure.
- Health care personnel may be at risk of off-gassing from patients.
- Decontaminate patients prior to arrival at the emergency department.
- Vapor exposures should be decontaminated by clothing removal and clothing storage in air-tight bags.

- Liquid exposures should be decontaminated by copious irrigation with tap water.
- Identify and treat hypotension with fluids and pressors, if needed.
- Administer oxygen, if needed.
- Treat bronchospasm, if identified.
- Treat arrhythmias, if identified.
- Treat seizures; drugs of choice are benzodiazepines.
- Treat intractable seizure aggressively; consider barbiturate coma.
- Modalities for accelerated elimination (hemodialysis, hemoperfusion) are not clinically useful.

REFERENCES

Hoizey G, Souchon PF, Trenque T, et al. An unusual case of methyl bromide poisoning. *J Toxicol Clin Toxicol.* 2002;40(6):817-821.

Lifshitz M, Gavrilov V. Central nervous system toxicity and early peripheral neuropathy following dermal exposure to methyl bromide. *J Toxicol Clin Toxicol.* 2000;38(7):799-801.

METHYL ISOCYANATE (C_2H_3NO)

SYNONYMS AND TRADE NAMES

Isocyanate de methyle, isocyanatomethane, isocyanic acid, iso-cyanomethane, methyl carbonimide, methyl ester, methylisocyanaat, methyl isocyanat, methylisokyanat, metil isocianato, MIC, RCRA waste number P064, TL 1450, and UN 2480. (CAS No. 624-83-9)

BACKGROUND

- Methyl isocyanate is a colorless liquid that exhibits a sharp, distinctive, pungent odor. Its vapor is nearly twice as dense as air and thus this chemical, when released into the atmosphere, tends to collect in low-lying areas.
- Methyl isocyanate is one of the chemicals released in 1984 from the Union Carbide plant in Bhopal, India, in what is widely considered one of the most serious industrial accidents in history. Tens of thousands were killed, and hundreds of thousands were injured in the event.

ROUTINE USE

Methyl isocyanate is used as a chemical intermediate in the synthesis of carbamate pesticides.

POTENTIAL TERRORIST USE

If methyl isocyanate were released by terrorists, it would probably involve aerosolization or dispersal of large quantities of the chemical in areas where large numbers of persons may congregate (e.g., theaters, sports venues, shopping malls, etc.). Severe injury to large numbers of people might occur, particularly if the release took place within a confined space or area with poor ventilation.

MECHANISM OF ACTION

Methyl isocyanate acts as a potent irritant to lungs, eyes, skin, and mucous membranes. This chemical reportedly binds covalently to proteins in the blood and various organs, although it is unclear to what degree this contributes to its toxicity.

POTENTIAL ROUTES FOR EXPOSURE

Patients may be exposed to methyl isocyanate by dermal absorption, ocular exposure, or inhalation.

TARGET ORGANS/SYSTEMS

Skin, eyes, and lungs.

CLINICAL FEATURES

- Burning of the eyes and lacrimation are often the symptoms first reported.
- With severe exposures, corneal destruction may result and lead to permanent impairment of vision or even blindness.
- Coughing, nausea, vomiting, and diarrhea have also been reported following exposure to methyl isocyanate.
- Inhalation of methyl isocyanate vapors at adequate concentrations may result in non-cardiogenic pulmonary edema. This is the most common cause of death in those so exposed.

- With higher concentrations and longer durations of exposure, extensive destruction of alveolae may result in permanent lung damage and subsequent permanent alteration of pulmonary function.

DIAGNOSIS

- There is no specific test to confirm exposure to methyl isocyanate. The diagnosis relies on clinical suspicion and/or a specific history of release and exposure.
- It is important to note that, despite the name of this chemical, clinical cyanide toxicity is not a feature of methyl isocyanate exposure, although it may occur if the methyl isocyanate is contaminated with other cyanide-containing chemicals.

LABORATORY TESTING AND IMAGING

- There are no diagnostic laboratory findings.
- Chest x-rays may demonstrate nonspecific abnormalities that include atelectasis, infiltrates, or pulmonary edema.
- Arterial blood gas analysis may reveal hypoxia, and peak flow measurement may demonstrate bronchospasm.
- Symptomatic patients should have renal and hepatic function evaluated, and should be monitored with continuous ECG and pulse oximetry.

TREATMENT AND DISPOSITION

- There is no specific antidote for methyl isocyanate. The mainstay of care is supportive.
- Immediate removal from exposure, as well as decontamination, are the initial steps in treatment. This includes removal of clothing and washing exposed areas of skin with soap and water.
- Supplemental oxygen should be provided for hypoxic patients.
- Beta agonists should be administered to patients with evidence of bronchospasm.
- Mechanical ventilation is necessary in the most severe cases.
- Ocular exposures should be evaluated by flourescein staining and treated with irrigation, topical anesthetics, and mydriatics for comfort.
- Hospitalization is recommended for exposed patients to detect delayed pulmonary edema.

REFERENCES

Departments of the Army, the Navy, the Air Force, and Commandant, Marine, Corps. *Treatment of Chemical Agent Casualties and Conventional Military Chemical Injuries: NAVMED P-5041, FMFM 11-11, AFJMAN 44-149, FM 8-285.* Washington, DC: Departments of the Army, the Navy, the Air Force, and Commandant, Marine, Corps, U.S. Government Printing Office; 1995. Available at: http://www.vnh.org/FM8285/cover.html. Accessed September 1, 2005.

Mehta PS, Mehta AS, Mehta SJ, et al. Bhopal tragedy's health effects. A review of methyl isocyanate toxicity. *JAMA.* 1990;264(21):2781-2787.

Rye WA. Human responses to isocyanate exposure. *J Occup Med.* 1973; 15(3):306-307.

OSMIUM TETROXIDE (OsO₄)

SYNONYMS AND TRADE NAMES

Osmic acid, osmium oxide, and perosmic acid. (CAS No. 20816-12-0)

BACKGROUND

Osmium tetroxide (OsO_4) exists as either a colorless crystalline or a yellowish solid at room temperature, and is slowly released when osmium is exposed to air.

ROUTINE USE

Osmium tetroxide is used as a biologic stain in histopathologic labs, in electron microscopy, and as a chemical intermediate and oxidizing agent. Osmium tetroxide was once used as a fingerprinting agent but was discontinued because of contact dermatitis.

POTENTIAL TERRORIST USE

- The primary concern is the potential for dispersal of this agent in conjunction with an explosive device.
- Terrorists could also potentially contaminate food or water with this agent, but these uses are currently considered to be low-risk events.
- Osmium tetroxide has come to the attention of experts as a terrorist weapon primarily through

a recently described plot to deploy this chemical as part of an improvised explosive device (IED). The plot was interrupted before the actors could obtain the chemical.

- It is important to note that heating osmium tetroxide would cause it to decompose into osmium metal or osmium dioxide—both much less toxic than the tetroxide form. As such, the likelihood of a successful attack using an IED containing osmium tetroxide is probably minimal.

MECHANISM OF ACTION

- Osmium tetroxide is an irritant to mucous membranes and lungs.
- At higher concentrations, burning and irritation of the eyes and throat, as well as bronchospasm and pulmonary edema, may result from irritation.
- At lower concentrations, effects may be delayed but nevertheless insidious.

POTENTIAL ROUTES FOR EXPOSURE

Inhalational, ingestion, and dermal contact.

TARGET ORGANS/SYSTEMS

Respiratory, dermal, ocular, and renal.

CLINICAL FEATURES

- Initial burning of the eyes and throat may be accompanied by headache and the appearance of halos around objects.
- Bronchospasm and wheezing may progress to noncardiogenic pulmonary edema.
- Chronic exposures may lead to accumulation in the liver and may result in both hepatic and renal damage.
- Contact with skin may cause dark discoloration.
- Ingestion may lead to mucosal damage due to caustic effects.

DIAGNOSIS

Clinical suspicion and a history of exposure are the means of diagnosis, as there are no distinctive laboratory findings.

LABORATORY TESTING AND IMAGING

In severe exposures, pulmonary infiltrates and hypoxemia may occur. Consequently, baseline chest x-ray, pulse oximetry, and arterial blood gases are indicated for severely affected individuals.

TREATMENT AND DISPOSITION

- There is no specific antidote for osmium tetroxide.
- Supportive care—with special attention to airway, hemodynamic, and cardiac monitoring—is essential.
- For a patient who has inhaled aerosolized particles, prehospital treatment starts with removal from exposure.
- This should be followed by decontamination with copious amounts of water and, if available, soap.
- Assess oxygen saturation using pulse oximetry and administer supplemental oxygen as needed.
- Beta agonists should be administered to patients with evidence of bronchospasm.
- Mechanical ventilation may be required in severe cases.
- Symptomatic patients should be admitted for observation, as pulmonary edema is a possibility.

REFERENCES

Division of Environmental and Occupational Epidemiology, Michigan Department of Community Health. *Osmium Tetroxide: Information for the Public.* Lansing, MI: Division of Environmental and Occupational Epidemiology, Michigan Department of Community Health; 2004. Available at: www.michigan.gov/documents/mdch-osmium_tetroxide_fs_109244_7.pdf. Accessed September 9, 2005.

PHOSGENE (CCl$_2$O)

SYNONYMS AND TRADE NAMES

Carbone, carbonic chloride, carbonic dichloride, carbon oxychloride, carbonyl chloride, carbonyl dichloride, chloroformyl chloride, and fosgene. (CAS No. 77-44-5)

BACKGROUND

- Phosgene is a colorless gas at room temperature with an odor reminiscent of green corn or moldy hay.

- Phosgene's vapor is three and a half times denser than air and tends to collect along low-lying areas.
- Phosgene is weakly soluble in water and slowly decomposes to form hydrochloric acid.

ROUTINE USE

Phosgene is used in a variety of industrial processes, including dye, resin, and pesticide manufacturing. It is also a product of combustion of a variety of synthetic materials that include polyvinyl chloride (PVC).

POTENTIAL TERRORIST USE

A terrorist release in an enclosed space would have the potential to injure large numbers of people, since exposure to low concentrations is not particularly noxious and olfactory fatigue occurs quickly.

MECHANISM OF ACTION

Phosgene is a pulmonary irritant. Its low water solubility allows it to enter the distal airways where it liberates hydrochloric acid (HCl). This causes direct injury to the lungs and results in delayed noncardiogenic pulmonary edema and ARDS.

POTENTIAL ROUTES FOR EXPOSURE

Inhalational.

TARGET ORGANS/SYSTEMS

Pulmonary and mucous membranes.

CLINICAL FEATURES

- Despite being a powerful irritant, low concentrations of phosgene may cause only minimal mucous membrane irritation.
- Many symptoms related to phosgene exposure have been described, including fatigue, headache, nausea, and sore throat.
- However, the lungs are the primary target organ for phosgene. After an asymptomatic period that may last hours, dyspnea develops, often accompanied by hypoxia. As lung injury progresses, pulmonary edema develops. This may occur up to a day following exposure and may require mechanical ventilation. Even after recovery from acute illness, permanent lung injury may follow severe exposures.

DIAGNOSIS

There is no specific test for phosgene. As such, the diagnosis relies on clinical suspicion and/or a history of exposure.

LABORATORY TESTING AND IMAGING

- There are no diagnostic laboratory findings.
- A baseline chest x-ray should be obtained in most exposed patients, although pathologic findings may take 24 hours to develop.
- Pulse oximetry is a useful tool for monitoring pulmonary function in exposed patients.

TREATMENT AND DISPOSITION

- There is no specific treatment for phosgene, and care provided to the patient is primarily supportive.
- Although some mass casualty settings may require more stringent triage decisions, most patients exposed to phosgene should probably be admitted due to the concern for delayed pulmonary edema.
- Decontamination and evacuation are the initial steps in treatment.
- Supplemental oxygen should be provided for hypoxic patients.
- Beta agonists should be administered to patients with evidence of bronchospasm.
- Mechanical ventilation is necessary in the most severe cases.
- While definitive evidence is lacking, there is theoretical and limited experimental support for treatment with N-acetylcysteine and/or aminophylline.
- Early administration of corticosteroids may reduce pulmonary edema.

REFERENCES

Lazarus AA, Devereaux A. Potential agents of chemical warfare. Worst-case scenario protection and decontamination methods. *Postgrad Med.* 2002;112(5):133-140.

Sciuto AM, Hurt HH. Therapeutic treatments of phosgene-induced lung injury. *Inhal Toxicol.* 2004;16(8):565-580.

U.S. Government Printing Office. *Treatment of chemical agent casualties and conventional military chemical injuries. Field Manual No. 8-285.* Washington, DC: U.S. Government Printing Office; 1995.

PHOSPHINE (PH₃)

SYNONYMS AND TRADE NAMES

Hydrogen phosphide, phosphorated hydrogen, phosphorus hydride, and phosphorus trihydride. (CAS No. 7803-51-2)

BACKGROUND

- Phosphine is a heavier-than-air, colorless, usually odorless gas.
- In some formulations, phosphine may emit a fishy or garlicky odor.
- Phosphine is primarily used as a fumigant chemical.
- Phosphine is generally formed when various phosphide-containing compounds (e.g., aluminum phosphide, magnesium phosphide, or zinc phosphide) become moist.

ROUTINE USE

Phosphine and phosphide salts are found in shipping containers, grain elevators, and foodstuff storage facilities.

POTENTIAL TERRORIST USE

If used as a terrorist weapon, phosphine would be expected to be released as a gas into closed-space environments where large numbers of people congregate, such as theaters, sports venues, shopping malls, office complexes, or airport terminals.

MECHANISM OF ACTION

The mechanisms of toxicity for phosphine gas have not been delineated as yet, but they may involve interference with mitochondrial-based electron transport systems.

POTENTIAL ROUTES FOR EXPOSURE

Inhalation is the primary route of concern. However, dermal and/or ocular contact may occur.

TARGET ORGANS/SYSTEMS

Pulmonary, CNS, renal, hepatic, and cardiac.

CLINICAL FEATURES

- Affected persons may experience various problems, including nausea, vomiting, dizziness, coughing, abdominal pain, diarrhea, chest discomfort, difficulty breathing, chills, syncope, and pulmonary edema.
- Skin exposure to liquid phosphine may cause local skin lesions, as well as frostbite.
- Severely affected individuals may develop ARDS and renal failure, as well as myocardial injury.
- ST-T wave ECG abnormalities may occur, along with a variety of other cardiac arrythmias.
- Methemoglobinemia may occur in some of the more severely exposed patients.

DIAGNOSIS

The diagnosis usually depends on obtaining a history of exposure from prehospital personnel who have identified a phosphine release.

LABORATORY TESTING AND IMAGING

- No lab studies are clearly diagnostic, and blood/body fluid levels are not clinically helpful.
- Patients requiring evaluation and supportive care should have baseline lab studies done, including CBC, electrolytes, and blood glucose.
- Other studies should be guided by the clinical setting. Consider obtaining methemoglobin levels in patients unable to maintain normal oxygenation.
- Due to the possibility of delayed pulmonary edema, consider obtaining baseline chest x-rays for admitted patients, as well as for patients selected for clinical observation pending the decision to admit or discharge.

TREATMENT AND DISPOSITION

- There are no specific antidotes available for phosphine gas.
- Administer supportive care (airway maintenance, ventilation, cardiac monitoring).
- Administer oxygen as needed.
- Health care personnel may be at risk if off-gassing from patients occurs. Decontaminate patients prior to arrival at the emergency department.
- Vapor exposures are decontaminated by clothing removal and storage in air-tight bags.
- Identify and treat hypotension with fluids and pressors, if needed.
- Watch for adrenal insufficiency manifested by unresponsive hypotension. If identified, treat with systemic corticosteroids.
- Treat arrhythmias when identified.
- Treat seizures; drugs of choice are benzodiazepines.
- Treat methemoglobinemia with IV methylene blue, if indicated.
- Admit all patients to watch for delayed pulmonary edema.
- Modalities for accelerated elimination (hemodialysis, hemoperfusion) are not clinically useful.

REFERENCES

Pepelko B, Seckar J, Harp PR, et al. Worker exposure standard for phosphine gas. *Risk Anal.* 2004;24(5):1201-1213.

Singh S, Singh D, Wig N, et al. Aluminum phosphide ingestion—A clinico-pathologic study. *J Toxicol Clin Toxicol.* 1996;34(6):703-706.

PHOSPHORUS

SYNONYMS AND TRADE NAMES

Hittorf's phosphorus, phosphorus-30, phosphorus tetramer, red phosphorus, UN 1338, violet phosphorus, and yellow phosphorus. (CAS No. 7723-14-0)

BACKGROUND

- Phosphorus is the fifteenth element in the periodic table, has an atomic weight of 30.97376 and exists in a highly purified form: P_4.
- Phosphorus exists in several forms, but the most hazardous is white (or yellow) phosphorus. The lethal dose is estimated to be 1 mg/kg or 50 mg.
- White phosphorus is a colorless or slightly yellow solid that is extremely flammable. It is sparingly soluble in water, but more so in oil.
- Phosphorus is unstable in the environment and may form less toxic substances in minutes to hours when placed in air or water.

ROUTINE USE

- Phosphorus is used in detergents, plasticizers, water treatment, and the striking surfaces of matches.

POTENTIAL TERRORIST USE

- While phosphorus has been used in military applications as a smoke generator, and has found terrorist application as an incendiary agent in phosphorus bombs, there are several other potential terrorist uses. Phosphorus is extremely dangerous when ingested, and its radioactive isotope, P_{32}, could be used in radiological terrorism.

MECHANISM OF ACTION

- Initial toxicity is related to direct tissue destruction.
- Burns to the skin, mucous membranes, and lungs occur when exposed to phosphorus or its vapors.
- Ingested phosphorus causes severe abdominal pain, vomiting, and diarrhea as a result of its caustic effects.
- Systemic toxicity may be mediated by several mechanisms, including depression of serum calcium.

POTENTIAL ROUTES FOR EXPOSURE

Phosphorus may be absorbed through the skin, inhaled, or ingested.

TARGET ORGANS/SYSTEMS

Skin, mucous membranes, lungs, kidneys, liver, hematologic system, and CNS are all targets of phosphorus toxicity.

CLINICAL FEATURES

- Patients will present with symptoms related to the route of exposure.
- Dermal application results in third-degree burns in a matter of minutes. Dermal burns are both chemical and thermal, since phosphorus applied to skin will ignite.
- Ocular burns may result from direct or vapor exposure.
- Abdominal pain and vomiting occur after ingestion and possibly after dermal absorption.
- Vomitus and stool characteristically have a garlic odor and have been reported to smoke.
- Inhalational exposure results in rapid pulmonary damage and dyspnea similar to phosphine toxicity. (See Phosphine)
- Neurologic toxicity ranging from anxiety and restlessness to confusion, delirium, or coma has been described following acute exposure. If present, these symptoms are poor prognostic indicators.
- If the patient survives, initial symptoms typically resolve or diminish, followed by a return of gastrointestinal symptoms, accompanied by hepatic and renal dysfunction, hemolysis, and jaundice.
- Cardiovascular collapse and dysrhythmias may occur.
- Seizures, delirium, or coma may result from neurologic toxicity.
- Death is typically delayed by several days.

DIAGNOSIS

- A garlic odor to the breath, vomitus, or feces is suggestive of phosphorus poisoning.
- Luminescent or smoking vomitus and stool are highly suggestive, but are not always present.
- An elevated phosphorus level may be seen, but is not always present.
- A history of exposure to an incendiary device, or continued combustion of the substance on skin, is also suggestive.

LABORATORY TESTING AND IMAGING

- A CBC may show anemia from hemolysis, thrombocytopenia, or pancytopenia following severe exposures.

- Depression of serum potassium, chloride, and calcium in particular has been described.
- Serum phosphorus may also be affected.
- Renal failure and hepatic dysfunction are common delayed effects of phosphorus poisoning, and baseline tests should be obtained.
- Coagulation studies are also recommended.
- The ECG may show a prolonged QT and ST-T wave changes.
- Chest x-rays may demonstrate pulmonary edema.
- Arterial blood gas analysis may reveal hypoxia. Symptomatic patients should be monitored with continuous pulse oximetry.

TREATMENT AND DISPOSITION

- There is no specific treatment for phosphorus, and care provided to patients is primarily supportive.
- Decontamination and evacuation are the initial steps in treatment. This includes removal of clothing and washing exposed areas of skin with soap and water.
- Avoid irrigation with a copper sulfate-containing solution. While this has been recommended in the past, it has been associated with intravascular hemolysis.
- Continued irrigation may be necessary to prevent ignition of phosphorus on skin or clothing.
- Charcoal may be administered following ingestion.
- Supplemental oxygen should be provided for hypoxic patients.
- Beta agonists should be administered to patients with evidence of bronchospasm.
- Mechanical ventilation is necessary in the most severe cases.
- Ocular exposures should be evaluated by flourescein staining and treated with irrigation, topical anesthetics, and mydriatics for comfort.
- Hypotension should be treated with isotonic fluids and pressors, if necessary.
- Anemia may require blood transfusion.
- Hemodialysis may be required for renal failure.
- Seizures should be treated with benzodiazepines.
- Hospitalization is recommended for exposed patients to detect delayed pulmonary edema.

REFERENCES

Agency for Toxic Substances and Disease Registry. *Toxicological Profile for White Phosphorus.* Atlanta, GA: Agency for Toxic Substances and Disease Registry; 1997.

Available at: http://www.atsdr.cdc.gov/toxprofiles/tp103.html. Accessed September 27. 2005.

Konjoyan TR. White phosphorus burns: Case report and literature review. *Mil Med.* 1983;148(11):881-884.

Simon FA, Pickering LK. Acute yellow phosphorus poisoning. "Smoking stool syndrome." *JAMA.* 1976;235(13):1343-1344.

Talley RC, Linhart JW, Trevino AJ, et al. Acute elemental phosphorus poisoning in man: Cardiovascular toxicity. *Am Heart J.* 1972;84(1):139-140.

SULFURYL FLUORIDE (F$_2$O$_2$S)

SYNONYMS AND TRADE NAMES

Fluorure de sulfuryle, sulfonyl fluoride, sulfur dioxide difluoride, sulfuric oxyfluoride, sulfuryl difluoride, UN 2191, and Vikane®. (CAS No. 2699-79-8)

BACKGROUND

- A colorless and odorless gas, sulfuryl fluoride is often used as a fumigant chemical.
- Sulfuryl fluoride is three and a half times as dense as air.
- While stable in water and light, sulfuryl fluoride is hydrolyzed by alkaline solutions.
- When sulfuryl fluoride is used as a fumigant, the National Institute for Occupational Safety and Health has designated a time-weighted average of 5 ppm.
- Sulfuryl fluoride is considered immediately dangerous to life and health in concentrations of 200 ppm.

ROUTINE USE

- Used as a structural and post-harvest fumigant and insecticide, sulfuryl fluoride is a restricted-use pesticide sold under the trade name Vikane®.
- Sulfuryl fluoride is also used in the synthesis of drugs and dyes.
- This chemical may be transported nationwide via rail or truck and stored where manufactured or used. Thus, sulfuryl fluoride may be readily available for theft by terrorists.

POTENTIAL TERRORIST USE

If sulfuryl fluoride were used as a terrorist weapon, the release would probably involve aerosolization or dispersal of large quantities of the chemical in areas where large numbers of persons may congregate (e.g., theaters, sports venues, shopping malls, etc.). Severe injury to large numbers of people might occur, particularly if release took place within a confined space or area with poor ventilation.

MECHANISM OF ACTION

While the mechanism of action is not completely understood, animal studies indicate that absorption of sulfuryl fluoride results in the release of fluoride, which inhibits several enzyme systems and interferes with cellular respiration and glycolysis.

POTENTIAL ROUTES FOR EXPOSURE

People may be exposed dermally or via the lungs or eyes. Traces of sulfuryl fluoride have been found in the food supply, presumably due to the fumigation use of this chemical.

TARGET ORGANS/SYSTEMS

Skin, mucous membranes, lungs, kidneys, heart, and CNS.

CLINICAL FEATURES

- Direct contact with sulfuryl fluoride may irritate the skin or eyes.
- Dyspnea and coughing may progress to pulmonary edema.
- Nausea, vomiting, and diarrhea are nonspecific symptoms.
- Following acute exposures, neurologic dysfunction may range from irritability, to seizures, to mental status depression.
- Cardiac dysrhythmias, as well as cardiac arrest, have been described following severe exposures.

DIAGNOSIS

There is no specific test that confirms exposure to sulfuryl fluoride. The diagnosis relies on clinical suspicion and/or a history of exposure.

LABORATORY TESTING AND IMAGING

- There are no diagnostic laboratory findings.
- Chest x-rays may be normal or demonstrate pulmonary edema.
- Arterial blood gas analysis may reveal hypoxia, and peak flow measurement may demonstrate bronchospasm.
- Symptomatic patients should be monitored with continuous pulse oximetry.
- Serum fluoride and calcium levels should be measured.

TREATMENT AND DISPOSITION

- There is no specific antidote for sulfuryl fluoride. The mainstay of care is supportive.
- Immediate removal from exposure, as well as decontamination, are the initial steps in treatment. This includes removal of clothing and washing exposed areas of skin with soap and water.
- Supplemental oxygen should be provided for hypoxic patients.
- Beta agonists should be administered to patients with evidence of bronchospasm.
- Mechanical ventilation is necessary in the most severe cases.
- Ocular exposures should be evaluated by flourescein staining and treated with irrigation, topical anesthetics, and mydriatics for comfort.
- Intravenous calcium should be administered for symptomatic hypocalcemia.
- Benzodiazepines are the drugs of choice for the treatment of seizures.
- Hospitalization is recommended for symptomatic patients.

REFERENCES

Calvert GM, Mueller CA, Fajen JM, et al. Health effects associated with sulfuryl fluoride and methyl bromide exposure among structural fumigation workers. *Am J Public Health.* 1998;88(12):1774-1780.

Centers for Disease Control and Prevention. Fatalities resulting from sulfuryl fluoride exposure after home fumigation—Virginia. *MMWR.* 1987;36(36):602-604, 609-611.

Scheffrahn RH, Hsu RC, Su NY. Fluoride residues in frozen foods fumigated with sulfuryl fluoride. *Bull Environ Contam Toxicol.* 1989;43(6):899-903.

Scheuerman EH. Suicide by exposure to sulfuryl fluoride. *J Forensic Sci.* 1986; 31(3):1154-1158.

INCAPACITATING AGENTS

ADAMSITE ($HN\text{-}(C_6H_4)_2\text{-}AsCl$)

SYNONYMS AND TRADE NAMES

10 chloro-5, 10-dihydrophenarsine, diphenylaminechloroarsine, and DM. (CAS No. 578-94-9)

BACKGROUND

- Adamsite is a "sneeze gas" developed by the United States and used during World War I.
- Adamsite also is known for inducing emesis, and was used to cause soldiers to precipitously remove their personal protective equipment.
- This incapacitating agent is a yellow-green crystal that, upon heating, vaporizes and condenses, creating an odorless yellow smoke.
- The most toxic of the incapacitating agents, adamsite has an estimated lethal median concentration (LCt) of 11,000 mg/min/m^3.
- Adamsite is generally disseminated as an aerosol; however, illness may also result from ingestion, skin exposure, or ocular exposure.

ROUTINE USE

Adamsite was initially used as a riot-control agent, but its use against civilians has been banned in the United States.

POTENTIAL TERRORIST USE

If used as a terrorist weapon, adamsite would be expected to be aerosolized in a densely populated area (such as busy downtown urban areas), at sporting events, or even in closed-space environments (such as shopping malls, office complexes or airport terminals).

MECHANISM OF ACTION

Adamsite is an arsenical that acts as an irritant to skin and mucous membranes. The precise mechanism of action is unknown.

TARGET ORGANS/SYSTEMS

Gastrointestinal, CNS, dermal, and ocular.

CLINICAL FEATURES

- Symptoms following exposure may include eye irritation, malaise, nausea, vomiting, diarrhea, abdominal cramps, severe headache, chest tightness, and sneezing.
- Severe exposures may result in necrosis of the corneal epithelium.
- Massive exposures may result in death.
- Symptoms may begin three to four minutes after exposure, and may last one to two hours.
- Minor sensory disturbances may persist for 24 to 48 hours.

DIAGNOSIS

The diagnosis is based on the history of exposure in conjunction with the specific clinical findings.

LABORATORY TESTING AND IMAGING

- There is no specific blood test available to test for an adamsite exposure.
- Patients who experience an inhalation exposure may require pulse oximetry monitoring.
- Additionally, patients who experience significant gastrointestinal distress may need electrolyte screening and monitoring.

TREATMENT AND DISPOSITION

- There are no specific antidotes for adamsite poisoning. Antiemetics, such as metoclopramide or ondansetron, may be effective, but there are no clinical data to support this.
- Prehospital treatment starts with removal from exposure and then decontamination with water or bicarbonate of soda solution. Dusting the skin with borated talcum may also be useful.
- Supportive care (airway maintenance, ventilation, and pulse oximetry as needed) is the

mainstay of treatment.

- Administer oxygen as needed.
- Replenish electrolytes as needed and administer intravenous fluids as needed for hypotension and hypovolemia.
- In the event of an ocular exposure, irrigate the eyes with copious amounts of fluid. A Morgan lens may facilitate this process.

REFERENCES

Williams KE. *General facts about vomiting agent adamsite (DM)*. Aberdeen Proving Ground, MD: U.S. Army for Health Promotion and Preventive Medicine. 218-41-1096.
Available at: http://chppm-www.apgea.army.mil/dts/docs/gendm.pdf. Accessed September 7, 2005.

BZ

SIMILAR AGENTS

"Agent 15."

SYNONYMS AND TRADE NAMES

1-azabicyclo(2.2.2)oct-3-yl ester, 1-azabicyclo (2.2.2)octan-3-ol, 3-chinuclidylbenzilate, 3-quinuclidinol, 3-quinuclidinol benzilate, 3-quinuclidinyl benzilate, 3-quinuclidinyl ester, benzeneacetic acid, benzilate, benzilate ester, benzilic acid, B-hydroxyphenyl, B-quinuclidinyl benzilate CS 4030, EA 2277, QNB, and RO 2-3308.
(CAS No. 6581-06-2)

BACKGROUND

- BZ is an anticholinergic glycolate compound similar to atropine and scopolamine.
- Agent 15 is an alleged Iraqi incapacitating agent that is likely to be either chemically identical to BZ or closely related to it.
- To date, no field detection is available for BZ and related agents.
- The U.S. had weaponized BZ, but demilitarization began in 1988 and has been completed.
- Agent 15 was reportedly stockpiled in large quantities prior to and during the 1991 Gulf War.

ROUTINE USE

BZ and related compounds are military weapons with no specific industrial or commercial use.

POTENTIAL TERRORIST USE

- It is anticipated that if BZ were used as a terrorist weapon, it would be disseminated as an aerosolized solid (inhalation threat) or dissolved in a solvent for ingestion or percutaneous absorption.
- Terrorist use might also include the introduction of this material into building ventilation systems, or spraying the material in areas where large numbers of people congregate.

MECHANISM OF ACTION

BZ competitively inhibits acetylcholine at postsynaptic and postjunctional muscarinic receptor sites in smooth muscle, brain, exocrine glands, and autonomic ganglia. Since BZ essentially decreases acetylcholine at receptors at these sites, it causes peripheral nervous system effects opposite of those seen in nerve-agent poisoning.

POTENTIAL ROUTES FOR EXPOSURE

Inhalational, mucous membrane, and ingestion.

TARGET ORGANS/SYSTEMS

Pulmonary and CNS.

CLINICAL FEATURES

- Clinical effects from ingestion or inhalation of BZ appear after an asymptomatic period ranging from a few minutes to as long as 20 hours.
- Following dermal exposures, the clinical effects may be delayed up to 36 hours.
- The clinical duration of symptoms ranges from 72 to 96 hours and are dose-dependent.
- The clinical course of BZ poisoning develops as follows:
  - Within four hours of exposure, parasympathetic blockade and mild CNS effects occur.
  - Four to 20 hours after exposure, stupor with

ataxia and hyperthermia are seen.
- Twenty to 96 hours after exposure, fluctuating delirium presents.
- Late symptoms include paranoid ideation, deep sleep, crawling or climbing automatisms, and slow clinical resolution.
- CNS effects may include altered mental status (e.g., stupor, confusion, confabulation with concrete and panoramic illusions, and hallucinations).
- Some patients will regress to automatic "phantom" behaviors such as plucking at skin and clothing.
- Disrobing behavior may be part of this regression and often characterizes anticholinergic toxidromes.

DIAGNOSIS

- The combination of anticholinergic PNS and CNS effects aids in the diagnosis of patients exposed to BZ or Agent 15.
- The diagnosis is based on situational recognition involving a possible BZ or Agent 15 release in which multiple casualties manifest one or more of the following symptoms:
  - Mydriasis
  - Dry mucous membranes
  - Dry skin (lack of axillary sweat is an important indicator)
  - Altered mental status
  - Disturbances in perception
  - Illusions
  - Hallucinations
  - Impaired reasoning
  - Impaired judgment

TREATMENT AND DISPOSITION

Physostigmine, which increases the concentration of acetylcholine in synapses and at neuromuscular and neuroglandular junctions, is a specific antidote.

REFERENCES

United States Army Medical Research Institute of Chemical Defense. Incapacitating Agents BZ, Agent 15. In: *Medical Management of Chemical Casualties Handbook*. 3rd ed. Aberdeen Proving Ground, MD: United States Army Medical Research Institute of Chemical Defense, Chemical Casualty Care Division;1999. Available at: http://www.vnh.org/CHEMCASU/06IncapacitatingAgents.html. Accessed September 13, 2005.

FENTANYL AND RELATED COMPOUNDS

SYNONYMS AND TRADE NAMES

Acetyl fentanyl ARS, Actiq®, Alfenta®, benzeylamide hydrochloride, butyryl fentanyl ARS, Duragesic®, fentanyl-N-oxide hydrochloride ARS, hyrolysis product base, N-(1-propionyl-4-piperioyl) propanamide, N-phenyl-(1-phenethyl-2-)piperidinyl amine ARS, propionanilide base, pyruval fentanyl ARS, Sufenta®, and Wildnil®.
(CAS No. 437-38-7)

BACKGROUND

- Fentanyl exhibits analgesic potency approximately 80 times that of morphine.
- Fentanyl was introduced into medical practice in the 1960s as an intravenous anesthetic under the trade name of Sublimaze®.
- Subsequently, other fentanyl analogs were introduced: alfentanil (Alfenta®), an ultra-short-acting (five to 10 minutes) analgesic, and sufentanil (Sufenta®). Alfentanil has about one quarter the analgesic and one tenth the respiratory depression potency of fentanyl, with approximately two thirds shorter duration of action. Sufentanil is an extremely potent analgesic with 2,000 times the potency of morphine.

ROUTINE USE

- Fentanyl-type drugs are usually found in hospitals, pharmacies, and veterinary clinics.
- Fentanyls are extensively used for anesthesia and analgesia. Duragesic® is a fentanyl transdermal patch used in chronic pain management. Actiq® is a solid formulation of fentanyl citrate on a stick that dissolves slowly in the mouth for transmucosal absorption. Actiq® is intended for opiate-tolerant individuals and is effective in treating breakthrough pain in cancer patients. Carfentanil (Wildnil®) is an analog of fentanyl with an analgesic potency 10,000 times that of morphine and is used in veterinary practice to immobilize certain large animals.
- Illicit fentanyl synthesis has been identified periodically in the U.S. In Pittsburgh, an individual

produced and distributed 3-methylfentanyl. This fentanyl analog has an opioid potency approximately 6,000 times that of morphine. Other fentanyl derivatives and analogs may currently be stockpiled by various countries for military or police use, as well as for deployment in covert operations.

POTENTIAL TERRORIST USE

Terrorists may use fentanyl-type drugs in aerosol form to attack large numbers of congregated people in such venues as stadiums, theaters, and shopping malls.

MECHANISM OF ACTION

Respiratory depression.

POTENTIAL ROUTES FOR EXPOSURE

Inhalational exposure is the primary route for contact.

TARGET ORGANS/SYSTEMS

CNS and cardiorespiratory system.

CLINICAL FEATURES

The clinical presentation following fentanyl exposure is the same as for any opioid toxidrome, and may include nausea, vomiting, severe respiratory depression, hypotension, bradycardia, chest wall rigidity, and seizures.

DIAGNOSIS

The diagnosis that fentanyl and/or its derivatives have been used in a terrorist attack is presumptive and hinges on the situational recognition of large numbers of people, all from the same location or venue, presenting with a profound opioid toxidrome.

LABORATORY TESTING AND IMAGING

There are no pathognomonic lab abnormalities for fentanyl casualties. However, the possibility of non-

cardiogenic pulmonary edema in these patients is significant. Consequently, consideration should be given to obtaining baseline chest x-rays in affected patients.

TREATMENT AND DISPOSITION

- All patients presenting with the opioid toxidrome require the prompt administration of naloxone, a specific antidote for the opioid toxidrome of any etiology, in addition to airway control and supportive care.
- Naloxone may be administered by the IV, IM, sublingual, or endotracheal routes, depending upon the clinical situation.
- Affected patients will require a minimum of six hours of observation following reversal of the opioid toxidrome.
- Selected patients probably requiring admission include those at the extremes of age, as well as debilitated persons and anyone with manifestations of noncardiogenic pulmonary edema.

REFERENCES

U.S. Drug Enforcement Administration Web site. Fentanyl. Available at: http://www.usdoj.gov/dea/concern/fentanyl.html. Accessed September 14, 2005.

OLEORESIN CAPSICUM (OC) AND CAPSAICIN

SYNONYMS AND TRADE NAMES

CapTor®, nonivamide, OC, and "pepper spray." (CAS No. 404-86-4)

BACKGROUND

- Isolated as a reddish-brown liquid from various hot pepper species, oleoresin capsicum and one of its active ingredients, capsaicin, are potent sensory irritants. Both natural and synthetic formulations have found use as personal defense and riot-control agents.
- OC-based agents have been increasing in popularity among civilians, military personnel, and law enforcement personnel. Personal self-defense

OC sprays are sold under a variety of names, including CapStun, Punch II, and CapTor.®

- In the color-coding system for handheld riot-control dispersion devices, OC is denoted by the color orange.

ROUTINE USE

OC is used as a harassment and incapacitating agent by police and military forces.

POTENTIAL TERRORIST USE

- Terrorists might release OC in crowded areas. This would be expected to transiently affect large numbers of people, causing incapacitation and panic. Large releases in confined spaces would be expected to cause fewer but more severe casualties.
- OC is typically deployed as a propelled aerosol when used by law enforcement for personal defense, but since it is less heat-stable than other lacrimators, mass release would require nonincendiary grenades, bombs, or a vehicle-mounted dispersion device.
- While many people exposed in open-air scenarios would not be expected to have serious injury, the emergency response system and health care facilities could be seriously taxed by large numbers of patients.
- In addition, fear and uncertainty among potentially exposed civilians could create psychological distress.

MECHANISM OF ACTION

Oleoresin capsicum is a sensory irritant that appears to act through activation of vanilloid receptors on certain neurons. Inflammation is mediated by several neuropeptides, including substance P. This leads to vasodilation, pain, bronchoconstriction, coughing, and vomiting, which are responsible for the incapacitating effects.

POTENTIAL ROUTES FOR EXPOSURE

The route of primary concern is inhalation and mucous membrane contact resulting from aerosol dissemination of this agent.

TARGET ORGANS/SYSTEMS

Eyes, skin, mucous membranes, and lungs are the primary targets of OC-based agents.

CLINICAL FEATURES

- Irritation of the eyes and throat occurs rapidly and at low concentrations.
- Lacrimation, burning in the oropharynx, and irritation of moist and sensitive areas of the skin are early effects.
- Nausea, vomiting, and headache are commonly reported.
- The above effects are of limited duration, and usually resolve within 30 to 60 minutes following evacuation and decontamination.
- Because OC is a natural irritant, some people, such as asthmatics, are expected to be more sensitive to the effects of pepper sprays.
- Deaths associated with OC use, rather than being caused by pulmonary edema, are usually attributed to asphyxia secondary to laryngospasm and victim proximity to the agent.
- When OC is applied to the skin, a burning sensation quickly develops. At high concentrations, edema and blister formation may result.

DIAGNOSIS

The diagnosis is based on the history of exposure as reported by prehospital personnel or by the presentation of multiple patients exposed to a tear gas-like agent in the field.

LABORATORY TESTING AND IMAGING

There is no specific test for this agent. Patients complaining of dyspnea or who present with clinical evidence of hypoxemia should be evaluated with chest radiography and pulse oximetry.

TREATMENT AND DISPOSITION

- Evacuation and decontamination are the first steps to treatment.
- Exposed clothing should be removed and the skin cleansed.
- Eyes should be liberally irrigated with sterile

saline or Lactated Ringers solution.

- Patients should be screened for corneal abrasions and, if found, these lesions should be treated with analgesics and topical antibiotics.
- If skin findings exceed simple erythema, lesions should be treated with comfort measures, local hygiene, and topical antibiotics on areas with denuded epithelium.
- Supplemental oxygen should be provided for hypoxic or dyspneic patients.
- A beta agonist may be beneficial for patients with clinical evidence of bronchospasm.
- Mechanical ventilation may be required for patients with severe exposures or underlying medical conditions.
- All patients with signs of hypoxemia should be observed in the hospital for 24 hours.

REFERENCES

Blain PG. Tear gases and irritant incapacitants. 1-chloroacetophenone, 2-chlorobenzylidene malononitrile and dibenz[b,f]-1,4-oxazepine. *Toxicol Rev.* 2003;22(2):103-110.

Department of the Army, the Navy, and the Air Force. *Air Force Joint Manual 44-151.* Washington, DC: Department of the Army, the Navy, and the Air Force; 1996.

Department of the Army, the Navy, and the Air Force. *Army Field Manual 8-9.* Washington, DC: Department of the Army, the Navy, and the Air Force; 1996.

Department of the Army, the Navy, and the Air Force. *NATO Handbook on the Medical Aspects of NBC Defensive Operations AMedP-6(B).* Washington, DC: Department of the Army, the Navy, and the Air Force; 1996.

Department of the Army, the Navy, and the Air Force. *Navy Medical Publication 5059.* Washington, DC: Department of the Army, the Navy, and the Air Force; 1996.

NIOSH and Department of Health and Human Services. *National Institute for Occupational Safety and Health (NIOSH) Pocket Guide to Chemical Hazards.* Washington, DC: NIOSH and Department of Health and Human Services. NIOSH Publication No. 97-140;1997: 60. Available at: http://www.cdc.gov/niosh/npg/npg.html. Accessed September 2, 2005.

LONG-ACTING ANTICOAGULANTS

SUPERWARFARINS

SYNONYMS AND TRADE NAMES

Coumarin group: brodifacoum, coumatetralyl (4-hydroxycoumarin derivatives), and difenacoum. Indandione derivatives: chlorophacinone, diphacinone, pindone, and rat poisons.
(CAS No. 56073-10-0)

BACKGROUND

- Prior to 1976, most rodenticides contained a small amount of warfarin. After prolonged exposure, however, rodents acquired resistance through transmission of an autosomal dominant gene.
- The so-called "superwarfarins" were designed as a response to this genetic adaptation.

ROUTINE USE

- Superwarfarin chemicals do not occur naturally.
- Used as rodenticides, the superwarfarins act by preventing the production of essential clotting factors.
- Both home and industrial use of these chemicals is quite common and they are widely available in essentially unlimited quantities.

POTENTIAL TERRORIST USE

With low dermal and no proven inhalational toxicity, superwarfarins would most likely be used by terrorists as food- or water-supply contaminants.

MECHANISM OF ACTION

- Superwarfarins are long-acting anticoagulants available in solid, oil-soluble liquid, and powder forms.
- The mechanism of action involves the inhibition of the active form of vitamin K by inhibiting vitamin K 2, 3-epoxide reductase. Vitamin K is a cofactor used in the synthesis of blood clotting factors II, VII, IX, and X. Inhibition of these cofac-

tors may lead to uncontrollable hemorrhage.
- Due to their high lipid solubility and concentration in the liver, superwarfarins are orders of magnitude more potent than warfarin.

POTENTIAL ROUTES FOR EXPOSURE

- Oral ingestion of superwarfarins is the most common route for exposure.
- However, the high-molecular-weight, polycyclic hydrocarbon side chains in these compounds renders them only poorly water-soluble.
- At this time the greatest terrorist threat would appear to be secondary exposure through contamination of food supplies.

TARGET ORGANS/SYSTEMS

Hematologic.

CLINICAL FEATURES

- Acute unintentional ingestions of superwarfarins are unlikely to cause prolongation of PT or INR. In fact, medically important anticoagulation is a rare sequela, as substantial ingestions of these chemicals are required before this toxicity is manifested. Most patients remain asymptomatic following single oral ingestions.
- The majority of cases involving clinically significant superwarfarin toxicity are related to what amounts to repetitive ingestions. Following substantial ingestions of a superwarfarin, clinical signs of toxicity typically occur within 24 to 72 hours.
- The patient may manifest bleeding from virtually any mucosal site, hematoma formation (with possible airway compromise if located on the neck), bleeding or eccymosis out of proportion to trauma, and intracranial hemorrhages.
- Common sites for bleeding include the gastrointestinal and genitourinary tracts.
- It is important to note that the anticoagulant effects of superwarfarins may be long-lasting, ranging from weeks to months, and patients

may be at risk for substantial blood loss during that time.

DIAGNOSIS

- The diagnosis is based primarily on a history of ingestion or possible contact with the offending agent, as well as a careful physical exam.
- Most patients with an unintentional ingestion will be asymptomatic; thus, the diagnosis may be suspected after routine laboratory screening.

LABORATORY TESTING AND IMAGING

- In any patient with hemorrhagic sequelae, a full evaluation of coagulation parameters should be undertaken including PT (INR), PTT, thrombin time, and fibrinogen concentration.
- Because superwarfarins primarily affect the extrinsic coagulation cascade, expect to see an abnormal PT (INR) as the sole laboratory manifestation of toxicity.
- INRs greater than 12 have been recorded with coagulopathies lasting more than 11 months.

TREATMENT AND DISPOSITION

- As with all toxicologic emergencies, initial care should consist of supportive measures with special attention to the ABCs.
- For patients with significant hemorrhage or hypotension with clinical signs of anemia, venous access should include two large-bore catheters, and patients should be blood-typed and cross-matched for packed red blood cells and FFP.
- A CBC with differential and coagulation studies should also be obtained, in addition to any other clinically relevant laboratory testing. The hypotensive patient should have up to 2 L normal saline solution or Lactated Ringers solution until the patient is normotensive or the appropriate blood products arrive at the bedside.
- It is imperative for the clinician to determine the amount and route of exposure. For single, unintentional oral ingestions, warfarin-containing

rodenticides pose only a minimal threat to normal or even previously anticoagulated patients.
- However, large ingestions, whether intentional or otherwise—or repeated ingestions—have the potential to manifest a severe, prolonged coagulopathy and possible hemorrhagic sequelae.
- Gastric decontamination should be reserved for patients who present within one hour of a potentially life-threatening ingestion. Any attempts at gastric decontamination in a severely anticoagulated patient may result in uncontrollable hemorrhage and are contraindicated.
- Data is limited on the use of single or multidose activated charcoal; however, most texts recommend the administration of at least one dose at 1 gm/kg.
- Patients with significant hemorrhage or anemia should receive blood products. Life-threatening hemorrhage should be controlled with fresh frozen plasma (10 mL/kg to 25 mL/kg), and vitamin K, as whole blood contains relatively small amounts of vitamin K-dependent factors.
- Ultimately, the correction of the coagulopathy is accomplished through the administration of vitamin K_1. Hematology consult is recommended but should not delay treatment. Vitamin K_1 should be initially administered parenterally, then switched to oral treatment for long-term care. In some cases, IV doses up to 60 mg/kg may be needed in the initial stages.
- In patients with medical conditions requiring long-term anticoagulation, heparin may be used for anticoagulation if the PT is completely reversed.
- Patients should be followed with a daily or twice daily INR until their coagulation studies are normal for several days while off vitamin K therapy.

REFERENCES

Belson MG, Schier JG, Patel MM. Case Definitions for Chemical Poisoning. *MMWR Recomm Rep.* 2005;54(RR01):1-24. Available at: http://www.cdc.gov/mmwr/preview/mmwrhtml/rr5401a1.htm. Accessed October 11, 2005.

Burkhart KK. Anticoagulant Rodenticides. In: Delaney KA, Ling LJ, Erickson T, et al, eds. *Clinical Toxicology.* Philadelphia, PA: W.B. Saunders; 2001:848-853.

Su M, Hoffman RS. Anticoagulants. In: Goldfrank LR, Flomenbaum NE, Lewin NA, et al, eds. *Goldfrank's Toxicologic Emergencies.* 7th ed. New York, NY: McGraw-Hill; 2002:635-640.

METALS

ARSENIC (As)

SYNONYMS AND TRADE NAMES

Arsen, arsenic-75, arsenicals, arsenic black, colloidal arsenic, Fowler's solution, grey arsenic, metallic arsenic, UN 1558. (CAS No. 7440-38-2)

BACKGROUND

- Arsenic is considered to be a heavy metal and shares many physical and chemical characteristics with other heavy metals.
- Arsenic is a naturally occurring element in the earth's crust. It exists in several forms, including organic, gaseous, elemental, and inorganic.
- Of the four forms of arsenic, the inorganic form is the most prevalent and the gaseous form (arsine) is the most potentially harmful. (See Arsine).

ROUTINE USE

- Arsenic finds its primary industrial uses in the production of glass and semiconductors. Some lawn products have small amounts of arsenic trioxide in their formulae, and arsenic trioxide is currently available as a pharmaceutical used to treat certain forms of leukemia.
- Poisoning typically occurs through industrial exposure. Soil, water, and food contaminated with arsenic are the primary sources for arsenic exposure in the general population.
- Clinically important toxicity has been associated with contaminated wine or "moonshine" whiskey, and herbal preparations or nutritional supplements, as well as with poisoning by malicious intent.

POTENTIAL TERRORIST USE

- Inorganic arsenic is water-soluble, tasteless, and readily absorbed by the respiratory, gastrointestinal, and mucosal routes. Though inorganic arsenic is considered to be potentially harmful, its oxidized counterpart diarsenic pentoxide, though less soluble in water, has the potential to be extremely harmful.
- Due to the difficulty in diagnosis, as well as the insidious health effects that may not be seen for days to months after exposure (depending on the dose), arsenic is considered to be an important terrorist threat agent.
- The most likely terrorist use of arsenic would involve the surreptitious contamination of food or water supplies.

MECHANISM OF ACTION

- Inorganic arsenic exists in two forms, trivalent and pentavalent arsenic.
- Trivalent arsenic is considered to be potentially the most harmful form. By binding the sulfhydryl groups of dihydrolipoamide, trivalent arsenic prevents the regeneration of lipoamide, a cofactor necessary in the conversion of pyruvate to Acetyl CoA. This, in turn, leads to decreased ATP production and hypoglycemia as a result of decreased gluconeogenesis.
- Trivalent arsenic also inhibits the production of porphyrins and amino acids and reduces glutathione, which contributes to cellular toxicity and may explain the anemia and wasting seen in chronic arsenic toxicity.
- Pentavalent arsenic toxicity occurs in two ways. First, pentavalent arsenic may be converted to trivalent arsenic and act as previously described.
- Second, pentavalent arsenic resembles inorganic phosphate and has the ability to uncouple oxidative phosphorylation by substituting for phosphate in glycolytic and cellular respiration pathways. Instead of the formation of ATP, ADP-arsenate is formed, which rapidly hydrolyzes and uncouples phosphorylation.

POTENTIAL ROUTES FOR EXPOSURE

- Inorganic arsenic is readily absorbed by the gastrointestinal, respiratory, and mucosal routes.

- GI absorption approaches 90% with trivalent and pentavalent arsenic; more toxic substances, such as arsenic trioxide and diarsenic pentoxide, are poorly soluble and less well absorbed.
- Respiratory absorption is inversely proportional to particulate size. However, larger particles are often cleared by the ciliary tract and swallowed, allowing GI absorption to occur.
- Arsenic exposure to intact skin poses no significant threat.

TARGET ORGANS/SYSTEMS

Arsenic may reach and affect virtually any organ system.

CLINICAL FEATURES

- Clinical features of arsenic toxicity are directly related to the amount and type of arsenic ingested.
- Arsenic greatly varies in its toxicity, depending on the form and dose encountered. A very highly toxic form such as diarsenic pentoxide is likely to manifest with an acute or subacute toxic syndrome, whereas pentavalent arsenic would be more prone to chronic manifestations.
- Acute toxicity may occur within 10 minutes to hours after oral exposure. Patients will typically complain of nausea, vomiting, abdominal pain, and severe diarrhea that has been described as "cholera-like" because of its rice-watery character.
- Patients with less severe exposure may present with complaints similar to gastroenteritis and mild hypotension refractory to days of IV fluids. This should alert the astute clinician to the possibility of arsenic poisoning.
- With repetitive exposures, the patient may give a history of multiple gastrointestinal illnesses.
- Patients with severe exposure are generally in acute distress and may present in hypovolemic shock. Cardiac arrhythmias may be present, including prolonged QT syndrome and ventricular fibrillation.
- Because arsenic may attack any organ system, the patient is also subject to pulmonary edema, ARDS, hemolytic anemia, acute renal failure, fever, hepatitis, and rhabdomyolysis.
- Subacute toxicity may appear in the days to weeks following an acute exposure. Patients may see prolonged or even new signs or symptoms involving the nervous, dermatologic, gastrointestinal, pulmonary, and cardiovascular systems.
- Neurologic symptoms may range from headache to encephalopathy to delirium, and many patients will develop a stocking-glove peripheral neuropathy that is painful to the touch.
- Dermatologic signs may include Mee's lines (1 mm to 2 mm-wide white nail bands that signify a disruption in nail matrix keratinization), patchy alopecia, and nonprurutic desquamation.
- Respiratory complaints commonly resemble chronic viral bronchitis. Typically the GI and cardiovascular symptoms are a less severe prolongation of those mentioned for acute toxicity.
- Chronic exposure, usually through environmental or occupational sources, has a more insidious presentation. Chronic hepatic and renal damage is common.
- Common neurologic manifestations include encephalopathy and peripheral neuropathy.
- Many dermatologic phenomena are seen, ranging from hyperpigmentation or hypopigmentation to squamous and basal cell carcinomas.
- Other systemic effects include restrictive lung disease, aplastic anemia, diabetes, and vascular disease.
- Arsenic is also a carcinogen. It has been associated with bladder, skin, and lung cancer.

DIAGNOSIS

- In the acute setting, the diagnosis may be made with a spot urine sample demonstrating an elevated arsenic level.
- However, a low arsenic level does not exclude the diagnosis, as arsenic is intermittently excreted from the urine. Therefore, a 24-hour urine collection for total arsenic excretion is necessary. Clearance of more than 50 mcg over a 24-hour period is diagnostic.
- It is imperative to specify than the laboratory speciate the arsenic into organic and inorganic moieties, as nutritional sources of organic arsenic are common.
- Urinary excretion varies inversely with postexposure time, but in suspected cases with urinary levels below the aforementioned 50 mcg, hair and nail specimens may demonstrate arsenic levels for up to nine months postexposure.

LABORATORY TESTING AND IMAGING

- Laboratory tests helpful in the evaluation of chronic toxicity include a CBC, which most commonly demonstrates a microcytic hypochromic anemia; leukocytosis followed by leukopenia; and thrombocytopenia.
- Urinalysis may show proteinuria, hematuria, and pyuria. Elevations in creatinine, amino-transferases, and bilirubin may also be seen.
- In acute ingestions, radiopaque material may be seen on an abdominal radiograph.

TREATMENT AND DISPOSITION

- As with all toxicologic emergencies, initial care should consist of supportive measures with special attention to the ABCs.
- For patients with significant hypotension, venous access should include two large-bore catheters with judicial infusion of crystalloid solution, as cerebral or pulmonary edema may be present.
- Acute arsenic toxicity has been associated with cardiac dysrhythmias. Therefore, ACLS monitoring should be in place, with special emphasis on maintaining potassium, magnesium, and calcium within normal ranges. Agents that prolong the QT interval should be avoided.
- The patient should be monitored for hypoglycemia. Glycogen stores should be maintained with enteral feedings or IV dextrose.
- As with other heavy metals, arsenic binds poorly to charcoal. However, data is lacking as to its exact binding characteristics. Therefore, it is recommended that one dose of activated charcoal be administered at 1gm/kg.
- Whole bowel irrigation and nasogastric suctioning may assist in bowel cleansing and is recommended, especially if radiopaque material is seen on abdominal radiographs.
- Chelation therapy remains the mainstay of treatment for removing arsenic from the blood and peripheral tissues, although it has limitations.
- BAL (dimercaprol) is the drug of choice for acute toxicity and is the only intracellular/extracellular chelator available in the U.S. It may be administered IV or IM. However, IM administration has been associated with sterile skin abscesses. Some animal studies have shown that BAL shifts arsenic into the brain and testes.
- Succimer (meso-2,3-dimercaptosuccinic acid) is the treatment of choice for subacute and chronic toxicity.
- In patients requiring prolonged therapy, liver function tests and essential metal levels should be monitored.
- DMPS (sodium 2,3-dimercapto-1-propane sulfonate) may be used for acute, subacute, or chronic toxicity. It has the advantage of oral, IV, or IM administration and intra/extra-cellular distribution.
- In patients with normal renal function, urinary arsenical clearance far exceeds that removed by hemodialysis. Therefore, dialysis should be reserved only for patients with acute renal failure. Significant clearance in dialysate should not be anticipated.

REFERENCES

Ford M. Arsenic. In: Goldfrank LR, Flomenbaum NE, Lewin NA, et al, eds. *Goldfrank's Toxicologic Emergencies*. 7th ed. New York, NY: McGraw-Hill; 2002:1183-1195.

Hryhorczuk D, Eng J. Arsenic. In: Delaney KA, Ling LJ, Erickson T, et al, eds. *Clinical Toxicology*. Philadelphia, PA: W.B. Saunders; 2001:716-722.

United States Environmental Protection Agency. Ground Water & Drinking Water: Arsenic Rule Implementation. 2005. Available at: http://www.epa.gov/safewater/ars/implement.html. Accessed October 11, 2005.

United States Environmental Protection Agency. Implementation Guidance for the Arsenic Rule: Drinking Water Regulations for Arsenic and Clarifications to Compliance and New Source Contaminants Monitoring. 2002. Available at: http://www.epa.gov/safewater/ars/pdfs/regguide/ars_final_!mainguide_9-13.pdf. Accessed October 11, 2005.

BARIUM (Ba)

SYNONYMS AND TRADE NAMES

UN 1399, UN 1400, and UN 1854.
(CAS No. 7440-39-3)

BACKGROUND

- Barium is classified as a metal. It is silver-white in color and it occurs naturally as a part of several compounds.
- The relevant water-soluble salts include barium carbonate, barium chloride, barium nitrate, barium sulfide, and barium hydroxide.
- Insoluble barium salts include barium sulfate, barium apatite, and barium hydroxyapatite.

- The solubility of the various salts affects their specific uses and potentials for toxicity.
- Solubility also affects how long barium remains persistent in the environment.

ROUTINE USE

- Barium salts are both commercially and medically important.
- Barium sulfate ore is mined and utilized as lubrication by the gas and oil industries for drilling.
- Barium sulfate is also used for automotive paint, plastic stabilizers, case-hardening steels, bricks, tiles, glass, and rubber.
- Barium carbonate, chloride, and hydroxide are used to manufacture ceramics and as additives to oil and fuel.
- Barium compounds are also used in pesticides, rodenticides, and depilatories.
- Due to its relative insolubility, chemically pure barium sulfate is nontoxic and frequently used as a radiopaque medium for radiologic examination, as it is not absorbed after oral administration.

POTENTIAL TERRORIST USE

- Due to barium sulfate and carbonate's insolubility, it would be unlikely that either would find use as a terrorist agent.
- However, soluble barium salts are readily absorbed, and there have been previous reports of intentional overdoses.
- Soluble barium salts may be used by terrorists to contaminate food or water supplies.

MECHANISM OF ACTION

- The adverse effects that may result from barium exposure vary, but barium is capable of interacting with potassium, calcium, and magnesium, which are important cations in processes such as cell respiration, muscle control, and nerve conduction.
- Barium acts as a competitive potassium-channel antagonist. At adequate doses, barium may cause an accumulation of intracellular potassium, resulting in extracellular hypokalemia.
- Barium may also stimulate insulin release by calcium displacement.

POTENTIAL ROUTES FOR EXPOSURE

Inhalational, ingestion, and dermal.

TARGET ORGANS/SYSTEMS

Cardiovascular, gastrointestinal, muscular, and neurological.

CLINICAL FEATURES

- The potential adverse health effects associated with barium exposure depend on the specific solubility of each barium compound.
- Acute barium toxicity usually affects the gastrointestinal system first; hypokalemia, hypertension, and heart-rhythm disturbances may result.
- Muscle weakness is frequently reported and may, at times, be followed by muscle paralysis.
- Abnormalities in nerve conduction may also occur, including perioral and extremity numbness, as well as loss of deep-tendon reflexes.
- Swelling of the brain has been reported, as well as injury to the liver, kidney, spleen, and heart (e.g., arrhythmias).

DIAGNOSIS

- The diagnosis is based on the history of exposure in conjunction with the specific clinical findings and syndromic recognition.
- Barium exposure may be suspected in some patients with symptomatic hypokalemia and hypertension and a history consistent with barium exposure.

LABORATORY TESTING AND IMAGING

- Measures of serum potassium concentration may indicate hypokalemia due to intracellular translocation of potassium.
- Barium may be measured in the blood, bone, urine, and feces, but these measurements may not be clinically useful following the terrorist use of barium.

TREATMENT AND DISPOSITION

- Initial care should consist of supportive measures, with special attention to the ABCs.
- GI decontamination with activated charcoal may be helpful.
- Early treatment may include enteral sodium sulfate administration. This may prevent digestive absorption by precipitating ions to insoluble barium sulfate. Intravenous administration is not recommended, as the ions may precipitate in the kidneys, resulting in acute renal failure.
- Large amounts of oral and/or intravenous potassium replacement may be needed to resolve hypokalemia.
- Patients with rhabdomyolysis should be treated with aggressive IV hydration.
- Hemodialysis may be effective in treating barium toxicity.
- In cases of intentional barium ingestion, psychiatric evaluation may be necessary.

REFERENCES

Agency for Toxic Substances and Disease Registry, Public Health Service, U.S. Department of Health and Human Services. *Toxicological Profile for Barium*. Atlanta, GA: Agency for Toxic Substances and Disease Registry, Public Health Service, U.S. Department of Health and Human Services; 1992. Available at: http://www.atsdr.cdc.gov/toxprofiles/tp24.html. Accessed October 10, 2005.

Koch M, Appoloni O, Haufroid V, et al. Acute barium intoxication and hemodiafiltration. *J Toxicol Clin Toxicol.* 2003;41(4):363-367.

Sigue G, Gamble L, Pelitere M, et al. From profound hypokalemia to life-threatening hyperkalemia: A case of barium sulfide poisoning. *Arch Intern Med.* 2000;160: 548-551.

THALLIUM (TI)

SYNONYMS AND TRADE NAMES

Ramor.
(CAS No. 7440-28-0)

BACKGROUND

- Thallium is a trace mineral in the earth's crust. In its pure form, thallium is bluish-white in color and is both odorless and tasteless. However, it is often found in combination with other elements such as halogens, oxygen, or sulfur. Thallium salts include thallous (Tl^{+1}) and thallic (Tl^{+3}) series.
- Thallium was historically recovered as a byproduct from coal burning or smelting, but has not been domestically produced since 1981, and is now either imported or obtained from reserves. Once released into the environment, thallium tends not to be biodegradable.

ROUTINE USE

- Thallium is predominantly used in the semiconductor industry as an ingredient of electronic devices, switches, and closures. It may also be found in the production of low-range thermometers, photoelectric cells, and low-melting glass, as well as a component of rodenticides and insecticides.
- Thallium was also used to treat tinea infections in the 1920s and 1930s, resulting in hundreds of cases of thallium toxicity (thallotoxicosis) and multiple deaths.
- Thallium's use as a pesticide still holds the potential for deleterious human exposure.

POTENTIAL TERRORIST USE

- In the 1990s, thallium was used as a terrorist agent against dissidents against the Iraqi government, with more than 80 cases of confirmed thallium poisoning.
- Thallium has also been used in domestic cases of intentional poisoning. It is most likely to be used by terrorists to contaminate food or water supplies.

MECHANISM OF ACTION

Exposure to thallium may result in the inhibition of cellular respiration and disruption of calcium homeostasis, as well as ligand formation with sulfhydryl groups and/or interaction with riboflavin and associated cofactors. This is due to similar ionic radii between thallium and potassium, making it possible for thallium to interfere with potassium pathways and alter potassium-dependent processes.

POTENTIAL ROUTES FOR EXPOSURE

Inhalational, ingestion, and dermal.

TARGET ORGANS/SYSTEMS

Gastrointestinal, neurologic, renal, hepatologic, and hair.

CLINICAL FEATURES

- Symptoms of thallium poisoning may occur from hours to days following exposure, with the classic presentation consisting of alopecia with an ascending peripheral neuropathy that begins in the lower extremities.
- Patients may experience extreme pain with only light touch. Such a presentation may arise from either a single acute exposure or from chronic exposure to limited amounts of thallium.
- A study of workers with chronic occupational exposure to thallium revealed finger and toe numbness from inhalation of thallium.
- Other symptoms of CNS involvement may include ataxia, seizure, delirium, sleep disturbances, optic neuropathy, and cranial-nerve dysfunction.
- Patients exposed to thallium may also report gastrointestinal symptoms, most commonly abdominal pain.
- Nausea, vomiting, constipation, tachycardia, hypertension, palmar erythema, anhydrosis, and Mee's lines may also occur.
- Severe cases will progressively worsen and may ultimately result in coma, respiratory paralysis, or death.

DIAGNOSIS

Thallium exposure should be strongly suspected in any patient with acute onset of patchy alopecia in conjunction with peripheral neuropathy.

LABORATORY TESTING AND IMAGING

- Laboratory confirmation of thallium exposure requires 24-hour urine collection and measurement.
- If multiple exposures have occurred, thallium may be seen microscopically as multiple bands of black deposits in the hair roots. This can be seen in approximately 95% of patients.
- Additionally, abdominal radiography may show metallic material in the gastrointestinal tract.

TREATMENT AND DISPOSITION

- Prussian blue (ferric hexacyanoferrate) should be administered as soon as possible, because it binds thallium and enhances elimination. However, Prussian blue may not be readily available.
- Limited supplies of Prussian blue (Radiogardase™)—enough to treat three to five victims—are available from the Radiation Emergency Assistance Center Training Site (865-576-1005). Delivery generally takes 12 to 24 hours. Limited quantitites may also be available at local pharmacies.
- For larger quantities of Prussian blue, contact your state department of health for the quantity available in your state's emergency medical stockpile, which is adequate in some states (such as New York and California) but small to nonexistent in others, because the cost of Prussian blue is expensive.
- For sufficient quantities of Prussian blue to treat mass casualties, your state governor must make a formal request to the Centers of Disease Control and Prevention's Strategic National Stockpile Coordination Center at 404-687-6656.
- Multidose activated charcoal also decreases thallium absorption and enhances elimination.
- Whole-bowel irrigation may be considered, especially if thallium has remained in the gastrointestinal tract.
- Charcoal hemoperfusion (with or without hemodialysis) may be helpful.
- The efficacy of chelating agents is questionable. It is generally thought that EDTA and BAL are not useful for treatment of thallium intoxication, but dithizon (diphenylthiocarbazone) has been effective.

REFERENCES

Centers for Disease Control and Prevention. *Thallium*. 2005. Available at: http://www.bt.cdc.gov/agent/thallium. Accessed October 11, 2005.

International Programme on Chemical Safety. *Thallium sulfate*. WHO and FAO Data Sheets on Pesticides No. 10; VBC/DS/75.10. 1975. Available at: http://www.inchem.org/documents/pds/pds/pest10_e.htm. Accessed October 11, 2005.

Mulkey JP, Oehme FW. A review of thallium toxicity. *Vet Hum Toxicol*. 1993;35(5):445-453.

NERVE AGENTS

SARIN

SYNONYMS AND TRADE NAMES

1-methylethyl, EA 1208, GB, IMPF, isopropoxy-methylphosphoryl fluoride, MFI, T-144, T-2106, TL 1618, trilone, trilone 46, and zarin. (CAS No. 107-44-8)

BACKGROUND

- Sarin is an organophosphate nerve agent developed in Germany in 1938 as a pesticide.
- Sarin is a clear, colorless liquid at room temperature.
- Sarin is generally described as odorless, but it has also been described as having a mild, fruity odor.
- The most volatile of the nerve agents, when it evaporates and condenses, sarin forms a gas that is heavier than air. As such, it will accumulate in low-lying areas.
- Sarin is highly soluble in water; however, sarin hydrolyzes and becomes much less toxic when mixed with water.

ROUTINE USE

- Sarin does not occur naturally and is not legal for use in any industry. It is manufactured solely for use as a military weapon.
- Most recently, sarin was used as a terrorist weapon in Japan in the Matsumoto incident of 1994 and the Tokyo subway sarin attack of 1995.
- In 2004, insurgents in Iraq detonated a shell containing two sarin precursors that were intended to mix together to form sarin in an attempt to kill American soldiers.

POTENTIAL TERRORIST USE

- Because of its high volatility, sarin could be used in any number of ways as a terrorist weapon.
- Contaminating a population's water supply with sarin is less likely, however, as sarin is less

toxic when mixed with water.
- In the Matsumoto incident, fans in the back of a truck were used to blow sarin vapor toward an apartment building.
- In the Tokyo subway sarin attack, four bags containing the nerve agent were placed in the subway system and simply punctured with umbrella tips, thereby releasing the agent into the subway cars.

MECHANISM OF ACTION

- Sarin is an organophosphate nerve agent that binds to and inhibits acetylcholinesterase in two phases.
- The first phase is reversible binding and inhibition.
- The second phase, also known as aging, is an irreversible chemical bond that permanently inhibits acetylcholinesterase.

POTENTIAL ROUTES FOR EXPOSURE

- Inhalation of sarin vapor and dermal absorption of sarin liquid are the primary routes of exposure.
- Ocular contact and ingestion of sarin may also occur.
- Of note, sarin vapor is not well absorbed through the skin.

TARGET ORGANS/SYSTEMS

Central and peripheral nervous systems, pulmonary, gastrointestinal, and musculoskeletal.

CLINICAL FEATURES

- Sarin will exert both muscarinic and nicotinic effects on the nervous system.
- The muscarinic effects are generally remembered by the mnemonic SLUDGEM (salivation, lacrimation, urination, defecation, gastrointestinal upset, emesis, and miosis).
- Another muscarinic effect is bronchosecretions.

- The nicotinic effects include muscle fasciculations, muscle weakness, tachycardia, hypertension, and mydriasis.
- Additional CNS effects may include anxiety, seizures, and coma.
- Patients who survive exposure to soman will often recover without sequelae.
- However, of concern are two distinct sequelae that have been seen after exposure to other organophosphates. One, the intermediate syndrome, which generally occurs two to three days after recovery, is categorized by a descending muscle paralysis that may result in respiratory depression secondary to diaphragmatic weakening.
- Another delayed complication of organophosphate poisoning is OPIDN, a delayed distal motor polyneuropathy that begins two to three weeks after organophosphate poisoning. This syndrome is thought to be a result of neuropathy target esterase (NTE) inhibition.

DIAGNOSIS

- The diagnosis is based on the history of exposure in conjunction with specific clinical findings and syndromic recognition.
- Decreased RBC and plasma cholinesterase levels may help confirm the diagnosis of soman poisoning. However, these tests are not useful in the acute management of soman-poisoned patients because they are not readily available at most facilities.

LABORATORY TESTING AND IMAGING

- Most patients who are exposed to soman will require pulse oximetry and continuous cardiac monitoring, as well as routine lab studies, including electrolyte panels and CBCs.
- Patients who are experiencing respiratory difficulty should have a chest x-ray.
- RBC and plasma cholinesterase levels may confirm soman poisoning but are not clinically helpful in the acute management of these patients.

TREATMENT AND DISPOSITION

- Supportive care with prompt attention to airway

is paramount for soman-poisoned patients.
- Decontamination is crucial, with complete clothing removal and washing with large amounts of water, as victims' clothing may off-gas soman vapor, thereby exposing prehospital care providers or emergency department personnel.
- Patients who are symptomatic after soman exposure require treatment with atropine and an oxime such as pralidoxime or obidoxime.
- Atropine may be given IV, IM, or endotracheally. Adults may initially require as much as 6 mg of atropine. The goal of treatment is drying of secretions. The recommended pediatric dose is 0.01 mg/kg to 0.02 mg/kg IV or IM.
- Pralidoxime (2-PAM) should be administered as soon as possible in order to prevent soman's second phase, aging. The recommended dose is 1 g to 2 g IV or IM. Continuous infusion may be necessary. The recommended pediatric dose is 15 mg/kg to 25 mg/kg IM or administered slowly intravenously. If given too rapidly, severe hypertension may be precipitated.
- Adults who seize should be given diazepam 10 mg IV or IM. Should patients continue to seize, treatment with barbiturates or propofol should be considered, along with intubation and mechanical ventilation.
- Seizing children should be administered diazepam 0.2 mg/kg to 0.5 mg/kg IV.
- Propofol should be avoided in children.
- Patients with bronchosecretions or respiratory difficulty should receive supplemental oxygen, inhaled beta agonists, and/or inhaled ipratropium.
- Patients in extremis may need intubation and mechanical ventilation.
- Ocular exposure requires prompt decontamination with copious amounts of water or saline. This process may be facilitated by use of a Morgan lens.
- Treat hypotension with saline or Lactated Ringers solution. If there is no improvement in blood pressure, consider pressors such as norepinephrine.
- Patients experiencing only miosis and mild rhinorrhea can most likely be discharged from the emergency department. However, patients with more severe symptoms should be admitted to the hospital for further management and close observation.

REFERENCES

Agency for Toxic Substances and Disease Registry. Medical management guidelines for nerve agents: Tabun (GA); Sarin (GB); Soman (GD); and VX. Atlanta, GA: Agency for Toxic Substances and Disease Registry; 2004. Available at: www.atsdr.cdc.gov/MHMI/mmg166.html. Accessed September 28, 2005.

De Bleecker J, Van Den Neucker K, Willems J. The intermediate syndrome in organophosphate poisoning: Presentation of a case and review of the literature. *J Toxicol Clin Toxicol.* 1992, 30(3):321-329; 331-332.

TABUN

SYNONYMS AND TRADE NAMES

Cyanophosphate, dimethylamidoethoxyphosphoryl-cyanide, ethylester-dimethylamid kyseliny kyanfos-fonove, ethyl phosphorodimethylamidocyanate, GA, Gelan I, Le-100, MCE, T-2104, Taboon A, TL 1578, and Trilon 83.
(CAS No. 77-81-6)

BACKGROUND

- Gerhard Schrader, a German chemist specializing in the development of new insecticides, synthesized tabun in 1936, the first of the so-called G-agents (precursors to modern nerve agents) to be developed.
- Considered by some authors to be the least potent but the easiest to synthesize of the G-agents, tabun is, under normal environmental conditions, a volatile liquid that will readily vaporize.
- When tabun vaporizes, it forms a gas that is heavier than air, and as such, will tend to accumulate in low-lying areas.

ROUTINE USE

Tabun does not occur naturally in the environment and has no known industrial use. It is manufactured only as a military weapon. Its production and stockpiling were outlawed in 1993.

POTENTIAL TERRORIST USE

- Because of its high volatility, tabun could have many uses as a terrorist weapon.
- Tabun could be dispersed onto a populace via crop dusters.
- Tabun vapor could be dispersed using fans or simply spilled onto the ground and allowed to disperse via air currents.
- Tabun hydrolyzes in water and when mixed with bleaching powder. When tabun hydrolyzes, gases such as cyanogen chloride, hydrogen cyanide, carbon monoxide, and oxides of nitrogen may be released.

MECHANISM OF ACTION

- Tabun is an organophosphate nerve agent that binds to and inhibits acetylcholinesterase in two phases.
- The first phase is reversible binding and inhibition.
- The second phase, also known as aging, is an irreversible chemical bond that permanently inhibits acetylcholinesterase.

POTENTIAL ROUTES FOR EXPOSURE

- Inhalation of tabun vapor and dermal absorption of tabun liquid are the primary routes of exposure.
- Ocular contact and ingestion of this nerve agent may also occur.
- Of note, tabun vapor is not well absorbed through the skin.

TARGET ORGANS/SYSTEMS

Central and peripheral nervous systems, pulmonary, gastrointestinal, and musculoskeletal.

CLINICAL FEATURES

- Tabun will exert both muscarinic and nicotinic effects on the nervous system.
- The muscarinic effects are generally remembered by the mneumonic SLUDGEM (salivation, lacrimation, urination, defecation, gastrointestinal upset, emesis, and miosis).
- Another muscarinic effect is bronchosecretions.
- Nicotinic effects include muscle fasciculations, muscle weakness, tachycardia, hypertension, and mydriasis.

- Additional CNS effects may include anxiety, seizures, and coma.
- Patients who survive exposure to tabun will often recover without sequelae.
- However, of concern are two distinct sequelae that have been seen after exposure to other organophosphates. One, the intermediate syndrome, which generally occurs two to three days after recovery, is characterized by a descending muscle paralysis that may result in respiratory depression secondary to diaphragmatic weakening.
- Another delayed complication of organophosphate poisoning is OPIDN, a delayed distal motor polyneuropathy that begins two to three weeks after organophosphate poisoning. This syndrome is thought to be a result of neuropathy target esterase (NTE) inhibition.

DIAGNOSIS

- The diagnosis is based on the history of exposure in conjunction with specific clinical findings and syndromic recognition.
- Decreased RBC and plasma cholinesterase levels may help confirm the diagnosis of tabun poisoning, but these tests are not useful in the acute management of tabun-poisoned patients because they are not readily available at most facilities.

LABORATORY TESTING AND IMAGING

- Most patients who are exposed to tabun will require pulse oximetry and continuous cardiac monitoring, as well as routine lab studies, including electrolyte panels and CBCs.
- Patients who are experiencing respiratory difficulty should have a chest x-ray.
- RBC and plasma cholinesterase levels may confirm tabun poisoning but are not clinically helpful in the acute management of these patients.

TREATMENT AND DISPOSITION

- Supportive care with prompt attention to airway is paramount for tabun-poisoned patients.
- Decontamination is crucial, with complete clothing removal and washing with large amounts of water, as victims' clothing may off-gas tabun

vapor, thereby exposing prehospital care providers or emergency department personnel.
- Patients who are symptomatic after tabun exposure require treatment with atropine and an oxime such as pralidoxime or obidoxime.
- Atropine may be given IV, or IM, or endotracheally. Adults may require as much as 6 mg of atropine initially. The goal of treatment is drying of secretions. The recommended pediatric dose is 0.01 mg/kg to 0.02 mg/kg IV or IM.
- Pralidoxime (2-PAM) should be administered as soon as possible in order to prevent tabun's second stage, aging. The recommended dose is 1 g to 2 g IV or IM. Continuous infusion may be necessary. The recommended pediatric dose is 15 mg/kg to 25 mg/kg IM or administered slowly intravenously. If given too rapidly, severe hypertension may be precipitated.
- Adults who seize should be given diazepam 10 mg IV or IM.
- Should the patient continue to seize, treatment with barbiturates or propofol should be considered, along with intubation and mechanical ventilation.
- Seizing children should also be administered diazepam 0.2 mg/kg to 0.5 mg/kg IV.
- Propofol should be avoided in children.
- Patients with bronchosecretions or respiratory difficulty should receive supplemental oxygen, inhaled beta agonists, and/or inhaled ipratropium.
- Patients in extremis may need intubation and mechanical ventilation.
- Ocular exposure requires prompt decontamination with copious amounts of water or saline. This process may be facilitated by use of a Morgan lens.
- Treat hypotension with saline or Lactated Ringers solution. If there is no improvement in blood pressure, consider pressors such as norepinephrine.
- Patients experiencing only miosis and mild rhinorrhea can most likely be discharged from the emergency department. However, patients with more severe symptoms should be admitted to the hospital for further management and close observation.

REFERENCES

Agency for Toxic Substances and Disease Registry. *Medical management guidelines for nerve agents: Tabun (GA); Sarin (GB); Soman (GD); and VX.* Atlanta, GA:

Agency for Toxic Substances and Disease Registry; 2004. Available at: www.atsdr.cdc.gov/MHMI/mmg166.html. Accessed September 28, 2005.

De Bleecker J, Van Den Neucker K, Willems J. The intermediate syndrome in organophosphate poisoning: Presentation of a case and review of the literature. *J Toxicol Clin Toxicol.* 1992;30(3):321-329; 331-332.

VX

SYNONYMS AND TRADE NAMES

EA 1701, methyl-, O-ethyl S-(2-diisopropy-laminoethyl) methylphosphonothioate, phospho-nothioic acid, and TX 60.
(CAS No: 50782-69-9)

BACKGROUND

- VX was first synthesized in England in the early 1950s.
- VX is an odorless, tasteless liquid under normal environmental conditions. Its color ranges from colorless to shades of amber, and is often described as having a consistency resembling that of motor oil. It has low viscosity and low volatility; therefore, VX would be expected to persist in the environment for prolonged periods.
- VX as a vapor is considered to be three times more potent than sarin, but as a skin agent is approximately 100 times more potent than sarin.
- In water, VX will hydrolyze to form O-ethyl S-(2-diisopropylaminoethyl) methylphospho-nothioic acid, a Class B poison. As such, it is presumed by the U.S. Department of Transportation to present a serious threat to health during transportation that is nearly as potent and harmful as VX.

ROUTINE USE

- VX does not occur naturally in the environment and has no known industrial use. It is manufac-tured solely as a military weapon.
- The U.S. government is currently in the process of destroying domestic stockpiles and is assisting Russia in destroying its stockpiles as well.
- There is one report of an accidental spill of VX in

Skull Valley, Utah, in 1968, where approximately 75% of 6,000 exposed sheep perished; the area remained contaminated for more than three months afterward.

POTENTIAL TERRORIST USE

- Because of its low volatility, VX would most likely be released as a liquid spray over and on large groups of people congregated at sporting events or other public venues.
- In addition to causing substantial morbidity and mortality shortly after release, VX would render an area uninhabitable until adequately decon-taminated or agent dissipation occurred natu-rally over many months.

MECHANISM OF ACTION

- VX is an organophosphate nerve agent that binds to and inhibits acetylcholinesterase in two phases.
- The first phase involves reversible binding and enzyme inhibition.
- The second phase, also known as aging, involves irreversible chemical bonding that permanently inhibits acetylcholinesterase.

POTENTIAL ROUTES FOR EXPOSURE

- Dermal absorption of VX liquid is the primary route of exposure.
- VX vapor inhalation, ocular contact, and inges-tion may also occur.

TARGET ORGANS/SYSTEMS

Central and peripheral nervous systems, pul-monary, gastrointestinal, and musculoskeletal.

CLINICAL FEATURES

- VX will exert both muscarinic and nicotinic effects on the nervous system.
- The muscarinic effects are generally remem-bered by the mneumonic SLUDGEM (saliva-tion, lacrimation, urination, defecation, gas-trointestinal upset, emesis, and miosis).
- Another muscarinic effect is bronchosecretions.

- The nicotinic effects include muscle fasciculations, muscle weakness, tachycardia, hypertension, and mydriasis.
- Additional CNS effects may include anxiety, seizures, and coma.
- Patients who survive exposure to VX will often recover without sequelae.
- However, of concern are two distinct sequelae that have been seen after exposure to other organophosphates. The first, the intermediate syndrome, which generally occurs two to three days after recovery, is characterized by a descending muscle paralysis that may result in respiratory depression secondary to diaphragmatic weakening.
- Another delayed complication of organophosphate poisoning is OPIDN, a delayed distal motor polyneuropathy that begins two to three weeks after organophosphate poisoning. This syndrome is thought to be a result of neuropathy target esterase (NTE) inhibition.

DIAGNOSIS

- The diagnosis is based on the history of exposure in conjunction with specific clinical findings and syndromic recognition.
- Decreased RBC and plasma cholinesterase levels may help confirm the diagnosis of VX poisoning. However, these tests are not useful in the acute management of VX-poisoned patients because they are not readily available at most facilities.

LABORATORY TESTING AND IMAGING

- Most patients who are exposed to VX will require pulse oximetry and continuous cardiac monitoring, as well as routine lab studies, including electrolyte panels and CBCs.
- Patients who are experiencing respiratory difficulty should have a chest x-ray.
- RBC and plasma cholinesterase levels may confirm VX poisoning but are not clinically helpful in the acute management of these patients.

TREATMENT AND DISPOSITION

- Supportive care with prompt attention to airway is paramount for VX-poisoned patients.

- Decontamination is crucial, with complete clothing removal and washing with large amounts of water, as victims' clothing may off-gas VX vapor, thereby exposing prehospital care providers or emergency department personnel.
- Patients who are symptomatic after VX exposure require treatment with atropine and an oxime such as pralidoxime or obidoxime.
- Atropine may be given IV, IM, or endotracheally. Adults may require as much as 6 mg of atropine initially. The goal of treatment is drying of secretions. The recommended pediatric dose is 0.01 mg/kg to 0.02 mg/kg IV or IM.
- Pralidoxime (2-PAM) should be administered as soon as possible in order to prevent VX's second phase, aging. The recommended dose is 1 g to 2 g IV or IM. Continuous infusion may be necessary. The recommended pediatric dose is 15 mg/kg to 25 mg/kg IM or administered slowly intravenously. If given too rapidly, severe hypertension may be precipitated.
- Adults who seize should receive diazepam 10 mg IV or IM. Should a patient continue to seize, treatment with barbiturates or propofol should be considered, along with intubation and mechanical ventilation.
- Seizing children should also receive diazepam 0.2 mg/kg to 0.5 mg/kg IV.
- Propofol should be avoided in children.
- Patients with bronchosecretions or respiratory difficulty should receive supplemental oxygen, inhaled beta agonists, and/or inhaled ipratropium.
- Patients in extremis may need intubation and mechanical ventilation.
- Ocular exposure requires prompt decontamination using copious amounts of water or saline. This process may be facilitated by use of a Morgan lens.
- Treat hypotension with saline or Lactated Ringers solution. If there is no improvement in blood pressure, consider pressors such as norepinephrine.
- Patients experiencing only miosis and mild rhinorrhea may be discharged from the emergency department in most cases. However, patients with more severe symptoms should be admitted to the hospital for further management and close observation.

REFERENCES

Agency for Toxic Substances and Disease Registry. *Medical management guidelines for nerve agents: Tabun (GA); Sarin (GB); Soman (GD); and VX.* Atlanta, GA: Agency for Toxic Substances and Disease Registry; 2004. Available at: www.atsdr.cdc.gov/MHMI/mmg166.html. Accessed September 28, 2005.

De Bleecker J, Van Den Neucker K, Willems J. The intermediate syndrome in organophosphate poisoning: Presentation of a case and review of the literature. *J Toxicol Clin Toxicol.* 1992;30(3):321-329, 331-332.

ORGANIC SOLVENTS

BENZENE (C₆H₆)

SYNONYMS AND TRADE NAMES

[6]annulene, benzin, benzine, benzol, benzole, benzolene, bicarburet of hydrogen, carbon oil, coal naphtha, cyclohexatriene, mineral naphtha, motor benzol, NCI-C55276, nitration benzene, phene, phenyl hydride, pyrobenzol, and pyrobenzole. (CAS No. 71-43-2)

BACKGROUND

- Benzene is a naturally occurring substance in fossil fuels. It is also produced during combustion of coal, wood, and petroleum products.
- In liquid form, benzene is colorless, has a sweet odor, and evaporates quickly into air. Benzene is only slightly water soluble. In addition, it is considered to be biodegradable and highly flammable.
- On the Agency for Toxic Substances and Disease Registry's Comprehensive Environmental Response, Compensation, and Liability Act Priority List of Hazardous Substances, benzene ranks sixth out of 275 hazardous substances listed.

ROUTINE USE

- Benzene is used mainly in the industrial setting as a feedstock material in the synthesis of other chemicals.
- Benzene is also used to make various types of rubbers, dyes, lubricants, detergents, pesticides, and drugs.
- Volcanoes and forest fires are some natural atmospheric sources for benzene.

POTENTIAL TERRORIST USE

Benzene could have potential terrorist use if it is used to contaminate food and/or water supplies.

MECHANISM OF ACTION

- In certain circumstances, benzene is a known carcinogen.
- Numerical as well as structural chromosome abnormalities have been noted in the peripheral blood cells of workers exposed to high concentrations of benzene.
- Epidemiologic evidence suggests that the risk for leukemia increases with increasing doses of benzene, becoming significantly elevated at cumulative exposures exceeding 50 ppm-years. Chronic toxicity has been ascribed to formation of reactive metabolites.

POTENTIAL ROUTES FOR EXPOSURE

- Benzene may be absorbed via all routes of exposure in humans and animals, although most exposures occur by inhalation.
- Dermal absorption is limited by benzene's rapid evaporation from the skin.
- In certain circumstances, ingestion may also occur.

TARGET ORGANS/SYSTEMS

CNS, ocular, dermatologic, pulmonary, hematopoietic, and bone marrow.

CLINICAL FEATURES

- Acute exposure to high levels of benzene vapors may cause irritation of the eyes, skin, and respiratory system, as well as CNS depression.
- There have been reports of deaths from arrhythmias and cardiac sensitization, as well as coma after contact with substantial concentrations.
- Short-term effects may include dizziness, lightheadedness, vomiting, and headache.
- Chronic exposure may lead to leukemia and bone marrow depression, specifically acute myeloid leukemia.

- Ocular exposure to liquid benzene may cause eye pain and corneal injury.
- Prolonged or repeated skin exposure to the liquid form may cause skin breakdown. While percutaneous absorption through intact skin is slow, dermal exposure has the potential to result in systemic toxicity.
- The ingestion of benzene may cause mucous membrane, stomach, and esophageal injury. This may lead to nausea, vomiting, and abdominal pain.

DIAGNOSIS

Diagnosis is based on history of exposure in conjunction with presenting signs and symptoms, as described above.

LABORATORY TESTING AND IMAGING

- Blood levels for benzene or its metabolite, phenol, may be obtained in order to document exposure; however, these tests are not very useful in the acute clinical setting.
- Various other factors may also cause elevated phenol levels—e.g., ingestion of certain medications like Pepto-Bismol® and Chloraseptic®, the ingestion of benzoate preservatives, and smoking. Urinary metabolites of benzene may also be obtained to document exposure.
- Routine laboratory studies—such as CBC, electrolytes, BUN, creatinine, UA, liver function tests, and glucose—should be considered for all people exposed to benzene.
- For patients with severe inhalational exposures, additional tests include pulse oximetry and ECG, as well as chest x-ray and ABG measurements.

TREATMENT AND DISPOSITION

- There is no antidote available for benzene exposure. Hemodialysis is not effective.
- After removal from the source and appropriate decontamination, supportive care is the mainstay of treatment.
- In cases of respiratory compromise, endotracheal intubation may be required. Otherwise, provide supplemental oxygen by mask.

- Use caution when treating bronchospasm with aerosolized bronchodilators.
- If possible, avoid using sympathomimetics, such as epinephrine, because benzene has a myocardial sensitizing effect.
- Patients with seizures or hypotension should be treated in the conventional manner.
- Patients with dermal exposure should be decontaminated with copious amounts of tap water. Injuries should be treated as thermal burns.
- For eye exposures, continue water irrigation for 15 minutes. Examine eyes for corneal damage and manage appropriately. For patients with severe corneal injuries, consult ophthalmology.
- For oral ingestions, consider gastric lavage with a small NG tube if a large amount of benzene has been consumed, or if the patient is being evaluated within 30 minutes of the ingestion. Also consider this management if there are oral lesions or persistent esophageal discomfort.
- Care must be taken when placing the NG tube to prevent further injury to the chemically damaged upper GI tract.
- For alert patients with oral ingestions, activated charcoal at a dose of 1mg/kg may be helpful, but should not be used if endoscopy is anticipated.
- Patients may require endoscopy for evaluation of injury to the GI tract.
- Most patients who remain asymptomatic for six to 12 hours after exposure may be discharged. They should be advised to rest and to seek medical care immediately if symptoms develop.
- Symptomatic patients with substantial inhalational exposure or ingestions should be admitted to the hospital for supportive care and observation. These patients should be observed for signs of acute tubular necrosis, dysrhythmias, and encephalopathy.
- Patients with inhalational exposures should be watched for signs of pulmonary edema.
- Those who have ingested benzene should be observed for signs of aspiration pneumonitis, which has reportedly occurred as long as 72 hours after exposure.

REFERENCES

Agency for Toxic Substances and Disease Registry. *Medical Management Guidelines for Benzene.* Atlanta, GA: Agency for Toxic Substances and Disease Registry; 2004. Available at: http://www.atsdr.cdc.gov/MHMI/mmg3.html. Accessed September 8, 2005.

Agency for Toxic Substances and Disease Registry. *ToxFAQs for Benzene.* Atlanta,

GA: Agency for Toxic Substances and Disease Registry; 2004. Available at: http://www.atsdr.cdc.gov/tfacts3.html. Accessed September 8, 2005.

National Industrial Chemicals Notification and Assessment Scheme. *Benzene: Priority existing chemical assessment report No. 21*. Sydney, Australia: National Industrial Chemicals Notification and Assessment Scheme; 2001. Available at: http://www.nicnas.gov.au/publications/CAR/PEC/PEC21/PEC21_whole.pdf. Accessed September 8, 2005.

National Safety Council. *Chemical Backgrounders: Benzene.** Itasca, IL: National Safety Council. 2005. Available at: http://www.nsc.org/library/chemical/benzene.htm. Accessed September 8, 2005.

* Permission to reprint granted by the National Safety Council, a membership organization dedicated to protecting life and promoting health.

RIOT CONTROL AGENTS

BROMOBENZYLCYANIDE (CA)

SYNONYMS AND TRADE NAMES

None.
(CAS No. 31938-07-5)

BACKGROUND

- This tear gas is a clear to white crystalline substance with the odor of sour fruit.
- Used by the French and Americans during World War I, CA was considered obsolete after the introduction of the newer riot control agents in the 1920s.
- It is no longer generally stockpiled in NATO arsenals.

ROUTINE USE

CA is no longer commonly used as a riot control agent.

POTENTIAL TERRORIST USE

This agent may be released by terrorists in crowded areas. This would be expected to transiently affect large numbers of people, causing incapacitation and panic. Large releases in confined spaces would be expected to cause fewer but more severe casualties.

MECHANISM OF ACTION

- Temporary interaction of the halogen group with sulfhydryl groups are thought to be the mechanism of action of CA.
- The dose that incapacitates 50% of exposed individuals is 30 mg/min/m^3, whereas the estimated lethal dose is 8,000 mg/min/m^3 to 11,000 mg/min/m^3.

POTENTIAL ROUTES FOR EXPOSURE

Inhalational and mucous membrane contact.

TARGET ORGANS/SYSTEMS

Eyes, skin, mucous membranes, and lungs.

CLINICAL FEATURES

- Irritation of the eyes and throat occurs rapidly.
- Lacrimation, burning in the oropharynx, and irritation of moist and sensitive areas of the skin are early effects.
- Nausea, vomiting, and headache are commonly reported.
- The above effects are of limited duration, and usually resolve within 30 to 60 minutes following evacuation and decontamination.
- With longer and more intense exposure, non-cardiogenic pulmonary edema may occur.

DIAGNOSIS

The diagnosis is based on the history of exposure as reported by prehospital personnel or the presentation of multiple patients exposed to a tear gas-like agent in the field.

LABORATORY TESTING AND IMAGING

- There is no specific test for this agent.
- Patients complaining of dyspnea or who present with hypoxia should be evaluated with chest radiography and pulse oximetry.

TREATMENT AND DISPOSITION

- Evacuation and decontamination are the first steps to treatment.
- Exposed clothing should be removed and the skin cleansed.
- Eyes should be liberally irrigated with sterile saline or Lactated Ringers solution.
- CA is poorly soluble in water and should be removed with soap. It is also slowly hydrolyzed in water, and therefore is only removed and not inactivated by washing. As such, decontamination effluent should be

kept out of contact with patients and health-care providers.

- Supplemental oxygen should be provided for hypoxic or dyspneic patients.
- Beta agonist may be beneficial for patients with clinical evidence of bronchospasm.
- Mechanical ventilation may be required for those with severe exposures or underlying medical conditions.

REFERENCES

Blain PG. Tear gases and irritant incapacitants. 1-chloroacetophenone, 2-chlorobenzylidene malononitrile and dibenz[b,f]-1,4-oxazepine. *Toxicol Rev.* 2003;22(2):103-110.

Centers for Disease Control and Prevention, Department of Health and Human Services. *Chemical Emergencies: Riot Control Agent Poisoning.* Washington, DC: Centers for Disease Control and Prevention, Department of Health and Human Services; 2005. Available at: http://www.bt.cdc.gov/agent/riotcontrol/casedefinition.asp. Accessed September 13, 2005.

Department of the Army, the Navy, and the Air Force. *Air Force Joint Manual 44-151.* Washington, DC: Department of the Army, the Navy, and the Air Force; 1996.

Department of the Army, the Navy, and the Air Force. *Navy Medical Publication 5059.* Washington, DC: Department of the Army, the Navy, and the Air Force; 1996.

Department of the Army, the Navy, and the Air Force. *NATO Handbook on the Medical Aspects of NBC Defensive Operations AMedP-6(B).* Washington, DC: Department of the Army, the Navy, and the Air Force; 1996.

Department of the Army, the Navy, and the Air Force. *Army Field Manual 8-9.* Washington, DC: Department of the Army, the Navy, and the Air Force; 1996.

NIOSH and Department of Health and Human Services. *National Institute for Occupational Safety and Health (NIOSH) Pocket Guide to Chemical Hazards.* Washington, DC: NIOSH and Department of Health and Human Services. NIOSH Publication No. 97-140; 1997:60. Available at: http://www.cdc.gov/niosh/npg/npg.html. Accessed September 2, 2005.

Olajos EJ, Stopford W, eds. *Riot Control Agents: Issues in Toxicology, Safety, and Health.* Boca Raton, FL: CRC Press; 2004.

CHLOROACETOPHENONE (CN)

SYNONYMS AND TRADE NAMES

2-Chloro-, acetophenone, CAF, CAP, Chemical Mace™, chloromethyl phenyl ketone, phenacyl chloride, phenyl chloromethyl ketone, and tear gas. (CAS No. 532-27-4)

BACKGROUND

- Along with chlorobenzylidenemalonitrile (CS), CN is one of the most frequently used riot-control agents.
- CN is a white to grayish crystalline solid that is typically dispersed as an aerosol.
- As a vapor at low concentrations, CN emits an odor that has been described as resembling apple blossoms.
- At higher concentrations, this odor reportedly becomes acrid and irritating.
- CN vapor is approximately five times as dense as air and tends to collect in low-lying areas.
- Chloroacetophenone, while considered more potent than other lacrimators, is still available without a license in the form of Chemical Mace.
- Chemical Mace is encountered far less frequently than "pepper spray" or Pepper Mace®, a capsaicin aerosol used for similar purposes.
- It is important to differentiate between CN and pepper spray or pepper mace, as their toxicity profiles are substantially different.
- In the color-coding system for handheld riot-control dispersion devices, CN is denoted by the color red.

ROUTINE USE

CN is used as an industrial chemical intermediate, as well as for personal protection by individuals and for riot control by law enforcement personnel in the form of Chemical Mace.

POTENTIAL TERRORIST USE

- Terrorists might release CN in crowded open-air areas. This could transiently affect large numbers of people, causing moderate incapacitation and panic. Large releases in confined spaces would be expected to cause fewer casualties because fewer people would be present, but the effects might be more severe.
- CN is typically deployed as a propelled aerosol when used in personal defense. However, CN deployed by the military or as a potential terrorist weapon would probably use an incendiary device (tear gas bomb or grenade) to disseminate this agent.
- While many people exposed in open-air scenarios would not be expected to have serious injury, the emergency response system and health care facilities could be overburdened by large numbers of patients. Fear and uncertainty among potentially exposed civilians also would be expected to create substantial psychological distress.

MECHANISM OF ACTION

- Chloroacetophenone is an alkylator that reacts readily with sulfydryl groups in enzymes. Inhibition of these enzymes may be responsible for tissue damage and necrosis.
- CN and other lacrimators are also potent sensory irritants, and the irritation and associated reflexes—such as coughing, vomiting, and blepharospasm—are primarily responsible for the incapacitating effects.
- The concentration of CN that is required to incapacitate one half of exposed persons is 20 mg/m^3 to 50 mg/m^3, while serious toxicity can be expected with exposures greater than 400 mg/m^3. The estimated lethal concentration is 850 ng/m^3.
- Handheld personal deployment devices are not thought to generate sufficient concentrations of CN to cause permanent injury in most circumstances.

POTENTIAL ROUTES FOR EXPOSURE

The route of primary concern is inhalation and mucous membrane contact resulting from aerosol dissemination.

TARGET ORGANS/SYSTEMS

Eyes, skin, mucous membranes, lungs, and respiratory tree.

CLINICAL FEATURES

- Irritation of the eyes and throat occurs rapidly.
- Lacrimation, burning in the oropharynx, and irritation on moist and sensitive areas of the skin are early effects.
- Nausea, vomiting, and headache are commonly reported.
- These effects are of limited duration, and usually resolve within 30 to 60 minutes following evacuation and decontamination.
- With more prolonged and more intense exposure, noncardiogenic pulmonary edema may occur, and there have been at least five deaths reported secondary to chloroacetophenone exposure.
- Tear gases are irritants that may cause chemical burns of the skin when directly applied. Chloroacetophenone is known to be a sensitizer of the skin, and thus may produce both a contact and an allergic dermatitis.

DIAGNOSIS

The diagnosis is based on the history of exposure as reported by prehospital personnel or by the presentation of multiple individuals exposed to a tear gas-like agent in the field.

LABORATORY TESTING AND IMAGING

- There is no specific diagnostic test for CN.
- However, a nonspecific leukocytosis has been described following CN exposure and may last several days.
- Patients complaining of dyspnea or who present with clinical evidence of hypoxemia should be evaluated with chest radiography and pulse oximetry.

TREATMENT AND DISPOSITION

- Evacuation and decontamination are the first steps to treatment.
- Exposed clothing should be removed and the skin cleansed.
- Eyes should be liberally irrigated with sterile saline or Lactated Ringers solution.
- CN is poorly soluble in water and should be removed with soap and a weakly alkaline solution.
- Vesicated skin should be washed with saline only. CN is slowly hydrolyzed in water, and therefore is only removed and not inactivated by washing. As such, decontamination effluent should be kept out of contact with patients and health care providers.
- Patients should be screened for corneal abrasions and, if found, these lesions should be treated with analgesics and topical antibiotics.
- If skin findings exceed simple erythema, lesions should be treated with comfort measures, local hygiene, and topical antibiotics for areas with denuded epithelium.

- Supplemental oxygen should be provided for hypoxic or dyspneic patients.
- Beta agonists may be beneficial for patients with clinical evidence of bronchospasm.
- Mechanical ventilation may be required for patients with severe exposures or underlying medical conditions.
- All patients with signs of hypoxemia should be observed in the hospital for 24 hours.

REFERENCES

Blain PG. Tear gases and irritant incapacitants. 1-chloroacetophenone, 2-chlorobenzylidene malononitrile and dibenz[b,f]-1,4-oxazepine. *Toxicol Rev.* 2003;22(2):103-110.

Centers for Disease Control and Prevention, Department of Health and Human Services. *Chemical Emergencies: Riot Control Agent Poisoning.* Washington, DC: Centers for Disease Control and Prevention, Department of Health and Human Services; 2005. Available at: http://www.bt.cdc.gov/agent/riotcontrol/casedefinition.asp. Accessed September 13, 2005.

Departments of the Army, the Navy, and the Air Force. *Air Force Joint Manual 44-151.* Washington, DC: Departments of the Army, the Navy, and the Air Force; 1996.

Departments of the Army, the Navy, and the Air Force. *Army Field Manual 8-9.* Washington, DC: Departments of the Army, the Navy, and the Air Force; 1996.

Departments of the Army, the Navy, and the Air Force. *Navy Medical Publication 5059.* Washington, DC: Departments of the Army, the Navy, and the Air Force; 1996.

Departments of the Army, the Navy, and the Air Force. *NATO Handbook on the Medical Aspects of NBC Defensive Operations AMedP-6(B).* Washington, DC: Departments of the Army, the Navy, and the Air Force; 1996.

National Institute for Occupational Safety and Health and Department of Health and Human Services. *NIOSH Pocket Guide to Chemical Hazards (NPG).* NIOSH Publication No. 97-140. Washington, DC: National Institute for Occupational Safety and Health and Department of Health and Human Services; 1997:60. Available at: http://www.cdc.gov/niosh/npg/npg.html. Accessed September 13, 2005.

CHLOROBENZYLIDENE-MALONITRILE (CS)

SYNONYMS AND TRADE NAMES

2-Chlorobenzylidene malononitrile and beta,beta-dicyano-O-chlorostyrene. (CAS No. 2698-41-1)

BACKGROUND

- Named for the two scientists, B.B. Carson and R.W. Sloughton, who first prepared it in 1928, CS is probably the most frequently used riot control agent.
- In 1959, CS supplanted CN (chloroacetophenone) as the riot control agent of choice for military operations due to its greater irritating effects as well as its reduced systemic toxicity, and it was

used during the Vietnam conflict.
- CS is a white to grayish crystalline solid that is typically dispersed as an aerosol or in conjunction with an incendiary device.
- As a vapor at low concentrations, its odor has been described as resembling that of pepper.
- The vapor is approximately three to four times as dense as air and collects in low-lying areas.
- In the color-coding system for handheld riot-control dispersion devices, CS is denoted by the color blue.

ROUTINE USE

CS is used as a harassment and incapacitating agent (i.e., riot control) by police and military forces.

POTENTIAL TERRORIST USE

- Terrorists might release this agent in crowded areas, and this would be expected to transiently affect large numbers of people, causing incapacitation and panic.
- Large releases in confined spaces would be expected to cause fewer but more severe casualties.
- While CS is typically deployed as a propelled aerosol when used by law enforcement as a personal defense device, CS is heat-stable. As a potential terrorist agent, deployment would probably utilize an incendiary device (such as tear gas bomb or grenade) or a vehicle-mounted dispersion device.
- While many people exposed in open-air scenarios would not be expected to have serious injury, the emergency response system and health care facilities could be seriously taxed by large numbers of patients.
- In addition, fear and uncertainty among potentially exposed civilians could create psychological distress.

MECHANISM OF ACTION

- Chlorobenzylidenemalonitrile is an alkylating agent that reacts readily with sulfydryl groups in enzymes.
- Inhibition of these enzymes may be responsible for tissue damage and necrosis.
- CS and other lacrimators are potent sensory irri-

tants, and the irritation—as well as associated reflexes, such as coughing, vomiting, and ble-pharospasm—are responsible for the incapacitating effects.

- In addition, metabolism and hydrolysis of CS liberate cyanide, although the contribution of the small amount of cyanide to the toxicity of CS is unclear.
- At concentrations above 3 mg/m^3, CS becomes intolerable, while the estimated lethal concentration is much higher—2,500 mg/m^3.
- Handheld personal deployment devices are not thought to generate sufficient concentrations of CS to cause permanent injury in normal use.

TARGET ORGANS/SYSTEMS

Ocular, dermal, mucous membranes, and lungs.

CLINICAL FEATURES

- Tear gases are irritants that may cause chemical burns when directly applied to the skin, and workers in plants producing chlorobenzylidene-malonitrile have reported dermatitis involving exposed areas of the arms.
- Irritation of the eyes and throat occurs rapidly and at low concentrations.
- Early effects include lacrimation, burning in the oropharynx, and irritation of moist and sensitive areas of the skin.
- Nausea, vomiting, and headache are common.
- These effects are of limited duration and usually resolve within 30 to 60 minutes following evacuation and decontamination.
- With longer and more intense exposure, non-cardiogenic pulmonary edema may occur.

DIAGNOSIS

The diagnosis is based on the history of exposure obtained from prehospital personnel or the presentation of multiple patients exposed to a tear gas-like agent in the field.

LABORATORY TESTING AND IMAGING

- There is no specific test for CS.

- Blood and urinary thiocyanate levels are not clinically useful.
- Patients complaining of dyspnea, or who present with clinical evidence of hypoxemia, should be admitted to the hospital and evaluated with chest radiography and pulse oximetry.

TREATMENT AND DISPOSITION

- Evacuation and decontamination are the first steps to treatment.
- Exposed clothing should be removed and the skin cleansed.
- Eyes should be liberally irrigated with sterile saline or Lactated Ringers solution.
- CS is poorly soluble in water and should be removed with soap and a weakly alkaline solution.
- Vesicated skin should be washed with sterile saline only. CS is slowly hydrolyzed in water; it is only removed but not inactivated by washing. Therefore, decontamination effluent should be kept out of contact with patients and health care providers.
- Patients should be screened for corneal abrasions. If found, these lesions should be treated with analgesics and topical antibiotics.
- If skin findings exceed simple erythema, lesions should be treated with comfort measures, local hygiene, and topical antibiotics for areas with denuded epithelium.
- Supplemental oxygen should be provided for hypoxic or dyspneic patients.
- Beta agonists may be beneficial for patients with clinical evidence of bronchospasm.
- Mechanical ventilation may be required for patients with severe exposures or underlying medical conditions.
- All patients with signs of hypoxemia should be observed in the hospital for 24 hours.

REFERENCES

Blain PG. Tear gases and irritant incapacitants. 1-chloroacetophenone, 2-chlorobenzylidene malononitrile and dibenz[b,f]-1,4-oxazepine. *Toxicol Rev.* 2003;22(2):103-110.

Centers for Disease Control and Prevention, Department of Health and Human Services. *Chemical Emergencies: Riot Control Agent Poisoning.* Washington, DC: Centers for Disease Control and Prevention. Department of Health and Human Services; 2005. Available at: http://www.bt.cdc.gov/agent/riotcontrol/agentpoisoning.asp. Accessed August 23, 2005.

Department of the Army, the Navy, and the Air Force. *Air Force Joint Manual 44-151.* Washington, DC: Department of the Army, the Navy, and the Air Force; 1996.

Department of the Army, the Navy, and the Air Force. *Army Field Manual 8-9.* Washington, DC: Department of the Army, the Navy, and the Air Force; 1996.

Department of the Army, the Navy, and the Air Force. *Navy Medical Publication 5059.* Washington, DC: Department of the Army, the Navy, and the Air Force; 1996.

Department of the Army, the Navy, and the Air Force. *NATO Handbook on the Medical Aspects of NBC Defensive Operations AMedP-6(B).* Washington, DC: Department of the Army, the Navy, and the Air Force; 1996.

NIOSH and Department of Health and Human Services. *National Institute for Occupational Safety and Health (NIOSH) Pocket Guide to Chemical Hazards.* Washington, DC: NIOSH and Department of Health and Human Services. NIOSH Publication No. 97-140; 1997: 60. Available at: http://www.cdc.gov/niosh/npg/npg.html. Accessed September 2, 2005.

CHLOROPICRIN (PS)

SYNONYMS AND TRADE NAMES

Acquinite®, chlor-o-pic, dolochlor, klop, larvacide, microlysin, nitrochloroform, nitrotrichloromethane, picfume, and trichloronitromethane.
(CAS No. 76-06-2)

BACKGROUND

- Chloropicrin (PS) belongs to a class of compounds known as riot-control agents. These chemicals are highly irritating agents usually disseminated as aerosols.
- Chloropicrin's primary use is as a soil fumigant. PS is a colorless liquid with an oily consistency and a strong, pungent odor. It is not soluble in water but is soluble in organic solvents, lipids, organophosphorus substances, mustards, phosgene, diphosgene, and chlorine.
- PS is denser than air, and thus may tend to concentrate in low-lying areas following atmospheric release.
- PS was extensively used in World War I and later stockpiled during World War II. It is potentially more harmful than chlorine, but somewhat less harmful than phosgene, depending on the specifics of the release in question.
- In small quantities, PS may be added to odorless fumigants to act as a warning agent.
- The photochemical decomposition of PS may result in the production and consequent dissemination of phosgene. (See Phosgene).

ROUTINE USE

- PS is no longer authorized for military use, and is predominantly used commercially as a fumigant, insecticide, and sterilizing agent.
- Cereal grains are the only foodstuffs routinely treated with PS.
- Chloropicrin is the fourth most commonly used soil fumigant in California, as it limits nematodes, microorganisms, and weed seeds.

POTENTIAL TERRORIST USE

- Chloropicrin may be harmful by all routes of exposure, making it a potentially important terrorist chemical weapon.
- If released as an aerosol into a confined area, PS may cause transient incapacitation and panic. Release into a closed space would be expected to cause fewer but more severe casualties.
- While many of those exposed in open-air situations would not be expected to sustain serious injury, local emergency response systems and health care facilities may be seriously overwhelmed by a large number of patients.
- Fear and uncertainty among those potentially exposed may cause psychological distress.
- PS is not combustible, but if heated under confinement, it may detonate and explode.
- Agricultural storage and transport of chloropicrin may be targeted as an opportunity to weaponize PS.

MECHANISM OF ACTION

As an oxidizing agent, chloropicrin is capable of reacting with free thiol groups, which then oxidize to disulfide groups, leading to protein alteration and enzyme-system inhibition.

POTENTIAL ROUTES FOR EXPOSURE

Inhalational, ingestion, dermal, and ocular.

TARGET ORGANS/SYSTEMS

Respiratory, mucous membranes, eyes, and skin.

CLINICAL FEATURES

- PS is a strong irritating lacrimator. Its vapors may cause skin, eye, nose, throat, and lung irritation.
- Coughing, a sensation of suffocation, nausea, and vomiting may also result following exposure.
- Methemoglobinemia has also been reported as a result of the strong oxidizing potential of this chemical.
- Following PS exposure, respiratory findings may include hoarseness, chest tightness, dyspnea, tachypnea, wheezing, hypoxemia, and cyanosis.
- Subsequent to the inhalation of PS at high concentrations, lung injury and pulmonary edema may result. Death from acute pulmonary edema has been reported following chloropicrin inhalation.
- Skin contact with PS may result in redness, dermal burns, blisters, or rash.
- Lacrimation, ocular irritation and redness, blurred vision, and corneal burns may also result following PS exposure.
- In addition, a variety of long-term ocular effects (corneal scarring, glaucoma, cataracts), as well as long-term respiratory effects (asthma, chronic pulmonary dysfunction), may occur.

DIAGNOSIS

The diagnosis will require situational recognition consistent with the release of PS in conjunction with examination findings as previously described. This would include a history of exposure obtained from prehospital personnel or the presentation of multiple patients subsequent to exposure to a tear gas-like agent in the field.

LABORATORY TESTING AND IMAGING

- There is no specific test for this agent.
- Patients complaining of dyspnea or who present with hypoxia should be evaluated with chest radiography and pulse oximetry.
- Baseline chest x-rays may be advisable for all patients with substantial exposure.

- At least six hours of close observation are indicated; however, longer periods may be appropriate in order to watch for delayed pulmonary edema.

TREATMENT AND DISPOSITION

- Evacuation and decontamination are the first steps to treatment.
- Exposed clothing should be removed and the skin cleansed.
- Eyes should be liberally irrigated with sterile saline or Lactated Ringers solution.
- PS is insoluble in water and should be removed with soap and a weakly alkaline solution.
- Vesicated skin should be washed with saline only. PS is slowly hydrolyzed in water, and is only removed and not inactivated by washing. Therefore, decontamination effluent should be kept out of contact with patients and health care providers.
- Patients should be screened for corneal abrasions and, if found, these lesions should be treated with analgesics and topical antibiotics.
- If skin findings exceed simple erythema, lesions should be treated with comfort measures, local hygiene, and topical antibiotics for areas with denuded epithelium.
- Supplemental oxygen should be provided for hypoxic or dyspneic patients.
- Beta agonists may be beneficial for patients with clinical evidence of bronchospasm.
- Mechanical ventilation may be required for those with severe exposures or underlying medical conditions.
- All patients with signs of hypoxemia should be observed in the hospital for a minimum of 24 hours.

REFERENCES

Centers for Disease Control and Prevention. CDC Chemical Emergencies Fact Sheet Interim Document: Facts About Riot Control Agents. 2005. Available at: http://www.bt.cdc.gov/agent/riotcontrol/pdf/riotcontrol_factsheet.pdf. Accessed October 12, 2005.

International Programme on Chemical Safety. *Evaluation of the hazards to consumers resulting from the use of fumigants in the protection of food.* FAO Meeting Report No. PL/1965/10/2; WHO/Food Add/28.65. International Programme on Chemical Safety. 1965. Available at: http://www.inchem.org/documents/jmpr/jmpmono/v65apr05.htm. Accessed October 11, 2005.

U.S. Army Center for Health Promotion and Preventive Medicine. *Detailed Facts about Tear Agent Chloropicrin (PS).* 218-22-1096. Aberdeen Proving Ground, MD: U.S. Army Center for Health Promotion and Preventive Medicine. Available at: http://chppm-www.apgea.army.mil/dts/docs/detps.pdf. Accessed October 11, 2005.

DIBENZOXAZEPINE (CR)

SYNONYMS AND TRADE NAMES

Dibenzo[b,f][1,4]oxazepine; dibenzoxazepine; dibenz(b,f)-1,4-oxazepin; and R (lacrimator). (CAS No. 257-07-8)

BACKGROUND

CR is a micro-particulate solid developed as a riot control agent and typically grouped with other such tear gas agents. It is usually dispersed as an aerosol.

ROUTINE USE

CR is used in the pharmaceutical industry as a parent compound for certain antipsychotic drugs, so stores of this chemical may exist at manufacturing facilities.

POTENTIAL TERRORIST USE

- Terrorists might release CR into crowded areas. This could transiently affect large numbers of people, causing incapacitation and panic. Large releases in confined spaces would be expected to cause fewer but more severe casualties.
- CR is typically deployed as a propelled aerosol when used in personal defense. However, CR deployed by the military or as a potential terrorist weapon would probably use an incendiary device (tear gas bomb or grenade) to disseminate this agent.
- While many of those exposed in open-air scenarios would not be expected to have serious injury, the emergency response system and health care facilities could be overburdened by large numbers of patients.
- In addition, fear and uncertainty among potentially exposed civilians would be expected to create substantial psychological distress.

MECHANISM OF ACTION

Dibenzoxazepine is a potent sensory irritant that affects the eyes, oropharynx, and skin. In higher concentrations, this agent can cause asphyxiation and pulmonary edema.

POTENTIAL ROUTES FOR EXPOSURE

The route of primary concern is inhalation and mucous membrane contact resulting from aerosol dissemination of this agent.

TARGET ORGANS/SYSTEMS

Mucous membranes, eyes, skin, and respiratory tract.

CLINICAL FEATURES

- Burning of eyes and lacrimation occur almost immediately following exposure.
- Throat irritation and coughing are accompanied by itching, pain, irritation, and redness of the skin.
- As exposure time and concentration of the agent increase, the lower respiratory tract can be affected and damage to the previously mentioned organ systems can become permanent.
- Corneal ulceration, blindness, glaucoma, and possibly asthma have been reported as long-term sequelae of CR exposure.
- Eye and respiratory irritation occurs at concentrations of 0.002 mg/m^3 to 0.004 mg/m^3, and incapacitation occurs at concentrations of 0.7 mg/m^3.
- Other effects of this agent may include nausea, vomiting, and chest tightness, as well as a sensation of suffocation.

DIAGNOSIS

The diagnosis is based on the history of exposure as reported by prehospital personnel or the presentation of multiple patients exposed to a tear gas-like agent in the field.

LABORATORY TESTING AND IMAGING

- There is no specific test for this agent.
- Patients complaining of dyspnea or who present with hypoxia should be evaluated with chest radiography and pulse oximetry.

TREATMENT AND DISPOSITION

- Evacuation and decontamination are the first steps in treatment.
- Exposed clothing should be removed and the skin cleansed.
- Eyes should be liberally irrigated with sterile saline or Lactated Ringers solution.
- CR is not hydrolyzed in water, and therefore is only removed and not inactivated by washing. As such, decontamination effluent should be kept out of contact with patients and health care providers.
- Supplemental oxygen should be provided for hypoxic or dyspneic patients.
- Beta agonists may be beneficial for patients with clinical evidence of bronchospasm.
- Mechanical ventilation may be required for those with severe exposures or underlying medical conditions.

REFERENCES

Centers for Disease Control and Prevention, Department of Health and Human Services. *Chemical Emergencies: Riot Control Agent Poisoning.* Washington, DC: Centers for Disease Control and Prevention, Department of Health and Human Services; 2005. Available at: http://www.bt.cdc.gov/agent/riotcontrol/casedefinition.asp. Accessed September 13, 2005.

Departments of the Army, the Navy, and the Air Force. *Air Force Joint Manual 44-151.* Washington, DC: Departments of the Army, the Navy, and the Air Force; 1996.

Departments of the Army, the Navy, and the Air Force. *Army Field Manual 8-9.* Washington, DC: Departments of the Army, the Navy, and the Air Force; 1996.

Departments of the Army, the Navy, and the Air Force. *NATO Handbook on the Medical Aspects of NBC Defensive Operations AMedP-6(B).* Washington, DC: Departments of the Army, the Navy, and the Air Force; 1996.

Departments of the Army, the Navy, and the Air Force. *Navy Medical Publication 5059.* Washington, DC: Departments of the Army, the Navy, and the Air Force; 1996.

URTICANTS (NETTLE AGENTS)

PHOSGENE OXIME (CHCl₂NO)

SYNONYMS AND TRADE NAMES

Dichloroformoxime and CX. (CAS No. 1794-86-1)

BACKGROUND

- Phosgene oxime (CX) belongs to a class of agents known as urticants or nettle agents. On dermal contact, it produces a profoundly itchy and intensely painful urticarial skin eruption.
- CX does not cause blistering of the skin, and thus is not technically classified as a vesicant.
- As a solid, CX is colorless. As a liquid, it is usually yellow to brown.
- CX has an intensely irritating odor and may act as a corrosive agent when it contacts skin or tissue in high concentrations. In concentrations less than about 8%, CX is relatively harmless; however, at higher concentrations, CX exposure may result in more severe injury than any of the vesicant agents.

ROUTINE USE

- CX does not occur naturally in the environment and finds no uses in industry or commerce.
- CX has been produced exclusively as a chemical warfare agent, although it has never been used during warfare.

POTENTIAL TERRORIST USE

- CX does not occur naturally in the environment and breaks down in soil in less than two hours at moderate temperatures.
- CX degrades and becomes inactive in water within a few days.
- CX vapor, heavier than air, tends to settle and accumulate in low-lying areas.
- It is expected that CX might be used by terrorists by release into the breathable air in spaces where large numbers of people may congregate. Once CX is released into the air, people may be exposed via inhalation and skin or eye contact.
- CX may also be released into potable water supplies; however, the dilutional effects of a large amount of water (such as in a reservoir) would tend to ameliorate adverse effects.
- In addition, CX degrades in water over a relatively brief period (several days). Nonetheless, ingestion or skin contact with water contaminated with CX has the potential to cause serious health effects.
- Terrorists may attempt to contaminate food supplies with CX liquid, and people may be exposed by eating contaminated food.

MECHANISM OF ACTION

The specific mechanisms associated with the production of adverse health effects have not yet been determined.

POTENTIAL ROUTES FOR EXPOSURE

Dermal contact, ocular contact, inhalation, and ingestion.

TARGET ORGANS/SYSTEMS

Skin, lungs, eyes, and gastrointestinal tract.

CLINICAL FEATURES

- Signs and symptoms occur immediately following contact with CX.
- On dermal exposure, intense and extreme pain and severe itching occur within seconds and are usually associated with blanching of the affected skin surrounded by circular erythema.
- The erythema develops within less than 60 seconds.
- Urticarial eruptions then follow within about 15 minutes.
- After 24 hours, the whitened areas of skin become brown and necrotic, followed by eschar formation.

- Itching and intense pain may continue for days to weeks following initial exposure.
- Subsequent to ocular exposure, corneal damage may result with severe pain, conjunctivitis, tearing, and temporary or permanent blindness.
- Following inhalational exposure, immediate irritation to the upper respiratory tract results and is manifested by runny nose, hoarseness, and sinus pain.
- Noncardiogenic pulmonary edema may develop following inhalational exposure. Noncardiogenic pulmonary edema may also result following substantial skin or ocular exposure.
- Inhalational exposure to high concentrations of CX may result in death.
- There are no data regarding the effects of CX ingestion in humans; however, studies in animals indicate that hemorrhagic inflammatory lesions in the GI tract may result following ingestion.
- There are no data regarding long-term health effects in humans following CX exposure.

DIAGNOSIS

- The diagnosis of CX exposure depends on situational recognition as well as identification of the clinical effects in conjunction with reports from prehospital personnel who may be aware of CX release at a given incident site.
- CX must be considered, when a large number of people present after a chemical exosure with immediate burning, irritation, and severe pain, followed by wheal-like skin lesions and with associated ocular and airway symptoms.

LABORATORY TESTING AND IMAGING

There is no specific laboratory assay to confirm or exclude exposure to CX.

TREATMENT AND DISPOSITION

- There is no specific antidote for CX.
- Supportive care—with special attention to airway and hemodynamic and cardiac monitoring—is paramount.
- Prehospital treatment begins with the removal of victims from exposure.
- This should be followed by rapid and immediate decontamination with copious amounts of water, and, if available, soap.
- Extreme care must be exercised by first responders and ED personnel as skin or clothing contaminated with CX may cross-contaminate rescuers via off-gassing or direct contact.
- Identify and treat hypotension with fluids and, if needed, direct pressors.
- Administer humidified oxygen, if needed.
- Parenteral opiate/opioid analgesics may be needed for pain control. Pain control may be augmented with sedation using benzodiazepines.
- If the patient begins to seize, administer benzodiazepines.
- If treatment with benzodiazepines fails, administer barbiturates or propofol and consider chemical paralysis, endotracheal intubation, and continuous EEG monitoring.
- Identify and treat electrolyte abnormalities.
- Treat bronchospasm with inhaled beta agonists, such as albuterol, as well as with parenteral or oral steroids.
- Treat arrhythmias, when identified.
- In the event of an ocular exposure, irrigate the eyes with copious amounts of water or saline. The use of a Morgan lens may facilitate this process.
- Skin lesions that become necrotic and ulcerate may require surgical resection and/or skin grafting.

REFERENCES

Agency for Toxic Substances and Disease Registry. *Medical Management Guidelines (MMGs) for Phosgene Oxime (CHCl$_2$NO)*. Atlanta, GA: Agency for Toxic Substances and Disease Registry; 2004. Available at: http://www.atsdr.cdc.gov/MHMI/mmg167.html. Accessed September 22, 2005.

Chemical Casualty Care Division, United States Army Medical Research Institute of Chemical Defense. Vesicants HD, H, L, CX. In: *Medical Management of Chemical Casualties Handbook*, 3rd ed. Aberdeen Proving Ground, MD: Chemical Casualty Care Division, United States Army Medical Research Institute of Chemical Defense; 1999. Available at: http://www.vnh.org/CHEMCASU/04 Vesicants.html. Accessed September 22, 2005.

VESICANTS (BLISTER AGENTS)

LEWISITE (C₂H₂AsCl₃)

LEWISITE ($C_2H_2AsCl_3$)

SYNONYMS AND TRADE NAMES

(2-Chloroethenyl)arsonous dichloride;
2-Chlorovinyldichloroarsine; arsine
(2-Chlorovinyl)dichloro-; arsine, dichloro
(2-Chlorovinyl)-; arsenous dichloride, arsenous
dichloride, (2-chloroethenyl) is a simple name
(2-Chloroethenyl); chlorovinylarsine dichloride;
L; lewisite I; and M-1.
(CAS No. 541-25-3)

BACKGROUND

- Lewisite is a colorless liquid with an oily consistency. It is a vesicant capable of damaging
  the eyes, skin, and airways as a result of direct
  contact.
- First synthesized in 1918, lewisite was never
  used in World War I.
- There is no documented use of lewisite in
  warfare to date, but this agent may be
  stockpiled by some nations today.
- Lewisite reportedly emits a faint odor reminiscent of geraniums. However, this scent is not
  reliable for agent identification.

ROUTINE USE

Lewisite does not occur naturally and has no
known industrial application. It is manufactured
only for use as a military weapon.

POTENTIAL TERRORIST USE

- If used as a terrorist agent, lewisite would be
  expected to be released as a liquid spray into
  large open areas or closed spaces where large
  numbers of people may congregate, either from
  a transport vessel, such as truck or train outfit-
  ted with a dissemination device, or via airplane
  spray (e.g., a crop duster).
- Once the liquid is disseminated, it may
  volatilize and then become a vapor threat.

- Alternatively, terrorists may attempt to contaminate food or water supplies with lewisite.

MECHANISM OF ACTION

- Lewisite is rapidly absorbed via the skin, eyes,
  or respiratory tree.
- Lewisite may also be absorbed into the body by
  ingestion or through open wounds.
- Following absorption, lewisite is distributed
  systemically to essentially all body tissues and
  organs.
- Lewisite contains trivalent arsenic and thus
  combines with thiol groups in a variety of
  enzymes. However, the precise mechanism of
  action of lewisite is undetermined.

POTENTIAL ROUTES FOR EXPOSURE

Dermal, ocular, inhalational, and via open wounds.

TARGET ORGANS/SYSTEMS

Skin, eyes, respiratory tree, and vascular
capillary beds.

CLINICAL FEATURES

- Immediate pain and irritation follow liquid or
  vapor lewisite exposures.
- In less than five minutes following skin contact
  with lewisite, gray-appearing areas of dead
  epithelium are visible.
- This is followed by redness and blister formation, with full lesion development occurring
  over 12 to 18 hours.
- Following ocular contact, eye injury occurs rapidly within minutes. These findings include eye
  pain, intense blepharospasm with lid and conjunctival edema, and iris and corneal injury.
- Airway contact with lewisite causes
  pseudomembrane formation as well as noncardiogenic pulmonary edema.
- Lewisite also causes an increase in capillary
  permeability with consequent intravascular fluid

loss, hypovolemia, and shock. This may result in necrosis of the liver and/or kidneys.

DIAGNOSIS

- The diagnosis is based on the history of exposure in conjunction with the specific clinical findings.
- While differences have been reported between the skin lesions caused by sulfur mustard and those of lewisite, this may be of no diagnostic help.
- The best way to differentiate clinically between sulfur mustard and lewisite is to recognize that lewisite causes immediate pain on contact.

LABORATORY TESTING AND IMAGING

- There are no specific laboratory tests or imaging studies helpful in diagnosing lewisite exposure.
- However, the nonspecific findings of leukocytosis and fever may be expected following exposure.
- Blood levels of arsenic or lewisite will not be available in time to be clinically useful.

TREATMENT AND DISPOSITION

- British anti-lewisite (BAL), also known as dimercaprol, is a partial antidote for lewisite. Early administration may help to ameliorate some of the systemic toxicity associated with lewisite. However, since systemic absorption is so rapid following exposure, BAL in this setting may only be partially effective.
- Very early and thorough decontamination is the only means to prevent or minimize lewisite-related injury. Unfortunately, effective decontamination must be accomplished very quickly, within two to four minutes, which may not be practical.
- Excellent supportive care is a mainstay of treatment for lewisite victims.
- Health care providers may be at risk for cross-contamination from victims.
- Skin blisters should be treated in the same manner as those blisters related to sulfur mustard exposure.
- Ocular exposures must be copiously irrigated with water; topical mydriatics and antibiotics are indicated, and ophthalmologic consultation is essential.

- Supplemental oxygen should be administered based on pulse oximetry measurements or findings of respiratory distress.
- Bronchodilators may be helpful if bronchospasm is identified.
- Prophylactic antibiotics should not be administered.
- Antibiotic therapy should be guided by clinical findings and culture and sensitivity lab results.
- Endotracheal intubation should be performed early.
- Minimally injured patients may be discharged, but close follow-up is essential.
- Patients with large areas of vesication, hypotension, hypoxemia, respiratory distress, and/or signs of systemic effects should be admitted to the hospital for observation, continuing care, and BAL administration.

REFERENCES

Chemical Casualty Care Division, United States Army Medical Research Institute of Chemical Defense. Vesicants HD, H, L, CX. In: *Medical Management of Chemical Casualties Handbook*. 3rd ed. Aberdeen Proving Ground, MD: Chemical Casualty Care Division, United States Army Medical Research Institute of Chemical Defense; 1999. Available at: http://www.vnh.org/CHEMCASU/04Vesicants.html. Accessed September 27, 2005.

SULFUR MUSTARD ($C_4H_8Cl_2S$)

SYNONYMS AND TRADE NAMES

Bis(2-chloroethyl)sulfide, bis(beta-chloroethyl)sulfide, dichlorodiethyl sulfide, distilled mustard, HD, iprit, mustard gas, senfgas, yellow cross gas, yellow cross liquid, and yperite.
(CAS No. 505-60-2)

BACKGROUND

- Sulfur mustard was first synthesized in the early 1800s. It was used as a chemical warfare agent in World War I on July 12, 1917, during a battle near Ypres, Belgium.
- Sulfur mustard does not occur naturally.
- Once used in the treatment of psoriasis, sulfur mustard has also been investigated as an antineoplastic agent, but it currently does not have

any medical or industrial applications.

- Sulfur mustard is generally described as a colorless, oily liquid at ambient temperatures. Some suggest that it has an odor resembling garlic, onions, or mustard.
- Sulfur mustard is not readily vaporized, but when this occurs, the vapor is heavier than air and accumulates in low-lying areas.

ROUTINE USE

Sulfur mustard does not occur naturally and is not used other than as a chemical warfare agent.

POTENTIAL TERRORIST USE

If used as a terrorist weapon, sulfur mustard would be expected to be released either as a liquid sprayed onto a population, presumably via an incendiary device or as a gas—the dispersal method used during World War I.

MECHANISM OF ACTION

- Sulfur mustard is a vesicant and alkylating agent that binds with DNA and key cellular proteins.
- One theory is that cell death is due to nicotinamide adenine dinucleotide (NAD) depletion, which eventually results in the release of proteases and causes cell death.
- Another theory is that cell death is secondary to glutathione depletion, which in turn results in free radical damage, lipid peroxidation, and eventually cell death.
- Sulfur mustard is also a known carcinogen.

POTENTIAL ROUTES FOR EXPOSURE

Inhalational, dermal, ingestion, and ocular.

TARGET ORGANS/SYSTEMS

Dermal, ocular, pulmonary, hematopoetic, CNS, and gastrointestinal.

CLINICAL FEATURES

- Sulfur mustard may affect virtually every part of the body.

- After an ocular exposure, a victim may initially experience a foreign body sensation, such as grittiness in the eyes, approximately one hour after the exposure.
- This is often followed by soreness and redness, then swelling.
- Two to six hours after an ocular exposure, the victim may experience eye pain, tearing, photophobia, and blindness that may be temporary or permanent.
- There may be vesication of the corneal epithelium, followed by its sloughing.
- Corneal opacification and ulcers have been reported, as has recurrent keratitis.
- Skin exposure to sulfur mustard or mustard gas generally results in blister formation. These blisters often resemble second-degree burns and are yellow in color. They are generally not painful. These blisters may not manifest for up to 24 hours after the exposure. They generally heal in four to six weeks.
- After an inhalational exposure, the victim may experience airway irritation and possibly pulmonary edema. Further chronic pulmonary effects, such as chronic bronchitis, asthma, pulmonary fibrosis, and tracheal and bronchial stenosis as a result of scar tissue formation, have been reported.
- Additionally, cancer of the lung, pharynx, and larynx has been associated with sulfur mustard exposure.
- One of the greatest concerns surrounding sulfur mustard is its hematopoietic effect. Leukopenia, thrombocytopenia, and anemia have been reported after sulfur mustard and mustard gas exposure. Leukopenia often starts three to four days after exposure, with a nadir approximately nine days after exposure. This carries associated risks, such as sepsis and opportunistic infections that may not be seen in a normally immunocompetent individual.
- Further effects after exposure to either sulfur mustard or mustard gas may include nausea, vomiting, diarrhea, and abdominal pain.
- Additionally, victims may experience dizziness, malaise, and lethargy.

DIAGNOSIS

The diagnosis is based on the history of exposure in conjunction with the specific clinical findings.

LABORATORY TESTING AND IMAGING

- Mustard or its metabolite thiodiglycol may be detected in the urine one week after an exposure to sulfur mustard.
- Additionally, beta-lyase metabolites of sulfur mustard, which are formed as a result of sulfur mustard combining with glutathione, may be detected in the exposed person's urine.
- It is unlikely that these laboratory studies will be of any clinical value.
- Patients who are exposed to sulfur mustard should have a baseline CBC drawn immediately after the exposure, if possible. The patient's blood counts may need to be monitored for at least two weeks after the exposure to look for evidence of bone marrow suppression.
- Other routine lab studies should be considered as clinically warranted after an acute exposure. Patients with respiratory complaints should have a chest x-ray performed.

TREATMENT AND DISPOSITION

- There is no specific antidote for sulfur mustard poisoning.
- Removal from the source is of utmost importance, as is complete decontamination by washing the skin with water.
- Some authors suggest that a dilute sodium hypochlorite solution may be of benefit.

- Other authors suggest that washing with a 2.5% sodium thiosulfate solution may also be beneficial, although evidence is lacking.
- After an ocular exposure, the eyes should be rinsed thoroughly with water or Lactated Ringers solution. This process may be facilitated by use of a Morgan lens.
- Supportive care remains the mainstay of treatment.
- Administer oxygen if needed.
- Treat hypotension with fluids and, if needed, pressors.
- Treat bronchospasm with inhaled beta agonists.
- Some authors recommend 1 mg/kg to 500mg/kg of sodium thiosulfate IV; however, evidence is lacking for the effectiveness of this measure.
- RBC and platelet transfusion may be necessary in the event of bone marrow suppression.
- There may also be a role for granulocyte colony stimulating factor and bone marrow transplant, but further studies must be done.
- Some authors recommend unroofing all blisters greater than 2 cm in diameter.
- Patients with more than mild exposures may need to be admitted/transferred to a burn unit.
- All patients exposed to sulfur mustard must have continuous physician follow-up for monitoring of blood counts.

REFERENCES

Agency for Toxic Substances and Disease Registry. *Medical Management Guidelines for Blister Agents: Sulfur Mustard Agent H or HD* ($C_4H_8Cl_2S$) and Sulfur Mustard Agent HT. Atlanta, GA: Agency for Toxic Substances and Disease Registry; 2004. Available at: http://www.atsdr.cdc.gov/MHMI/mmg165.html. Accessed October 11, 2005.

Balali-Mood M, Hefazi M. The pharmacology, toxicology, and medical treatment of sulphur mustard poisoning. *Fundam Clin Pharmacol.* 2005;19(3):297-315.

MEDICAL MANAGEMENT IN AN INCENDIARY ATTACK

ABC OF BURNS

INITIAL MANAGEMENT OF A MAJOR BURN: I—OVERVIEW

A major burn is defined as a burn covering 25% or more of total body surface area, but any injury over more than 10% should be treated similarly. Rapid assessment is vital. The general approach to a major burn can be extrapolated to managing any burn. The most important points are to take an accurate history and make a detailed examination of the patient and the burn, to ensure that key information is not missed.

This article outlines the structure of the initial assessment. The next article will cover the detailed assessment of burn surface area and depth and how to calculate the fluid resuscitation formula.

HISTORY TAKING

The history of a burn injury can give valuable information about the nature and extent of the burn, the likelihood of inhalational injury, the depth of burn, and probability of other injuries. The exact mechanism of injury and any prehospital treatment must be established. A patient's history must be obtained on admission, as this may be the only time that a first hand history is obtainable. Swelling may develop around the airway in the hours after injury and require intubation, making it impossible for the patient to give a verbal history. A brief medical history should be taken, outlining previous medical problems, medications, allergies, and vaccinations. Patients' smoking habits should be determined as these may affect blood gas analyses.

INITIAL ASSESSMENT OF A MAJOR BURN

- Perform an ABCDEF primary survey
  A—Airway with cervical spine control,
  B—Breathing
  C—Circulation
  D—Neurological disability
  E—Exposure with environmental control
  F—Fluid resuscitation
- Assess burn size and depth (see later article for detail)
- Establish good intravenous access and give fluids
- Give analgesia
- Catheterize patient or establish fluid balance monitoring
- Take baseline blood samples for investigation
- Dress wound
- Perform secondary survey, reassess, and exclude or treat associated injuries
- Arrange safe transfer to specialist burns facility

PRIMARY SURVEY

The initial management of a severely burnt patient is similar to that of any trauma patient. A modified "advanced trauma life support" primary survey is performed, with particular emphasis on assessment of the airway and breathing. The burn injury must not distract from this sequential assessment, otherwise serious associated injuries may be missed.

KEY POINTS OF A BURN HISTORY

Exact mechanism
- Type of burn agent (scald, flame, electrical, chemical)
- How did it come into contact with patient?
- What first aid was performed?
- What treatment has been started?
- Is there risk of concomitant injuries (such as fall from height, road traffic crash, explosion)?
- Is there risk of inhalational injuries (did burn occur in an enclosed space)?

Exact timings
- When did the injury occur?
- How long was patient exposed to energy source?
- How long was cooling applied?
- When was fluid resuscitation started?

Exact injury
Scalds
- What was the liquid? Was it boiling or recently boiled?
- If tea or coffee, was milk in it?
- Was a solute in the liquid? (Raises boiling temperature and causes worse injury, such as boiling rice)

Electrocution injuries
- What was the voltage (domestic or industrial)?
- Was there a flash or arcing?
- Contact time

Chemical injuries
- What was the chemical?

Is there any suspicion of non-accidental injury?

A—AIRWAY WITH CERVICAL SPINE CONTROL

An assessment must be made as to whether the airway is compromised or is at risk of compromise.

The cervical spine should be protected unless it is definitely not injured. Inhalation of hot gases will result in a burn above the vocal cords. This burn will become edematous over the following hours, especially after fluid resuscitation has begun. This means that an airway that is patent on arrival at hospital may occlude after admission. This can be a particular problem in small children. Direct inspection of the oropharynx should be done by a senior anesthetist. If there is any concern about the patency of the airway then intubation is the safest policy. However, an unnecessary intubation and sedation could worsen a patient's condition, so the decision to intubate should be made carefully.

AIRWAY MANAGEMENT

Signs of inhalational injury
- History of flame burns or burns in an enclosed space
- Full thickness or deep dermal burns to face, neck, or upper torso
- Singed nasal hair
- Carbonaceous sputum or carbon particles in oropharynx

Indications for intubation
- Erythema or swelling of oropharynx on direct visualization
- Change in voice, with hoarseness or harsh cough
- Stridor, tachypnea, or dyspnea

B—BREATHING

All burn patients should receive 100% oxygen through a humidified non-rebreathing mask on presentation. Breathing problems are considered to be those that affect the respiratory system below the vocal cords. There are several ways that a burn injury can compromise respiration.

Mechanical restriction of breathing—Deep dermal or full thickness circumferential burns of the chest can limit chest excursion and prevent adequate ventilation. This may require escharotomies (see **article 2**).

Signs of Carboxyhemoglobinemia

COHb levels	Symptoms
0-10%	Minimal (normal level in heavy smokers)
10-20%	Nausea, headache
20-30%	Drowsiness, lethargy
30-40%	Confusion, agitation
40-50%	Coma, respiratory depression
>50%	Death

COHb = Carboxyhemoglobin

Blast injury—If there has been an explosion, blast lung can complicate ventilation. Penetrating injuries can cause tension pneumothoraces, and the blast itself can cause lung contusions and alveolar trauma and lead to adult respiratory distress syndrome.

Smoke inhalation—The products of combustion, though cooled by the time they reach the lungs, act as direct irritants to the lungs, leading to bronchospasm, inflammation, and bronchorrhea. The ciliary action of pneumocytes is impaired, exacerbating the situation. The inflammatory exudate created is not cleared, and atelectasis or pneumonia follows. The situation can be particularly severe in asthmatic patients. Noninvasive management can be attempted, with nebulizers and positive pressure ventilation with some positive end-expiratory pressure. However, patients may need a period of ventilation, as this allows adequate oxygenation and permits regular lung toileting.

Carboxyhemoglobin—Carbon monoxide binds to deoxyhemoglobin with 40 times the affinity of oxygen. It also binds to intracellular proteins, particularly the cytochrome oxidase pathway. These two effects lead to intracellular and extracellular hypoxia. Pulse oximetry cannot differentiate between oxyhemoglobin and carboxyhemoglobin, and may therefore give normal results. However, blood gas analysis will reveal metabolic acidosis and raised carboxyhemoglobin levels but may not show hypoxia. Treatment is with 100% oxygen, which displaces carbon monoxide from bound proteins six times faster than does atmospheric oxygen. Patients with carboxyhemoglobin levels greater than 25-30% should be ventilated. Hyperbaric therapy is rarely practical and has not been proved to be advantageous. It takes longer to shift the carbon monoxide from the cytochrome oxidase pathway than from hemoglobin, so oxygen therapy should be continued until the metabolic acidosis has cleared.

C—CIRCULATION

Intravenous access should be established with two large bore cannulas preferably placed through unburnt tissue. This is an opportunity to take blood for checking full blood count, urea and electrolytes, blood group, and clotting screen. Peripheral circulation must be checked. Any deep or full thickness circumferential extremity burn can act as a tourniquet, especially once edema develops after fluid resuscitation. This may not occur until some hours after the burn. If there is any suspicion of decreased perfusion due to circumferential burn, the tissue must be released with escharotomies (see next article). Profound hypovolemia is not the normal initial response to a burn. If a patient is hypotensive then it is may be due to delayed presentation, cardiogenic dysfunction, or an occult source of blood loss (chest, abdomen, or pelvis).

D—NEUROLOGICAL DISABILITY

All patients should be assessed for responsiveness with the Glasgow coma scale; they may be confused because of hypoxia or hypovolemia.

E—EXPOSURE WITH ENVIRONMENT CONTROL

The whole of a patient should be examined (including the back) to get an accurate estimate of the

Algorithm for Primary Survey of a Major Burn Injury.

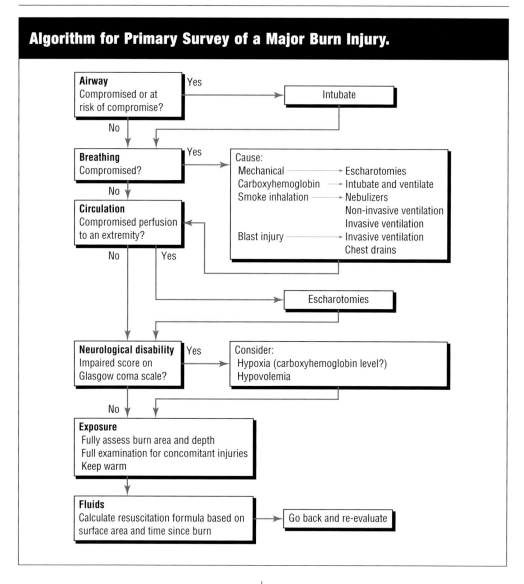

burn area and to check for any concomitant injuries. Burn patients, especially children, easily become hypothermic. This will lead to hypoperfusion and deepening of burn wounds. Patients should be covered and warmed as soon as possible.

F—FLUID RESUSCITATION

The resuscitation regimen should be determined and begun. This is based on the estimation of the burn area, and the detailed calculation is covered in the next article. A urinary catheter is mandatory in all adults with injuries covering >20% of total body surface area to monitor urine output. Children's urine output can be monitored with external catchment devices or by weighing nappies provided the injury is <20% of total body area. In children the interosseous route can be used for fluid administration if intravenous access cannot be obtained, but should be replaced by intravenous lines as soon as possible.

ANALGESIA

Superficial burns can be extremely painful. All patients with large burns should receive intravenous morphine at a dose appropriate to body weight. This can be easily titrated against pain and respiratory depression. The need for further doses should be assessed within 30 minutes.

INVESTIGATIONS

The amount of investigations will vary with the type of burn.

INVESTIGATIONS FOR MAJOR BURNS*

General
- Full blood count, packed cell volume, urea and electrolyte concentration, clotting screen
- Blood group, and save or crossmatch serum

Electrical injuries
- 12 lead electrocardiography
- Cardiac enzymes (for high tension injuries)

Inhalational injuries
- Chest x ray
- Arterial blood gas analysis
  Can be useful in any burn, as the base excess is predictive of the amount of fluid resuscitation required
  Helpful for determining success of fluid resuscitation and essential with inhalational injuries or exposure to carbon monoxide

*Any concomitant trauma will have its own investigations

SECONDARY SURVEY

At the end of the primary survey and the start of emergency management, a secondary survey should be performed. This is a head to toe examination to look for any concomitant injuries.

DRESSING THE WOUND

Once the surface area and depth of a burn have been estimated, the burn wound should be washed and any loose skin removed. Blisters should be deroofed for ease of dressing, except for palmar blisters (painful), unless these are large enough to restrict movement. The burn should then be dressed. For an acute burn which will be referred to a burn centre, cling film is an ideal dressing as it protects the wound, reduces heat and evaporative losses, and does not alter the wound appearance. This will permit accurate evaluation by the burn team later. Flamazine should not be used on a burn that is to be referred immediately, since it makes assessment of depth more difficult.

INDICATIONS FOR REFERRAL TO A BURNS UNIT

All complex injuries should be referred

A burn injury is more likely to be complex if associated with:
- Extremes of age—under 5 or over 60 years
- Site of injury
  - Face, hands, or perineum
  - Feet (dermal or full thickness loss)
  - Any flexure, particularly the neck or axilla
  - Circumferential dermal or full thickness burn of limb, torso, or neck
- Inhalational injury
  - Any substantial injury, excluding pure carbon monoxide poisoning
- Mechanism of injury
  - Chemical injury >5% of total body surface area
  - Exposure to ionizing radiation
  - High pressure steam injury
  - High tension electrical injury
  - Hydrofluoric acid burn >1% of total body surface area
  - Suspicion of nonaccidental injury
- Large size (dermal or full thickness loss)
  - Pediatric (<16 years old) >5% of total body surface area
  - Adult (≥16 years) >10% of total body surface area
- Coexisting conditions
  Any serious medical conditions (cardiac dysfunction, immunosuppression, pregnancy)
  Any associated injuries (fractures, head injuries, crush injuries)

REFERRAL TO A BURNS UNIT

The National Burn Care Review has established referral guidelines to specialist units. Burns are divided into complex burns (those that require specialist intervention) and non-complex burns (those that do not require immediate admission to a specialist unit). Complex burns should be referred automatically. If you are not sure whether a burn should be referred, discuss the case with your local burns unit. It is also important to discuss all burns that are not healed within two weeks. [Editor's note: The preceding is based on information from the British Burns Association. U.S.-based healthcare providers should use similar criteria for determining when to refer a burn victim.)

KEY POINTS

- Perform a systematic assessment as with any trauma patient (don't get distracted by the burn)
- Beware of airway compromise
- Provide adequate analgesia
- Exclude any concomitant injuries
- Discuss with a burns unit early
- If in doubt, reassess

FURTHER READING

- Sheridan R. Burns. *Crit Care Med* 2002;30:S500-514
- British Burn Association. Emergency management of severe burns course manual, UK version. Wythenshawe Hospital, Manchester, 1996
- Herndon D. *Total burn care*. 2nd ed. London: WB Saunders, 2002
- Kao CC, Garner WL. Acute burns. *Plast Reconstr Surg* 2000;105:2482-2493
- Burnsurgery.org. *www.burnsurgery.org*

Shehan Hettiaratchy is specialist registrar in plastic and reconstructive surgery, Pan-Thames Training Scheme, London; Remo Papini is consultant and clinical lead in burns, West Midlands Regional Burn Unit, Selly Oak University Hospital, Birmingham. The ABC of burns is edited by Shehan Hettiaratchy; Remo Papini; and Peter Dziewulski, consultant burns and plastic surgeon, St. Andrews Centre for Plastic Surgery and Burns, Broomfield Hospital, Chelmsford.

Competing interests: RP has been reimbursed by Johnson & Johnson, manufacturer of Integra, and Smith & Nephew, manufacturer of Acticoat and TransCyte, for attending symposia on burn care.

Source: *BMJ.* Shehan Hettiaratchy and Remo Papini 2004;328;1555-1557. Reprinted with permission.

ABCs of Burns

INITIAL MANAGEMENT OF A MAJOR BURN: II—ASSESSMENT AND RESUSCITATION

ASSESSMENT OF BURN AREA

Assessment of burn area tends to be done badly, even by those who are expert at it. There are three commonly used methods of estimating burn area, and each has a role in different scenarios. When calculating burn area, erythema should not be included. This may take a few hours to fade, so some overestimation is inevitable if the burn is estimated acutely.

Palmar surface—The surface area of a patient's palm (including fingers) is roughly 0.8% of total body surface area. Palmar surface are can be used to estimate relatively small burns (<15% of total surface area) or very large burns (>85%, when unburned skin is counted). For medium sized burns, it is inaccurate.

Wallace Rule of Nines—This is a good, quick way of estimating medium to large burns in adults. The body is divided into areas of 9%, and the total burn area can be calculated. It is not accurate in children.

Lund and Browder chart—This chart, if used correctly, is the most accurate method. It compensates for the variation in body shape with age and therefore can give an accurate assessment of burns area in children.

It is important that all of the burn is exposed and assessed. During assessment, the environment should be kept warm, and small segments of skin exposed sequentially to reduce heat loss. Pigmented skin can be difficult to assess, and in such cases it may be necessary to remove all the loose epidermal layers to calculate burn size.

RESUSCITATION REGIMENS

Fluid losses from the injury must be replaced to maintain homeostasis. There is no ideal resuscitation regimen, and many are in use. All the fluid formulas are only guidelines, and their success relies on adjusting the amount of resuscitation fluid against monitored physiological parameters. The main aim of resuscitation is to maintain tissue perfusion to the zone of stasis and hence prevent the burn deepening. This is not easy, as too little fluid will cause hypoperfusion whereas too much will lead to edema that will cause tissue hypoxia.

The greatest amount of fluid loss in burn patients is in the first 24 hours after injury. For the first eight to 12 hours, there is a general shift of fluid from the intravascular to interstitial fluid compartments. This means that any fluid given during this time will rapidly leave the intravascular compartment. Colloids have no advantage over crystalloids in maintaining circulatory volume. Fast fluid boluses probably have little benefit, as a rapid rise in intravascular hydrostatic pressure will just drive more fluid out of the circulation. However, much protein is lost through the burn wound, so there is a need to replace this oncotic loss. Some resuscitation regimens introduce colloid after the first eight hours, when the loss of fluid from the intravascular space is decreasing.

Burns covering more than 15% of total body surface area in adults and more than 10% in children warrant formal resuscitation. Again these are guidelines, and experienced staff can exercise some discretion either way. The most commonly used resuscitation formula is the Parkland formula, a pure crystalloid formula. It has the advantage of being easy to calculate and the rate is titrated against urine output. This calculates the amount of fluid required in the first 24 hours. Children require maintenance fluid in addition to this. The starting point for resuscitation is the time of injury, not the time of admission. Any fluid already given should be deducted from the calculated requirement.

Wallace Rule Of Nines

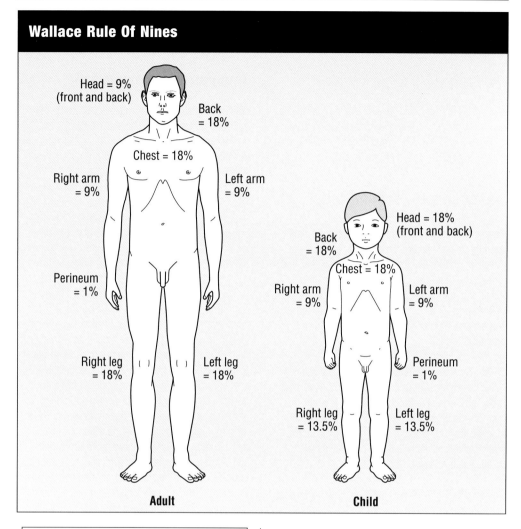

Head = 9%
(front and back)

Back = 18%

Chest = 18%

Right arm = 9%

Left arm = 9%

Perineum = 1%

Right leg = 18%

Left leg = 18%

Adult

Head = 18%
(front and back)

Back = 18%

Chest = 18%

Right arm = 9%

Left arm = 9%

Perineum = 1%

Right leg = 13.5%

Left leg = 13.5%

Child

PARKLAND FORMULA FOR BURNS RESUSCITATION

Total fluid requirement in 24 hours
  4 mL x (total burn surface area (%)) x (body weight (kg))
  50% given in first 8 hours
  50% given in next 16 hours
Children receive maintenance fluid in addition, at hourly rate of
  4 mL/kg for first 10 kg of body weight *plus*
  2 mL/kg for second 10 kg of body weight *plus*
  1 mL/kg for >20 kg of body weight
End point
Urine output of 0.5-1.0 mL/kg/hour in adults
Urine output of 1.0-1.5 mL/kg/hour in children

At the end of 24 hours, colloid infusion is begun at a rate of 0.5 mL x (total burn surface area (%)) x (body weight (kg)), and maintenance crystalloid (usually dextrose-saline) is continued at a rate of 1.5 mL x (burn area) x (body weight). The end point to aim for is a urine output of 0.5-1.0 mL/kg/hour in adults and 1.0-1.5 mL/kg/hour in children.

High tension electrical injuries require substantially more fluid (up to 9 mL x (burn area) x (body weight) in the first 24 hours) and a higher urine output (1.5-2 mL/kg/hour). Inhalational injuries also require more fluid.

In Britain, Hartman's solution (sodium chloride 0.6%, sodium lactate 0.25%, potassium chloride 0.04%, calcium chloride 0.027%) is the most

Lund And Browder Chart

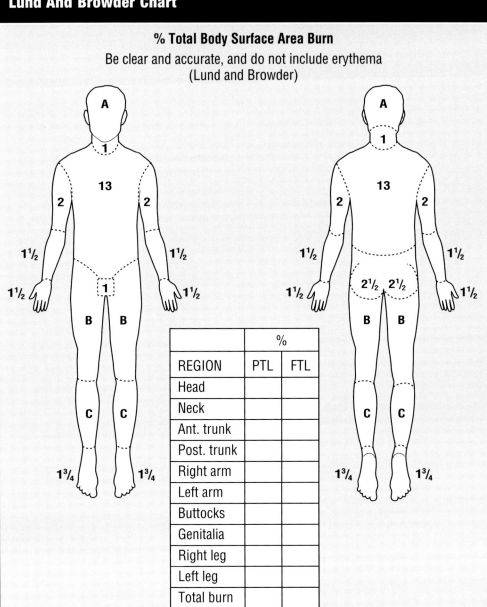

% Total Body Surface Area Burn

Be clear and accurate, and do not include erythema
(Lund and Browder)

	%	
REGION	PTL	FTL
Head		
Neck		
Ant. trunk		
Post. trunk		
Right arm		
Left arm		
Buttocks		
Genitalia		
Right leg		
Left leg		
Total burn		

AREA	Age 0	1	5	10	15	Adult
A = ½ OF HEAD	9½	8½	6½	5½	4½	3½
B = ½ OF ONE THIGH	2¾	3¼	4	4½	4½	4¾
C = ½ OF ONE LOWER LEG	2½	2½	2¾	3	3¼	3½

Worked examples of burns resuscitation

Fluid resuscitation regimen for an adult

A 25-year-old man weighing 70 kg with a 30% flame burn was admitted at 4 pm. His burn occurred at 3 pm.

1) Total fluid requirement for first 24 hours

4 mL×(30% total burn surface area)×(70 kg) = 8400 mL in 24 hours

2) Half to be given in first 8 hours, half over the next 16 hours

Will receive 4200 mL during 0-8 hours and 4200 mL during 8-24 hours

3) Subtract any fluid already received from amount required for first 8 hours

Has already received 1000 mL from emergency services, and so needs further 3200 mL in first 8 hours after injury

4) Calculate hourly infusion rate for first 8 hours

Divide amount of fluid calculated in (3) by time left until it is 8 hours after burn

Burn occurred at 3 pm, so 8 hour point is 11 pm. It is now 4 pm, so need 3200 mL over next 7 hours:
3200/7 = 457 mL/hour from 4 pm to 11 pm

5) Calculate hourly infusion rate for next 16 hours

Divide figure in (2) by 16 to give fluid infusion rate
Needs 4200 mL over 16 hours: 4200/16 = 262.5 mL/hour from 11 pm to 3 pm next day

Maintenance fluid required for a child

A 24 kg child with a resuscitation burn will need the following maintenance fluid:
4 mL/kg/hour for first 10 kg of weight = 40 mL/hour *plus*
2 mL/kg/hour for next 10 kg of weight = 20 mL/hour *plus*
1 mL/kg/hour for next 4 kg of weight = 1×4 kg = 4 mL/hour
Total = 64 mL/hour

commonly used crystalloid. Colloid use is controversial: some units introduce colloid after eight hours, as the capillary leak begins to shut down, whereas others wait until 24 hours. Fresh frozen plasma is often used in children, and albumin or synthetic high molecular weight starches are used in adults.

The above regimens are merely guidelines to the probable amount of fluid required. This should be continuously adjusted according to urine output and other physiological parameters (pulse, blood pressure, and respiratory rate). Investigations at intervals of four to six hours are mandatory for monitoring a patient's resuscitation status. These include packed cell volume, plasma sodium,

base excess, and lactate. Burns units use different resuscitation formulas, and it is best to contact the local unit for advice.

ESCHAROTOMIES

A circumferential deep dermal or full thickness burn is inelastic and on an extremity will not stretch. Fluid resuscitation leads to the development of burn wound edema and swelling of the tissue beneath this inelastic burnt tissue. Tissue pressures rise and can impair peripheral circulation. Circumferential chest burns can also cause problems by limiting chest excursion and impairing ventilation. Both of these situations require escharotomy, division of the burn eschar. Only the burnt tissue is divided, not any underlying fascia, differentiating this procedure from a fasciotomy.

Incisions are made along the midlateral or medial aspects of the limbs, avoiding any underlying structures. For the chest, longitudinal incisions are made down each mid-axillary line to the subcostal region. The lines are joined up by a chevron incision running parallel to the subcostal margin. This creates a mobile breastplate that moves with ventilation. Escharotomies are best done with electrocautery, as they tend to bleed. They are then packed with Kaltostat alginate dressing and dressed with the burn.

Although they are an urgent procedure, escharotomies are best done in an operating room by experienced staff. They should be discussed with the local burns unit, and performed under instruction only when transfer is delayed

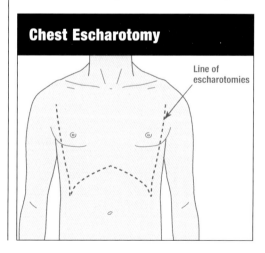

Chest Escharotomy

Line of escharotomies

by several hours. Initially, at risk limbs should be elevated and observed.

ASSESSMENT OF BURN DEPTH

The depth of burn is related to the amount of energy delivered in the injury and to the relative thickness of the skin (the dermis is thinner in very young and very old people).

CLASSIFICATION OF BURN DEPTHS

Burns are classified into two groups by the amount of skin loss. Partial thickness burns do not extend through all skin layers, whereas full thickness burns extend through all skin layers into the subcutaneous tissues. Partial thickness burns can be further divided into superficial, superficial dermal, and deep dermal (see diagram on next page):

- Superficial—The burn affects the epidermis but not the dermis (such as sunburn). It is often called an epidermal burn
- Superficial dermal—The burn extends through the epidermis into the upper layers of the dermis and is associated with blistering
- Deep dermal—The burn extends through the epidermis into the deeper layers of the dermis but not through the entire dermis.

ESTIMATION OF BURN DEPTH

Assessing burn depth can be difficult. The patient's history will give clues to the expected depth: a flash burn is likely to be superficial, whereas a burn from a flame that was not rapidly extinguished will probably be deep. On direct examination, there are four elements that should be assessed—bleeding on needle prick, sensation, appearance, and blanching to pressure.

Bleeding—Test bleeding with a 21-gauge needle. Brisk bleeding on superficial pricking indicates the burn is superficial or superficial dermal. Delayed bleeding on a deeper prick suggests a deep dermal burn, while no bleeding suggests a full thickness burn.

Sensation—Test sensation with a needle also. Pain equates with a superficial or superficial dermal burn, non-painful sensation equates with deep dermal injury, while full thickness injuries are insensate. However, this test is often inaccurate as edema also blunts sensation.

Appearance and blanching—Assessing burn depth by appearance is often difficult as burns may be covered with soot or dirt. Blisters should be de-roofed to assess the base. Capillary refill should be assessed by pressing with a sterile cotton bud (such as a bacteriology swab):

- A red, moist wound that obviously blanches and then rapidly refills is superficial
- A pale, dry but blanching wound that regains its color slowly is superficial dermal
- Deep dermal injuries have a mottled cherry red color that does not blanch (fixed capillary staining). The blood is fixed within damaged capillaries in the deep dermal plexus
- A dry, leathery or waxy, hard wound that does not blanch is full thickness. With extensive burns, full thickness burns can often be mistaken for unburned skin in appearance.

Most burns are a mixture of different depths. Assessment of depth is important for planning treatment, as more superficial burns tend to heal spontaneously whereas deeper burns need

Assessment of Burn Depth

	Burn type			
	Superficial	Superficial dermal	Deep dermal	Full thickness
Bleeding on pin prick	Brisk	Brisk	Delayed	None
Sensation	Painful	Painful	Dull	None
Appearance	Red, glistening	Dry, whiter	Cherry red	Dry, white, leathery
Blanching to pressure	Yes, brisk return	Yes, slow return	No	No

Diagram of Burn Depths

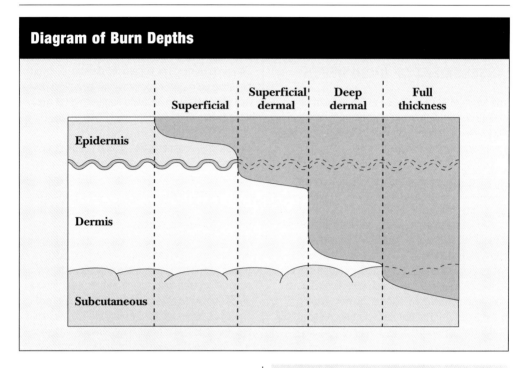

surgical intervention, but is not necessary for calculating resuscitation formulas. Therefore, in acute situations lengthy depth assessment is inappropriate. A burn is a dynamic wound, and its depth will change depending on the effectiveness of resuscitation. Initial estimates need to be reviewed later.

KEY POINTS

- Accurate assessment of burn area is crucial to calculate resuscitation formula
- Resuscitation formulas are only guidelines—monitor the patient
- Discuss resuscitation with a burns unit
- Be aware of the need for escharotomies
- Burn depth is difficult to estimate and changes with resuscitation

FURTHER INFORMATION

Clarke J. Burns. *Br Med Bull* 1999;55:885-94

Herndon D. *Total burn care.* 2nd ed. London: WB Saunders, 2002

Kao CC, Garner WL. Acute burns. *Plast Reconstr Surg* 2000;105:2482{93

Yowler CJ, Fratianne RB. The current status of burn resuscitation. *Clin Plast Surg* 2000;1:1-9

Collis N, Smith G, Fenton OM. Accuracy of burn size estimation and subsequent fluid resuscitation prior to arrival at the Yorkshire Regional Burns Unit. A three-year retrospective study. *Burns* 1999;25: 345-51 Burnsurgery.org (see *www.burnsurgery.org*)

Shehan Hettiaratchy is specialist registrar in plastic and reconstructive surgery, Pan-Thames Training Scheme, London; Remo Papini is consultant and clinical lead in burns, West Midlands Regional Burn Unit, Selly Oak University Hospital, Birmingham. The ABC of burns is edited by Shehan Hettiaratchy; Remo Papini; and Peter Dziewulski, consultant burns and plastic surgeon, St. Andrews Centre for Plastic Surgery and Burns, Broomfield Hospital, Chelmsford.

Competing interests: RP has been reimbursed by Johnson & Johnson, manufacturer of Integra, and Smith & Nephew, manufacturer of Acticoat and TransCyte, for attending symposiums on burn care.

Source: *BMJ.* Shehan Hettiaratchy and Remo Papini 2004;329;101-103. Reprinted with permission.

ABC OF BURNS

INTENSIVE CARE MANAGEMENT AND CONTROL OF INFECTION

INTENSIVE CARE MANAGEMENT

The goal in management of an acute burn is to limit the extent of the systemic insult. Intensive care management should not be seen as rescue for failed initial treatment but as a preventive measure in patients at high risk of organ failure. Intensive care units have the resources for improved monitoring and expertise in managing acute physiological changes. Intensive care management should not, however, become an obstacle to early aggressive surgical excision of the burn wound, which is associated with improved outcome.

AIRWAY BURNS

The term "inhalational injury" has been used to describe the aspiration of toxic products of combustion, but also more generally any pulmonary insult associated with a burn injury. Patients with cutaneous burns are two to three times more likely to die if they also have lower airway burns. Death may be a direct result of lung injury but is usually due to the systemic consequences of such injury. It may be impossible to distinguish lung injury caused at the time of the burn directly to the lungs by a burn from injury due to the systemic consequences of the burn.

Diagnosis of lower airway burns is largely based on the patient's history and clinical examination. Clinicians should have a high index of suspicion of airway burns in patients with one or more of the warning signs. Special investigations will support clinical suspicion. However, severity of injury or prediction of outcome is not aided by additional tests.

WARNING SIGNS OF AIRWAY BURNS
Suspect airway burn if:
- Burns occurred in an enclosed space
- Stridor, hoarseness, or cough
- Burns to face, lips, mouth, pharynx, or nasal mucosa
- Soot in sputum, nose, or mouth
- Dyspnea, decreased level of consciousness, or confusion
- Hypoxemia (low pulse oximetry saturation or arterial oxygen tension) or increased carbon monoxide levels (>2%)

Onset of symptoms may be delayed

The pathophysiology of airway burns is highly variable, depending on the environment of the burn and the incomplete products of combustion. The clinical manifestations are often delayed for the first few hours but are usually apparent by 24 hours. Airway debris—including secretions, mucosal slough, and smoke residue—can seriously compromise pulmonary function.

There is no specific treatment for airway burns other than ensuring adequate oxygenation and minimizing iatrogenic lung insult. Prophylactic corticosteroids or antibiotics have no role in treatment.

Control of the airway, by endotracheal intubation, is essential before transporting any patient with suspected airway burn. Rapid fluid administration, with inevitable formation of edema, may lead to life threatening airway compromise if control of the airway is delayed. Endotracheal intubation before edema formation is far safer and simpler. Oxygen (100%) should be given until the risk of carbon monoxide toxicity has been excluded, since high concentrations of oxygen will clear carbon monoxide from the body more rapidly than atmospheric concentrations. Importantly, carbon monoxide toxicity may result in a falsely elevated pulse oximetry saturation.

MECHANISMS OF PULMONARY INSULT AFTER LOWER AIRWAY BURNS

- Mucosal inflammation
- Mucosal burn
- Bronchorrhea
- Bronchospasm
- Ciliary paralysis
- Reduced surfactant
- Obstruction by debris
- Systemic inflammatory response

Airway burns are associated with a substantially increased requirement for fluid resuscitation. Reducing the fluid volume administered, to avoid fluid accumulation in the lung, results in a worse outcome. Invasive monitoring may be required to guide fluid administration, especially with failure to respond to increasing volumes of fluid. Adequate oxygen delivery to all the tissues of the body is essential to prevent multi-organ failure.

AIRWAY BURNS— KEY CLINICAL POINTS

- Restricting fluids increases mortality
- If in doubt, intubate
- Give 100% oxygen until carbon monoxide toxicity excluded
- Ventilatory strategies to avoid lung injury (low volume or pressure)
- Aggressive airway toilet
- Early surgical debridement of wounds
- Early enteral feeding

Aggressive airway toilet is essential. Diluted heparin and acetyl cystine nebulization may be helpful. Early surgical debridement, enteral feeding, mobilization of the patient, and early extubation are desirable. Antibiotics should be reserved for established infections and guided by regular microbiological surveillance.

Several ventilatory strategies have been proposed to improve outcome following airway burns. Adequate systemic oxygenation and minimizing further alveolar injury is the primary clinical objective. Prolonging survival will permit spontaneous lung recovery.

POSSIBLE VENTILATORY STRATEGIES FOR PATIENTS WITH AIRWAY BURNS

- Low volume ventilation
- Permissive hypercapnia
- High frequency percussive ventilation
- Nitric oxide
- Surfactant replacement
- Partial liquid ventilation (experimental)
- Extracorporeal membrane oxygenation (limited application)

Intensive monitoring—The intensive care environment facilitates rapid, graded response to physiological disturbance. Frequent reassessment, based on a range of clinical and monitored parameters, should guide treatment. Fluid administration should not be guided by calculated fluid requirements alone. Failure to respond to treatment should trigger an escalation in the invasiveness of the monitoring.

END POINTS TO GUIDE FLUID ADMINISTRATION

- Vital signs (blood pressure, heart rate, capillary refill)
- Urine output
- Peripheral perfusion (temperature gradient)
- Gastric mucosal pH
- Serum lactate or base deficit
- Central venous pressure or pulmonary capillary wedge pressure
- Cardiac output—oxygen delivery and consumption

HEART FAILURE

Myocardial dysfunction is a potential consequence of major burn injury. It has been attributed to a circulating myocardial depressant factor, primarily causing myocardial diastolic dysfunction. It may also be caused by myocardial edema.

Administration of an inotropic agent is preferable to overloading a failing myocardium with large volumes of fluid. However, the inotropic drug can produce vasoconstriction in the burn wound, reducing the viability of critically injured tissue. Inotropic drugs should not be used until adequate fluid resuscitation has been ensured (usually by invasive monitoring). Inotropic drugs that do not produce vasoconstriction (such as dopexamine or dobutamine) will preserve wound viability, providing they do not produce unacceptable hypotension.

KIDNEY FAILURE

Early renal failure after burn injury is usually due to delayed or inadequate fluid resuscitation, but it may also result from substantial muscle break down or hemolysis. Delayed renal failure is usually the consequence of sepsis and is often associated with other organ failure.

A reduced urine output, despite adequate fluid administration, is usually the first sign of acute renal failure. This will be followed by a rise in serum creatinine and urea concentrations. Early renal support (hemodialysis or hemodiafiltration) will control serum electrolytes and accommodate the large volumes of nutritional supplementation required in a major burn.

CEREBRAL FAILURE

Hypoxic cerebral insults and closed head injuries are not uncommonly associated with burn injuries. Fluid administration for the burn injury will increase cerebral edema and intracranial pressure. Monitoring intracranial pressure may help in minimizing the adverse effects of trying to achieve two contradictory treatment goals.

NUTRITION

Burn injury is associated with a considerable hypermetabolic response, mediated by the systemic response to the burn and related to the extent of the burn injury. The hypermetabolism may result in a resting energy expenditure increase in excesses of 100% of basal metabolic rate. Even small burns can be associated with hyperpyrexia directly due to hypermetabolism.

Only limited success has been achieved in reducing the hypermetabolic state, which may persist for many months. Close attention to nutritional needs is critical to prevent protein breakdown, decreased wound healing, immune suppression, and an increase in infective complications.

MANAGEMENT OF THE HYPERMETABOLIC RESPONSE
- Reduce heat loss—environmental conditioning
- Excision and closure of burn wound
- Early enteral feeding
- Recognition and treatment of infection

Energy requirements are proportional to the size of the burn and should be met by enteral nutrition, and this should be established as soon as possible after the burn injury. Total parenteral nutrition is associated with immunosuppression, an increase in infective complications, and reduced survival. Glutamine, arginine, and omega 3 fatty acid supplementation may improve immunity and gut function.

TUBE FEEDING IN BURNS PATIENTS
- In all patients with burns covering more than 20% of total body surface area
- Established during initial resuscitation
- Early enteral feeding improves success in establishing feeding
- Nasojejunal feeding will bypass gastric stasis

RISK FACTORS FOR PNEUMONIA
- Inhalational injury:
  - *a)* Destruction of respiratory epithelial barrier
  - *b)* Loss of ciliary function and impaired secretion clearance
  - *c)* Bronchospasm
  - *d)* Mucus and cellular plugging
- Intubation
- Circumferential, full thickness chest wall burns
- Decreased chest wall compliance
- Immobility
- Uncontrolled wound sepsis can lead to secondary pneumonia from hematogenous spread of organisms from wound

Potential Infection Sites.

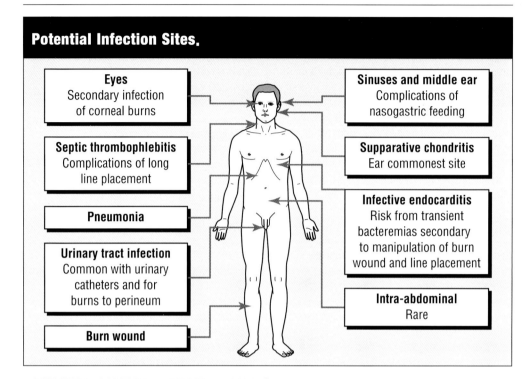

Eyes
Secondary infection
of corneal burns

Septic thrombophlebitis
Complications of long
line placement

Pneumonia

Urinary tract infection
Common with urinary
catheters and for
burns to perineum

Burn wound

Sinuses and middle ear
Complications of
nasogastric feeding

Supparative chondritis
Ear commonest site

Infective endocarditis
Risk from transient
bacteremias secondary
to manipulation of burn
wound and line placement

Intra-abdominal
Rare

INFECTION IN BURNS PATIENTS

After the initial resuscitation, up to 75% of mortality in burns patients is related to infection. Preventing infection, recognizing it when it occurs, and treating it successfully present considerable challenges. Infective pulmonary complications are now the most common types of infection seen in burns patients, but infection is common in many other sites. Several factors contribute to the high frequency and severity of infection at multiple sites in burns patients:

- Destruction of the skin or mucosal surface barrier allows microbial access
- Presence of necrotic tissue and serosanguinous exudate provides a medium to support growth of microorganisms
- Invasive monitoring provides portals for bacterial entry
- Impaired immune function allows microbial proliferation.

Deciding whether infection is present can be difficult. Burns patients have an inflammatory state from the injury itself that can mimic infection. Extensive microbial colonization of wounds makes interpretation of surface cultures difficult.

Patients may have open wounds and repeated episodes of infection over weeks. Excessive use of antibiotics will encourage the appearance of resistant colonizing organisms. A sensible approach is to limit antibiotic use to short courses of drugs with as narrow a spectrum of activity as is feasible.

PATHOGENESIS

The burn injury destroys surface microbes except for Gram positive organisms located in the depths of the sweat glands or hair follicles. Without prophylactic use of topical antimicrobial agents, the wound becomes colonized with large numbers of Gram positive organisms within 48 hours. Gram negative bacteria appear from three to 21 days after the injury. Invasive fungal infection is seen later.

The microbiology reflects the hospital environment and varies from centre to centre. In general there has been a change in the main infective organisms over time from β-hemolytic streptococci to resistant Gram negative organisms including pseudomonas, resistant Gram positive organisms, and fungi.

CAUSATIVE AGENTS OF WOUND INFECTION

Bacteria

β-hemolytic streptococci—Such as: *Streptococcus pyogenes*. Cause acute cellulitis, and occasionally associated with toxic shock syndrome

Staphylococci—Such as methicillin-resistant *Staphylococcus aureus* (MRSA). Cause abscesses and subeschar pus

Gram-negative bacteria—Such as *Pseudomonas aeruginosa, Acinetobacter baumanii, Proteus species*. Mini epidemics seen in specialized centers secondary to antibiotic pressure

Fungi

Candida—Most common fungal isolate, act as surface colonizers but have low potential for invasion

Filamentous fungi—Such as *Aspergillums, Fusarium*, and phycomycetes. Can be aggressive invaders of subcutaneous tissues. Treatment must include debridement of infected tissue

Viruses

Herpes simplex—Characterized by vesicular lesions

PREVENTING INVASIVE WOUND INFECTION

One aim of initial wound management is to prevent invasive infection. To this end, aggressive surgery and the use of topical antimicrobial agents are effective. Topical antimicrobial treatment slows wound colonization and is of use early, before definitive surgery. A wide selection of agents are available: silver sulfadiazine is the most frequently used. Early closure of the burn wound by surgical techniques then lessens the surface area available for further microbial colonization and subsequent infection.

Prophylactic use of systemic antibiotics is controversial. Most agree that prophylactic penicillin against group A streptococcal sepsis is not indicated, and broad spectrum antibiotics to cover wound manipulation are not required in patients with burns covering less than 40% of total body surface area.

DIAGNOSING INVASIVE WOUND INFECTION

Surface swabs and cultures cannot distinguish wound infection from colonization. Wound biopsy, followed by histological examination and quantitative culture, is the definitive method. However, it is time consuming and expensive, making it impractical as a routine diagnostic technique. Diagnosis of infection therefore relies heavily on clinical parameters, with the aid of blood, surface, or tissue cultures to identify likely pathogens.

TREATMENT

When invasive infection of a burn wound is suspected, empirical systemic antimicrobial treatment must be started. Topical treatment alone is not sufficient, as it does not effectively penetrate the eschar and damaged tissue. The choice of antibiotic depends on the predominant flora on the unit. This can be adjusted later depending on culture and sensitivity results of relevant specimens. Necrotic and heavily infected material must be removed by surgical excision.

INFECTION CONTROL

Infection control measures help to minimize cross infection between patients and acquisition of nosocomial pathogens (such as MRSA or multiresistant Gram negative bacteria). Strict isolation of every patient is impractical, but universal precautions are an absolute necessity.

SIGNS OF WOUND INFECTION

- Change in wound appearance:
  a) Discoloration of surrounding skin
  b) Offensive exudate
- Delayed healing
- Graft failure
- Conversion of partial thickness wound to full thickness

ADVANTAGES AND ADVERSE EFFECTS OF TOPICAL ANTIMICROBIALS

Silver sulfadiazine
- Water soluble cream
- *Advantages*—Broad spectrum, low toxicity, painless
- *Adverse effects*—Transient leucopenia, methemoglobinemia (rare)

Cerium nitrate-silver sulfadiazine
- Water soluble cream
- *Advantages*—Broad spectrum, may reduce or reverse immunosuppression after injury
- *Adverse effects*—As for silver sulfadiazine alone

Silver nitrate
- Solution soaked dressing
- *Advantages*—Broad spectrum, painless
- *Adverse effects*—Skin and dressing discoloration, electrolyte disturbance, methemoglobinemia (rare)

Mafenide
- Water soluble cream
- *Advantages*—Broad spectrum, penetrates burn eschar
- *Adverse effects*—Potent carbonic anhydrase inhibitor—osmotic diuresis and electrolyte imbalance, painful application

KEY POINTS

- Fluid resuscitation must be based on frequent reassessment. Formulas are only a guide
- Pulse oximetry readings may be normal in carbon monoxide toxicity
- Unnecessary intubation is preferable to systemic hypoxia
- Early enteral nutrition in major burns may improve survival
- Burn patients are at high risk of infection, and there are many sites for infective complications
- Antibiotics should be used wisely to limit emergence of multiresistant organisms: close liaison with a clinical microbiologist is crucial

FURTHER READING

Still JM Jr, Law EJ. Primary excision of the burn wound. *Clin Plast Surg* 2000;27:23-8

Desai MH, Micak R, Richardson J, Nichols R, Herndon DN. Reduction in mortality in pediatric patients with inhalation injury with aerosolized heparin/N-acetylcystine [correction of acetylcystine] therapy. *J Burn Care Rehabil* 1998;19:210-2

Pruitt BA, Mc Manus AT, Kim SH, Goodwin MD. Burn wound infections.*World J Surg* 1998;22:135-45

Monafo WM,West MA. Current treatment recommendations for topical therapy. *Drugs* 1990;40:364-73

Warren S, Burke JF. Infection of burn wounds: evaluation and management. *Curr Clin Top Infect Dis* 1991;11:206-17

Mark Ansermino is pediatric anesthesiologist, British Columbia's Children's Hospital, Vancouver, Canada. Carolyn Hemsley is specialist registrar in infectious diseases and microbiology, John Radcliffe Hospital, Oxford. The ABC of burns is edited by Shehan Hettiaratchy, specialist registrar in plastic and reconstructive surgery, Pan-Thames Training Scheme, London; Remo Papini, consultant and clinical lead in burns, West Midlands Regional Burns Unit, Selly Oak University Hospital, Birmingham; and Peter Dziewulski, consultant burns and plastic surgeon, St Andrew's Centre for Plastic Surgery and Burns, Broomfield Hospital, Chelmsford.

Source: Mark Ansermino, Carolyn Hemsley BMJ; 2004; 329;220-223 Reprinted with permission.

WHERE THERE'S FIRE, THERE'S SMOKE: ASSESSING AND MANAGING INHALATION INJURY IN THE ED

Now that mass casualty awareness is widespread, the staff of most EDs is more likely to be prepared for a range of disasters. Still, the simultaneous arrival of several burned and injured patients quickly taxes the resources of any ED. Within hours, victims of a fire that erupted in 2003 at The Station nightclub in Rhode Island filled area hospitals. Events like the Coconut Grove fire (492 killed), the Cleveland Clinic fire (125 killed), and the Happy Land Social Club fire (87 killed, mostly from smoke inhalation injury)[1-3] are terrifying. Though the sight of most cutaneous burns is jarring, the real killer in these fires is smoke inhalation. As the treatment of burns has improved, the importance of inhalation injury in burn mortality has become increasingly apparent. Emergency physicians need to be familiar with the assessment and management of smoke inhalation. Our responses to this clinical problem should be as immediate as our approach to acute myocardial infarction, so even the chaos of mass casualty will not slow us down.

CRITICAL APPRAISAL OF THE LITERATURE

There are few extensive clinical trials involving smoke inhalation injury.[4] In 2001, the American Burn Association published practice guidelines for burn care.[5] After evaluation of the literature, which contained mostly small prospective samples or retrospective analyses, the editors concluded that there was insufficient Class I evidence to delineate a treatment standard or guidelines for smoke inhalation injury, and instead published general consensus recommendations.[5] Currently, research using animal models of inhalation injury is ongoing. These efforts could lead to future human trials involving experimental therapies.[6-9]

EPIDEMIOLOGY

Smoke comes from fire, and most of our current understanding of smoke inhalation injury is contained under the larger heading of burn injury. There are more than 1 million burn injuries per year, accounting for 700,000 annual ED visits in the United States.[10] In 1991-1993, there were an estimated 1.29 million burns.[10] As the incidence of burn injury has decreased since the 1950s, so too has mortality from burns declined, by more than 60% in this same period.[10] This trend is credited to advances in fluid resuscitation, improved wound management, and innovations in skin grafting procedures. The impact of pulmonary complications on the morbidity and mortality of burn injury is underscored by the fact that, of burn patients who die, the majority have concomitant inhalation injuries.[10,11]

Because of differences in diagnostic criteria, the actual incidence of smoke inhalation injury is difficult to determine. Though the American Burn Association and related agencies track burn incidence, there is little information regarding the incidence and severity of inhalation injury. Case definitions of inhalation injury in the academic literature are variable: some have adhered to bronchoscopic and pathologic evidence, whereas others have required only the discharge diagnosis of "inhalation injury" on retrospective review of charts. With no gold standard for diagnosis, it is no wonder that the incidence of inhalation injury ranges from 13% in some studies up to 30% in others.[12-14] Groups shown to be at higher risk of inhalation injury are patients at the extremes of age, intoxicated patients, and those with coexistent medical problems.[15]

MORBIDITY

Morbidity due to inhalation injury is just as difficult to quantify as the epidemiology is.

Short-term morbidity can be approximated to some extent by length of hospital stay. Length of stay is increased threefold in burned patients with inhalation injury compared to those without inhalation injury. This is independent of age and TBSA.[12,13] In patients who survive to discharge, long-term morbidity from inhalation injury itself is generally thought to be minimal, although data on this subject is lacking.[16-18] Long-term follow-up studies have shown that cough, dyspnea on exertion, airway hyper-responsiveness, dysphagia, bronchiectasis, and bronchiolitis obliterans are all potential complications of smoke inhalation.[18,19] There is also evidence of long-term increase in pulmonary and systemic inflammatory markers, which, in theory, may contribute to an excess of illnesses like emphysema, asthma, and even lung cancer in these patients. However, data is scarce. Furthermore, other studies indicate that pulmonary function tests fall within normal limits after 2 years, so the effect of these changes is uncertain.[18,20]

MORTALITY

Patients with burns and inhalation injuries have an estimated mortality of 30% to 50%.[12,14,21] One study of burn victims reported 1.7% mortality in patients without concomitant inhalation injury, compared with 34.7% mortality in patients with inhalation injury.[12] Indeed, inhalation is a major factor in estimating mortality from burns and has been included with age and TBSA to predict individual patient outcomes. Ryan et al showed that inhalation injury, age greater than 60, and TBSA greater than 40% corresponded to mortality of 0.3, 3, 30 or 90%, depending on whether 0, 1, 2, or 3 of these risk factors was present.[13] Clearly, inhalation injury significantly contributes to burn mortality; some suggest its contribution is independent of age and TBSA.[12] Still, patients with very high TBSA or those at the extremes of age have a poorer prognosis, regardless of inhalation injury.[22] Accordingly, the impact of inhalation injury is most significant in patients with moderate, "survivable" burns. In one study, 30% of burn deaths associated with smoke inhalation occurred in patents with less than 50% TBSA.[21]

PATHOPHYSIOLOGY

Smoke has a diverse composition that depends on the materials in the blaze, with each compound having a unique toxicity profile. Regardless, the final common pathway of smoke inhalation injury is tissue hypoxia. Many animal models have been used to simulate and quantify the effects of inhalation.[23-29] These investigations demonstrate that inhalation injury causes an acute inflammatory cascade. Activated inflammatory mediators lead to increased vascular permeability at the site of injury, which can progress to pulmonary edema, atelectasis, decreased perfusion, and impaired gas exchange.[30] Smoke inhalation has also been shown to cause an immediate, intense pulmonary venoconstriction, with the potential for large pressure differentials as evidenced in experimental models. This characteristic of smoke inhalation may exacerbate pulmonary edema.[31]

In addition to the above mechanisms, inhalation of smoke produces tissue hypoxia in other ways. Edema of the burned upper airway leads to impaired respiratory mechanics and may deteriorate to ventilatory failure. Bronchopulmonary toxins cause bronchiolar edema and obstruction. Surfactant disruption leads to atelectasis. Carbon monoxide and methemoglobinemia result in decreased oxygen-carrying capacity of blood. At the cellular level, carbon monoxide and cyanide poison biochemical pathways.

THERMAL INJURY

The upper airway contains moist mucous membranes, which effectively protect the lower airways from thermal injury. Air is a poor conductor of heat, and the body is very efficient at dissipating it. Unless steam is inhaled, thermal injury does not directly affect the lungs. Direct thermal injury is limited to supraglottic structures.[33-35] This is not to say, however, that the effect of thermal injury is negligible. Supraglottic burns lead to increased capillary permeability and edema, which may rapidly give way to upper airway obstruction. Laryngeal edema begins 2 to 8 hours after injury.[23] Airway edema may begin before the patient arrives at the hospital and may progress in the intervening 24 hours.[23,36,37]

HYPOXIC GAS INHALATION

Hypoxia is the common endpoint of smoke inhalation. To compound the problem, smoke-filled air has lower oxygen content compared with "room" air. In other words, smoke-filled air is hypoxic. This is due to the presence of environmental asphyxiants found in smoke. Environmental asphyxiants are gases that displace oxygen in the air we breathe. High carbon dioxide, low oxygen (secondary to its consumption by fire), and high concentrations of other gases, eg, methane, create a hypoxic environment. To the patient breathing this mixture of gases, hypoxemia may quickly ensue, causing CNS depression and hyperventilation. This has the potential to increase both the length and the amount of a victim's smoke exposure. If the degree of hypoxic gas inhalation is severe and the patient is "overcome by smoke," the result is usually fatal at the scene.

CHEMICAL INHALATION INJURY

The exact composition of smoke is rarely known. Besides a few notable chemicals—among them carbon monoxide, cyanide, and phosgene—the specific makeup of smoke will not alter the emergency care. However, a general understanding of the pathologic effects of these chemicals is useful.[38]

Combustion produces chemicals that act as environmental asphyxiants (see preceding section), irritants, or chemical asphyxiants. (**Table 1**) Irritants are chemical by-products that lead to local lung injury. Chemical asphyxiants damage a wide variety of cells and thereby impair oxygen utilization at the tissue level. Often, a single type of material generates by-products that fall into all three categories. Also, many combustion products, while not toxic themselves, act as conduits for other chemical toxins. For example, carbonaceous soot can absorb toxic chemicals and deposit them directly in the alveoli, where they exert their harmful effects.[37]

Chemical irritants, like ammonia, acrolein, chlorine, sulfur dioxide, and phosgene, cause a local respiratory irritation. Most of these chemicals react to form caustic substances when they contact the respiratory epithelium. Caustic burning of the bronchopulmonary tree causes ulceration, sloughing of respiratory epithelium, and disruption

Table 1. Toxic Combustion Products
Environmental Asphyxiants
Carbon dioxide
Methane
Oxygen deprived environment
Chemical Asphyxiants
Carbon monoxide
Hydrogen cyanide
Hydrogen sulfide
Oxides of nitrogen
Irritants
High water solubility (upper airway injury)
Acrolein
Sulfur dioxide
Ammonia
Hydrogen chloride
Intermediate water solubility (upper and lower airway injury)
Chlorine
Isocyantates
Poor water solubility (pulmonary parenchymal injury)
Oxides of nitrogen
Phosgene

Source: *Goldfrank LR, Flomenbaum NE, Lewin NA, Weisman R, Howland MA, Hoffman R. Goldfrank's Toxicologic Emergencies. 6th ed. Stamford: Appleton & Lange; 1998.*

of the bronchociliary chain. Local damage to the lower respiratory tract causes increased susceptibility to bacterial infection.[39] The chemical's solubility determines the part of the respiratory tree it is likely to damage. For example, ammonia is highly water-soluble, thus rapidly absorbed in the upper airways. Phosgene, on the other hand, has low water solubility and mainly affects the terminal airways and pulmonary parenchyma.[37] Phosgene, a combustion product of wool, polyvinyl chloride (PVC), and some plastics, is of particular concern, because it can produce a delayed injury at the alveolar level. Because PVC and other plastic materials are ubiquitous in modern constructions, phosgene deserves special mention. In one case report, a firefighter, seemingly asymptomatic after fighting a small office fire, died suddenly, nearly 24 hours later, due to severe pulmonary hemorrhage and edema. For these reasons, a prolonged period of observation is recommended for patients suspected of having phosgene exposure during smoke inhalation.[40-42]

CARBON MONOXIDE

Carbon monoxide (CO), an extremely important constituent of smoke, is a colorless, tasteless, odorless gas that is produced by the incomplete combustion of organic matter.[43,44] CO poisoning is responsible for approximately 80% of the mortality from smoke inhalation. CO has a very high affinity for hemoglobin and displaces oxygen in pulmonary venous blood. CO binds hemoglobin approximately 250 times more than oxygen. The creation of carboxyhemoglobin also shifts the oxygen-dissociation curve to the left, which further reduces oxygen delivery to the tissues. At the cellular level, CO binds to mitochondrial cytochromes and reduces oxygen utilization. The sum of these pathopyshiologic effects is tissue hypoxia, manifest most notably in the myocardium and central nervous system. CO is thought to cause additional damage to the brain by the process of lipid peroxidation.[45]

Clinical features of carbon monoxide poisoning include headache, dizziness, nausea, vomiting, cardiac ischemia, arrhythmia, seizures, coma, and cardiovascular collapse. Delayed neuropsychiatric sequelae (DNS) are cognitive and psychiatric disturbances that occur between 2 and 240 days after CO exposure. DNS encompass a range of complaints, such as malaise, memory disturbances, depression, personality changes, anxiety, focal neurologic findings, Parkinsonism, ataxia, and other symptoms.[45-47] The severity of these symptoms is variable. Reliable estimates of the incidence of DNS are hindered by the lack of a case definition. Numerous studies have used different methodologies to identify patients with DNS, and have reported rates between 2% and 50 %.[45-48]

CYANIDE

Like carbon monoxide, cyanide is produced by the combustion of common substances—specifically, those containing nitrogen, such as wool, silk, vinyl, polyurethane, and plastics.[49,50] Cyanide forms a complex with ferric ions in the electron transport chain and inhibits oxidative phosphorylation. This leads to anaerobic metabolism and subsequent tissue hypoxia. Several authors have suggested that cyanide toxicity in smoke inhalation patients is underestimated.[51,52] A confirmatory test for cyanide is not easily available, and the signs of intoxication are similar to CO poisoning. The severity and type of symptoms depend on the source and amount of cyanide exposure. Significant exposure leads to metabolic acidosis, bradycardia, tachycardia, dyspnea, anxiety, agitation, seizures, and coma.[53] A pulse oximetry reading is usually normal.

DIFFERENTIAL DIAGNOSIS

Patients with smoke inhalation injury may also have cutaneous burns and other traumatic injuries. One of the keys in managing the patient with smoke inhalation is to avoid premature closure on the diagnosis. As will be discussed below, smoke inhalation patients with altered mental status require a careful evaluation for hypoxia secondary to either pulmonary injury or oxygen utilization at the cellular level. However, since common things happen commonly, other causes of altered mental status must be considered, including hypoglycemia, traumatic brain injury, seizures, and drug overdose.

PREHOSPITAL CARE

The prehospital care of the patient with inhalation injuries follows the same principles that govern the stabilization of any critically ill patient. The initial focus is on airway, breathing, and circulation. Management of these patients may be complicated by associated cutaneous burns or trauma. Intubation should be considered for patients in severe respiratory distress; however, since significant airway edema may complicate the intubation, the benefit of field intubation must be carefully weighed against rapid transport of the patient. All patients should be placed on high-flow oxygen via nonrebreather face mask.[54] Adjunctive airway devices, such as the esophageal-tracheal Combitube or laryngeal mask airway (LMA), can be used to assist in oxygenation when traditional bag-valve mask ventilation is difficult due to oropharyngeal edema. These devices cannot protect the airway from aspiration or increasing upper airway edema, but they may help maintain the patient's oxygen saturation during transport to the hospital. Bronchodilators may be used if the patient manifests evidence of bronchoconstriction, such as wheezing. Prehospital providers should suspect other traumatic injuries and be prepared to address them according to the usual protocols.

ED EVALUATION

INITIAL EVALUATION

Any patient with suspected inhalation injury and signs of imminent airway obstruction, including drooling, stridor, or hoarseness, should be immediately triaged to the critical care area of the ED, so the airway can be secured and resuscitation initiated. A pulse oximetry reading of 100% is not necessarily reassuring, because significant carbon monoxide poisoning may still be present. Tachypnea is a potential early sign of thermal airway injury or chemical injury, especially carbon monoxide. Hypotension should alert the physician to the potential for concomitant thoracoabdominal trauma, carbon monoxide exposure, or cyanide poisoning. Once the patient is stabilized, the assessment proceeds in a systematic manner.

HISTORY

The history may be difficult to obtain from a patient in distress, but is integral in making some treatment decisions. The diagnosis of smoke inhalation injury is made mainly on the basis of history.[34] If the patient is unable to provide historical information, prehospital personnel and family members may be helpful in this regard. Important points include the type of burning material, length of exposure, presence of explosion, and the odor of smoke. If the patient has a history of being burned in a closed space, smoke inhalation injury is highly probable.[34] Hanston et al retrospectively evaluated 64 patients with inhalation injury without burns and found that 32% of the patients reported a loss of consciousness at the scene.[39] Carbon monoxide should be strongly considered in all patients exposed to smoke, particularly if they lost consciousness, or if there were deaths at the scene.[37] Burnt plastic, silk, and nylon increase the risk of cyanide toxicity.[55,56] Phosgene exposure can occur in fires involving certain chlorinated organic compounds found in many household solvents, paint removers, and dry cleaning fluids, or wool,

PVC, and other plastics. Patients may report the characteristic smell of "newly mowed hay."[42] Another factor to consider is that premorbid conditions, especially chronic lung disease and heart disease, can affect the patient's response to inhalation injury.

PHYSICAL EXAMINATION

Airway

Early management of the airway is crucial in inhalation injury. A few patients arrive in the ED with respiratory failure and a decreased level of consciousness, making the need for immediate airway protection obvious. Recognizing that the patient may have a difficult airway should prompt a plan for adjuncts to standard endotracheal intubation.[57,58] The best technique for intubation is dependent on operator expertise. Proper preparation is paramount and includes an array of airway equipment: several sizes of ET tubes, rigid laryngoscope blades of various sizes and designs, forceps to manipulate the tip of the ET tube, flexible fiberoptic laryngoscope, laryngeal mask airways, an intubation stylet, and fiberoptic intubating laryngoscopes.[59] MacLennan et al suggest considering an awake intubation with intravenous opioids and local anesthesia, when a difficult airway is anticipated.[58] Early involvement of anesthesia may be lifesaving in these challenging situations. The emergency physician should also be prepared to perform a surgical airway, if the upper airway is damaged and orotracheal intubation is not possible.

Other patients present with signs of respiratory distress, including stridor, accessory muscle use, and hoarseness. Drooling or difficulty swallowing suggests significant injury and impending airway compromise. To prevent the rapid deterioration of these patients, they should be managed aggressively with early, elective endotracheal intubation.[34,37,54]

If the patient does not manifest obvious signs of thermal injury to the upper airway, secondary signs should be sought. The damage from burns is usually limited to the oropharyngeal area. Patients may report throat or neck pain, or odynophagia. Other signs of smoke exposure include conjunctivitis, tearing, and rhinitis.[60] The oropharynx should be checked for erythema, edema, or blisters. Laryngoscopy (indirect or direct) can be used to help assess the upper airway.[34] Any patient with visible burns or edema of the oropharynx, full thickness nasolabial burns, or circumferential neck burns should be considered for early endotracheal intubation.[61,62] Patients may manifest symptoms of obstruction secondary to laryngeal edema in a delayed fashion, up to 24 hours.[34]

The signs of inhalation injury to the lower airway can be subtle. Conventional teaching emphasizes the classic, indirect signs of inhalation injury, such as singed nasal hairs, facial burns, soot in the mouth, and carbonaceous sputum. While carbonaceous sputum is a reliable indicator of inhalation injury,[34,54,63] it is important to realize that patients may have significant airway injury without any of these signs.[34,64,65] Clark et al gathered statistics on 108 patients diagnosed with inhalation injury. They found that physical signs were not sensitive in predicting inhalation injury; less than 50% of the patients had facial burns, carbonaceous sputum, or soot in the nose or mouth. Furthermore, less than 15% of the patients had singed nasal hairs, cough, stridor, or dyspnea. On the other hand, patients with 3 or more findings had a 56% chance of inhalation injury.[66]

In summary, indirect signs of damage, such as burned face or singed nasal hairs, should prompt a more comprehensive airway examination; however, the absence of these signs does not reliably exclude airway injury.[32]

Breathing

Once impending airway obstruction is excluded, other factors to consider include lung injury, poisoning due to carbon monoxide or cyanide, and complications of traumatic injuries. The patient should be placed on continuous cardiac and pulse oximetry monitoring. Supplemental oxygen should be given immediately. If lung auscultation demonstrates unilateral absence of breath sounds, suspect pneumothorax and either empirically treat or obtain a CXR, depending on the patient's clinical presentation. Patients with lung injury may have adventitious sounds on exam, such as wheezing, rhonchi, or rales, which will help to direct immediate diagnostic testing and therapies. Circumferential chest-wall burns prompt an immediate surgical consultation and are an indication for an escharotomy.[34]

Circulation

Assess level of consciousness, heart rate, blood pressure, and capillary refill. Tachycardia may signify blood loss due to thoracoabdominal or extremity trauma. If the patient has associated burns, fluid resuscitation should be based on burn guidelines.

Disability

The patient should be completely undressed and systematically evaluated for other injuries. Trauma from falls or explosions should be suspected and evaluated. If the patient is burned, the percentage of total body surface area involved must be estimated.

The patient's mental status should be carefully evaluated, and a full neurologic examination performed. While the etiology of impaired consciousness may be multifactorial in these patients, this finding is considered by many authorities to be an indication for hyperbaric oxygen (HBO) therapy in the setting of carbon monoxide (CO) exposure.[48] Furthermore, neurologic signs, in addition to more subtle neuropsychiatric impairments, can identify patients who also may benefit from HBO.[48] Batteries of psychometric tests have been designed specifically for CO-poisoned patients and can detect abnormalities in attention/concentration, fine motor function, processing speed, problem solving, and new learning.[48] A trained examiner can generally administer the test in 30 minutes. Lack of testing materials and trained personnel may limit the use of this formal neuropsychiatric evaluation in many emergency departments.

DIAGNOSTIC STUDIES

ARTERIAL BLOOD GAS (ABG)

Initial ABG can provide information about metabolic acidosis secondary to decreased tissue perfusion. Touger demonstrated that using a venous blood sample is as accurate as an arterial sample, limiting the need for an arterial puncture.[67] Serial measurements can help identify patients with worsening hypoxemia.[37] Oxygen saturation on an ABG should be evaluated with caution. If measured using ABG analysis, the saturation reported may be falsely high. Measurement with a co-oximeter will accurately report the percentage of oxygenated hemoglobin. Communicating to the lab that there may be associated CO or CN poisoning will direct them to use the co-oximeter. Co-oximeters transmit 4 wavelengths of light through a blood sample and can detect methemoglobin and carboxyhemoglobin.

The PaO2/FiO2 ratio suggests the degree of transpulmonary shunting and is a gauge of impending respiratory failure. A ratio of less than 300 may predict subsequent respiratory failure.[68] The measurement of carboxyhemoglobin is readily available in most emergency departments. Because the symptoms of carbon monoxide poisoning are nonspecific and may be overlooked in the multiply-injured and burned patient, routine documentation of the carboxyhemoglobin level can alert the physician to this additional clinical problem. Normal levels are less than 5% in nonsmokers and up to 12% in heavy smokers.[74] Venous blood samples are adequate, but arterial samples may be desirable, since arterial blood gas analysis and co-oximetry can be performed.[67] The carboxyhemoglobin (COHb) level does not correlate with the severity of carbon monoxide toxicity.[48] Although patients demonstrate signs of toxicity with levels above 25%, they may still have significant CO poisoning with normal levels. Oxygen exposure and duration of exposure make COHb levels unreliable.[75]

PULSE OXIMETRY

Transcutaneous reading of oxygen saturation is unreliable in the setting of associated CO poisoning. Since the pulse oximeter uses 2 wavelengths of light, this method detects only oxygenated and deoxygenated hemoglobin and does not distinguish carboxyhemoglobin.[37,69] Bozeman et al reviewed 124 patients who had arterial blood gas and pulse oximetry readings. The pulse oximeter readings continued to be high, even as the percentage of carboxyhemoglobin increased. In patients with possible CO poisoning, pulse oximeter readings can be falsely reassuring.[76]

CHEST RADIOGRAPH

Initially, radiographs are usually normal for patients with inhalation injury.[70,71] If abnormalities are present, such as perivascular haziness, peribronchial cuffing, bronchial wall thickening, and subglottic edema, the prognosis is worse. Besides detecting lung injury from smoke inhalation, the chest radiograph can provide other useful clinical information, such as findings suggestive of chronic lung disease, or the presence of rib fractures and other traumatic injuries. Since it is relatively inexpensive, quick and noninvasive, a baseline chest radiograph is a reasonable test in the majority of patients who are suspected of inhalation injury.[71] After 24 hours, the chest radiographs of patients who develop widespread injury may demonstrate progressive changes secondary to ARDS, aspiration, or volume overload.[72,73]

CYANIDE

Treatment of cyanide toxicity should not be dependent on cyanide levels. Cyanide is cleared rapidly from the body, and no quick tests are available.[77,51] Lactic acid levels have been proposed as a surrogate marker, with levels of greater than 8 mmol/L indicating potential exposure.[51] Initially, case reports suggested that carboxyhemoglobin levels could be used to extrapolate cyanide levels.[52,78] Multiple studies have not supported this correlation.[79,51,80]

LACTIC ACID

Although the study was small, Baud et al retrospectively looked at 109 patients with inhalation injuries. They found that a plasma lactate level above 10 mmol/L was 87% sensitive for cyanide poisoning.[51] That study was followed up by a small cohort of 11 patients admitted for cyanide poisoning, though fire victims were excluded. This led the authors to conclude that a plasma lactate level greater than 8 mmol/L was 94% sensitive for a toxic cyanide level. Lactic acid is elevated in patients with impaired tissue oxygenation. In a victim of smoke inhalation, an elevated level may be secondary to methemoglobinemia, CO poisoning, volume depletion, or hypoxia, not just cyanide poisoning. Benaissa et al looked at 146 patients diagnosed with only carbon monoxide poisoning and reported that the plasma lactate was minimally elevated.[81] The studies supporting lactic acid levels as a surrogate marker for cyanide poisoning are small, but in a patient with a suspicion of cyanide poisoning, checking lactate levels is reasonable.

ELECTROLYTES AND OTHER SERUM TESTS

A serum chemistry analysis can identify an anion gap acidosis. In a smoke inhalation victim, this finding can signify hypoxemia, hypovolemia, CO, and CN exposure, or a combination of these derangements. A BUN/Cr can be helpful if there is associated trauma leading to shock or rhabdomyolysis. If rhabdomyolysis is suspected, a serum creatine kinase level (CK) should be measured. Toxicology screening may identify drugs or alcohol that could depress the patient's mental status. Along these lines, a bedside glucose determination should be obtained in any patient with altered mental status.

ECG

Hypoxia secondary to carbon monoxide poisoning can cause myocardial ischemia or arrythmias.82 ECG should be obtained in patients with known heart disease, patients with a history of loss of consciousness, or those complaining of chest pain or palpitations. Like the chest radiograph, there are many potential indications for this test. In addition, the ECG may provide important information that could significantly alter patient management, as in the case of carbon monoxide poisoning (**Table 4**). If a patient is suspected of inhalation injury, a low threshold for obtaining an ECG is a reasonable approach.

PREGNANCY TEST

A pregnancy test should always be obtained in women of child-bearing age, since pregnancy can impact many diagnostic and management decisions. Specifically, in pregnant patients with CO poisoning, hyperbaric therapy may be considered with a lower carboxyhemoglobin level.[83]

BRONCHOSCOPY

Inhalation injury can be subtle, and, in rare cases, patients may be asymptomatic for up to 72 hours.[33] As discussed, classical signs such as facial burns, hoarseness, stridor, or soot are suggestive of upper airway injury, but are poor predictors of the extent of injury to the lower airways and lung parenchyma.[34] In the absence of these signs, patients are still at risk for significant lung injury.[54,63,64] Masanes et al performed bronchoscopy and biopsies on 130 patients with suspected inhalation injury.[33] Of the patients with bronchoscopic evidence of inhalation injury, 25% had no dysphonia, 16% had no facial burns, 29% had normal ABGs, and 84% had normal chest radiographs. Patients diagnosed with lung injury by bronchoscopy had a significantly higher risk of ARDS and death.

Fiberoptic bronchoscopy allows for direct evaluation of the airway from the oropharynx to the lobar bronchi and is considered the "gold standard" for the diagnosis of inhalation injury.[4,63] With direct visualization, signs of lung damage, including airway edema, inflammation, mucosal necrosis, and the presence of soot, can be identified.[34] Bronchoscopy confirms that the patient has been exposed to smoke, but the findings do not correlate with mortality, the potential for respiratory failure, or the duration of subsequent endotracheal intubation.[84] Still, the advantages of early recognition of injury are clear-cut: a controlled, elective intubation as opposed to the emergent management of a rapidly deteriorating patient.[33,54]

Bronchoscopy can also be used to detect late pulmonary sequelae, including tracheobronchial stenosis and polyps,[85] as well as used therapeutically, to clear obstruction secondary to necrotic mucosa, exudates, and inflammatory cells.[63] The limitations of bronchoscopy are that bronchioles and pulmonary parenchyma cannot be evaluated by this method. Additionally, the availability of the study may be limited at certain institutions due to a lack of qualified operators.[63]

Bronchoscopy is indicated in any person who is suspected of having inhalation injury based on risk factor analysis or abnormal physical exam findings. Bronchoscopy can be used to confirm injury, clear debris, and document resolution of injuries after serial studies.[54] There is some controversy as to the optimal time for bronchoscopy.[33] Early pulmonary

Table 2. Ventilation Management

Tidal volume	6-8mL/kg
Respiratory rate	8-12 breaths/minute
I:E ratios	1:1-1:3
FiO2	100%
PEEP	5 cm H2O

All are starting values that should be adjusted to achieve adequate oxygenation and ventilation.

Source: Fitzpatrick JC, Cioffi WG. In: Herndon D, ed. Total Burn Care. 2nd ed. Philadelphia, Pa: WB Saunders; 2002.

Table 3. Arterial Blood Gas Goals

Variable	Goal
pH	7.25-7.45
pO2	55-80 mmHg or Sao2 of 88-95%
pCO2	35-55 mm Hg (permissive hypercapnia can be used as long as pH is >7.25

Source: Fitzpatrick JC, Cioffi WG. In: Herndon D, ed. Total Burn Care. 2nd ed. Philadelphia, Pa: WB Saunders; 2002.

consultation is advised in patients with suspected inhalation injury, but it is reasonable for the patient to have a bronchoscopic exam on admission to the hospital, rather than in the ED.

OTHER TESTS

Xenon ventilation-perfusion scans have been studied as adjuncts in the diagnosis of smoke inhalation injury.[57] Bronchoscopy examination fails to detect injury to the terminal bronchioles, which may be significant.[63] Studies have suggested xenon scanning to evaluate patients with a high suspicion of inhalation injury despite a negative bronchoscopy, but there are no data to support this practice.[63,86,87] The logistical difficulty of xenon scanning combined with the lack of evidence makes it impractical for the ED.

TREATMENT

AIRWAY SUPPORT

The choice of paralytics varies at different institutions. Succinylcholine can be used safely up to 24 hours postburn.[88] The largest ETT size possible should be used to allow for pulmonary toilet and bronchoscopy.[54] Some authors recommend allowing for a slight leak in the cuff to prevent damage of the already injured tracheal mucosa.[54] The risks are usually long-term with erosion of the tracheal cartilages, subglottic stenosis, and tracheomalacia.[89] In the acute setting, the cuff should be inflated to the pressure necessary to allow for adequate ventilation.

Securing the ET tube can be troublesome in patients with facial burns. A circumferential tie, securing the tube with wire to a tooth or dental arch bar, can be considered for improved stabilization.[58]

After smoke inhalation injury, lungs are less compliant.[90] Airway resistance is also increased by tracheal edema. Further damage can occur if the airway pressures exceed the mucosal capillary perfusion pressure, leading to ischemia.[89] In a volume control ventilator, minimizing tidal volumes, increasing the respiratory rate, and adequate PEEP can reduce airway pressures and barotraumas.[91]

Fitzpatrick suggests that ventilating the patient to achieve a normal blood gas may be detrimental and instead advocates permissive hypercapnia, which is usually well tolerated and allows for

Clinical Pathway: Assessment of Smoke Inhalation Injury

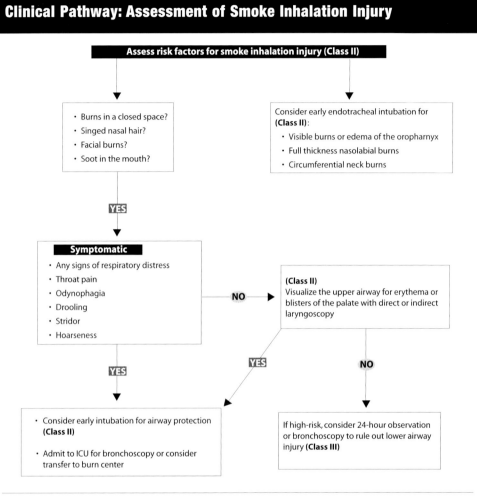

Assess risk factors for smoke inhalation injury (Class II)

- Burns in a closed space?
- Singed nasal hair?
- Facial burns?
- Soot in the mouth?

Consider early endotracheal intubation for **(Class II)**:
- Visible burns or edema of the oropharynx
- Full thickness nasolabial burns
- Circumferential neck burns

YES

Symptomatic
- Any signs of respiratory distress
- Throat pain
- Odynophagia
- Drooling
- Stridor
- Hoarseness

NO →

(Class II)
Visualize the upper airway for erythema or blisters of the palate with direct or indirect laryngoscopy

YES **NO**

YES

- Consider early intubation for airway protection **(Class II)**

- Admit to ICU for bronchoscopy or consider transfer to burn center

If high-risk, consider 24-hour observation or bronchoscopy to rule out lower airway injury **(Class III)**

The **evidence for recommendations** is graded using the following scale. **Class I:** Definitely recommended. Definitive, excellent evidence provides support. **Class II:** Acceptable and useful. Good evidence provides support. **Class III:** May be acceptable, possibly useful. Fair-to-good evidence provides support. **Indeterminate:** Continuing area of research.

This clinical pathway is intended to supplement, rather than substitute for, professional judgment and may be changed depending upon a patient's individual needs. Failure to comply with this pathway does not represent a breach of the standard of care.

reduced airway pressures. (**Table 2** and **Table 3**)[89]

Animal studies have demonstrated that inhalation injury leads to V/Q mismatch secondary to inflammatory occlusion of the small airways. Managing atelectasis is extremely important in this setting, so as to prevent further mismatching. Positive end-expiratory pressure (PEEP) is beneficial in preventing further atelectasis in mechanically ventilated patients, though its use must be adjusted depending on the presence or absence of bronchospasm.[54]

Trials with high frequency percussive ventilation (HFPV) for inhalation injury have been promising.[92-94] Cioffi et al prospectively studied 54 patients who were prophylactically placed on HFPV and compared those patients to a historical cohort. The group found that there was an increase in survival rate and a decrease in infection in patients treated with HFPV. Cioffi also retrospectively reviewed the charts of 1,256 burn patients and concluded that improved survival was associated with the use of HFPV.[87] Reper et al published

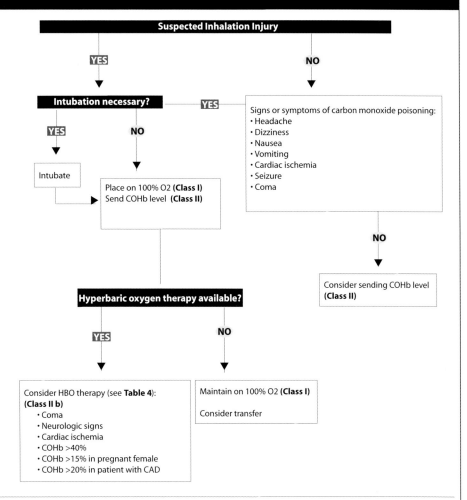

Clinical Pathway: Assessment of Carbon Monoxide Poisoning

Suspected Inhalation Injury

YES → **Intubation necessary?** → YES →

NO →

Signs or symptoms of carbon monoxide poisoning:
• Headache
• Dizziness
• Nausea
• Vomiting
• Cardiac ischemia
• Seizure
• Coma

Intubation necessary?
YES → Intubate
NO → Place on 100% O2 **(Class I)** / Send COHb level **(Class II)**

NO → Consider sending COHb level **(Class II)**

Hyperbaric oxygen therapy available?

YES → Consider HBO therapy (see **Table 4**):
(Class II b)
• Coma
• Neurologic signs
• Cardiac ischemia
• COHb >40%
• COHb >15% in pregnant female
• COHb >20% in patient with CAD

NO → Maintain on 100% O2 **(Class I)**
Consider transfer

The **evidence for recommendations** is graded using the following scale. **Class I:** Definitely recommended. Definitive, excellent evidence provides support. **Class II:** Acceptable and useful. Good evidence provides support. **Class III:** May be acceptable, possibly useful. Fair-to-good evidence provides support. **Indeterminate:** Continuing area of research.

This clinical pathway is intended to supplement, rather than substitute for, professional judgment and may be changed depending upon a patient's individual needs. Failure to comply with this pathway does not represent a breach of the standard of care.

the first randomized controlled trial comparing HFPV and conventional ventilation in patients. They found that HFPV improved blood oxygenation during the acute phase following inhalation injury, but there were no significant differences between the observed groups for mortality or infectious complications.[92] In patients that are difficult to ventilate with conventional methods, HFPV may be an alternative, but there are no consistent data to support HFPV as the first line of treatment.[95,96]

Nonintubated patients should be managed aggressively, as well. All patients should be provided with humidified oxygen.[34,54] Incentive spirometry helps to prevent atelectasis.[54] Continuous positive airway pressure (CPAP) may prevent shunting and mismatch, but has not been extensively studied in inhalation injury.[97] Until

---

Table 4. Guidelines For Hyperbaric Oxygen Therapy In Carbon Monoxide Poisoning.

- Coma
- Neurological impairment as evidenced by neuropsychiatric testing or other means
- Cardiovascular involvement
- Serum carboxyhemoglobin (COHb) level >40%, or COHb level >15% in pregnancy
- Ischemic heart disease in association with serum COHb levels >20%
- Recurrent symptoms up to 3 weeks after original treatment with NBO
- Symptoms that do not resolve after 6 hours of continuous 100% NBO therapy

Source: Minogue MF. Hyperbaric Oxygen Therapy and Carbon Monoxide Toxicity. *Clin Toxicol Rev.* 1998 Aug;20(11).

---

further evidence has accrued, patients who are thought to be candidates for CPAP should be strongly considered for intubation instead, since respiratory distress can be rapidly progressive.

BRONCHODILATORS

Wheezing in patients with inhalation injury can be secondary to multiple mechanisms, including bronchospasm, mucosal edema, or bronchial obstruction from sloughed mucosa.[89] Therapy needs to be tailored to the cause of wheezing. A trial of bronchodilators may help with bronchospasm, but if there is no response, the wheezing may be due edema or partial obstruction.[89]

FLUID RESUSCITATION

Some studies have shown that smoke inhalation injury increased fluid requirements independent of the cutaneous burn injury.[98,99] In contrast, experimental models have shown that smoke inhalation increases pulmonary vascular permeability, thus fluid infusion may amplify the risk of pulmonary edema.[54] A prospective study investigated the resuscitation of sheep with inhalation injury. One group received fluid at a normal maintenance rate, while the other group was resuscitated at twice the normal rate. Mortality was increased in the latter.[23] However, there is no support for limiting

fluid to prevent pulmonary edema.[23,100] Monitoring urine output and, in some cases, pulmonary artery catheter measurements, can help balance fluid resuscitation.[36]

TREATMENT OF CARBON MONOXIDE EXPOSURE

The goal in the treatment of carbon monoxide poisoning is to maximize oxygen delivery to the tissues. To this end, patients should be placed on 100% supplemental oxygen by nonrebreather face mask. Immediate administration of high-flow, normobaric oxygen (NBO) enhances the removal of carbon monoxide from hemoglobin. Faster elimination of carboxyhemoglobin can be accomplished with hyperbaric oxygen (HBO) therapy.[46] The half-life of COHb is 320 minutes when patients are breathing room air, 60 minutes when breathing 100% NBO, and 23 minutes when breathing 100% HBO at 2.8 atm. HBO therapy may have other benefits beyond hastening the removal of carbon monoxide from blood, such as prevention of lipid peroxidation in the brain, or reducing delayed neurologic symptoms.[101] (See "Controversies")

TREATMENT OF CYANIDE EXPOSURE

If there is a strong suspicion of cyanide toxicity based on the features of the history (materials burned) or laboratory data (lactic acid level greater than 8mml/L), treatment can be initiated. The most important intervention is 100% oxygen therapy. There have been reports of successful treatment with just supportive care.[102] However, a specific antidote for cyanide poisoning is widely available. The Lilly Cyanide Antidote Kit™ contains amyl nitrate, sodium nitrite, and sodium thiosulfate.

Amyl nitrite and sodium nitrite produce methemoglobinemia, which can be problematic, if the oxygen-carrying capacity of blood is already reduced by COHb and other factors. Due to these concerns, administration of sodium thiosulfate alone is the safest intervention. Some authors have suggested that fire victims treated with sodium nitrite have not demonstrated deleterious effects.[103] Still, the safest treatment is 100% oxygen and sodium thiosulfate.

Ten tips for effective patient care

1. **Although external signs may indicate lower airway injury, absence of these findings does not rule out injury.**

   Other risk factors should be sought, such as loss of consciousness or death of another victim. Also, other physical exam features should be considered, specifically lung auscultation. Patients with any of these risk factors should be admitted for a 24-hour observation period and possible bronchoscopy, even if physical signs are lacking. Only asymptomatic patients without risk factors for inhalation injury and a normal physical exam can safely be discharged after an observation period in the ED.

2. **Laryngeal edema and inflammation may not progress to respiratory distress for several hours — up to 24 hours.**

   Patients with an abnormal exam should be admitted for monitoring and possible bronchoscopy.

3. **Consider early intubation of a patient who will be transferred for further care.**

   Progressive edema makes intubation difficult under the best conditions; imagine the procedure in the back of a speeding ambulance!

4. **Always consider additional traumatic injury in patients.**

   Because of altered mental status or respiratory difficulty, the patient may not be able to provide a history. Head injury or cervical spine injury may be due to a fall or explosion. Always maintain c-spine precautions and do the appropriate tests to rule out additional injury.

5. **Always consider carbon monoxide poisoning.**

   Pulse oximetry does not differentiate between HbO_2 and $COHb$. The SaO_2 should be measured with a co-oximeter.

6. **Patients who are treated with 100% oxygen by prehospital personnel may have a normal CO level when it is measured in the ED.**

   Carboxyhemoglobin levels do not correlate with the degree of poisoning or risk of delayed neurologic sequelae. Consider further therapy in high-risk patients, such as those with comorbid conditions and pregnancy (see **Table 4**).

7. **Give female patients a pregnancy test.**

   Pregnant patients may benefit from HBO with lower CO levels. Fetal hemoglobin has a greater affinity with CO, leading to greater hypoxemia and acidosis.

8. **Do not underestimate cyanide poisoning in inhalation injury.**

   Treatment should not be based a CN levels but on history and physical. CN poisoning can cause a significant acidosis that cannot be explained by CO poisoning alone.

9. **Consider the appropriate ward for the patients.**

   Patients may present with minimal complaints and can "go south" easily, especially if they have comorbid conditions like COPD.

10. **The treatment should be based not on CN levels, but on the history.**

    Some studies have suggested that sodium nitrate can be safe in inhalation injury; but, to be safe, only sodium thiosulfate can be administered.

Hydroxocobalamin has been used in Europe as an antidote for cyanide toxicity but is not approved in the United States. Hydroxocobalamin binds with cyanide to form cyanocobalamin and thereby attenuates its toxic effects. There are side effects to the medication, including anaphylaxis, hypertension, and tachycardia, but it is considered relatively safe. The recommended dose is 4 to 5 grams.[104,105] Two notes of caution: this treatment is not approved in the United States, and a large volume is required to infuse the 1mg/ml concentration.[106]

STEROIDS

In the setting of smoke inhalation, steroids have been studied as a way to decrease initial airway inflammation. They have not proved to be beneficial. Levine et al found no benefit in 60 patients who were randomized to receive dexamethasone for inhalation injury.[107] Neiman et al documented no change in lung parameters, including lung compliance or gas exchange, when anesthetized dogs were exposed to wood smoke and subsequently treated with methylprednisolone.[108] Robinson et al studied patients from a Las Vegas hotel fire who were randomized to receive dexamethasone. This investigation showed no survival benefit in the steroid-treated group.[85]

CONTROVERSIES

The most important controversy in smoke inhalation scholarship concerns the role of hyperbaric oxygen (HBO) therapy for the treatment of carbon monoxide poisoning. Identifying patients who might benefit from HBO therapy is challenging. This is because of conflicting patient outcomes in studies where normobaric oxygen (NBO) and HBO therapy have been directly compared. A review published in 2000 by the Cochrane Database examined 6 randomized controlled trials where NBO and HBO were included in the primary analysis. Although the severity of CO poisoning was not consistent between the trials, and there was no uniform definition of delayed neurologic sequelae, the authors concluded there was "no evidence that unselected use of hyperbaric oxygen in the treatment of CO poisoning reduces the frequency of neurologic symptoms at one month."[109] After that writing, a double-blind, randomized clinical trial compared the rate of neurologic symptoms in patients treated with NBO to those treated with HBO.[101] Patients in this study were administered a battery of neuropsychological tests before, and at various intervals after, treatment. Sham dives were included in the study design to ensure blinding of investigators. The rates of cognitive sequelae were significantly different at the 12-month follow-up; 18.4% in the HBO group and 32.9% in the NBO group. Unfortunately, the groups were not equivalent at baseline. There were a greater number of patients with cerebellar dysfunction in the NBO group relative to the HBO group. The authors minimized the impact of this discrepancy, but 10 out of 14 patients (71.4%) with cerebellar dysfunction developed neurologic symptoms, regardless of their method of treatment. This unintended bias detracts from the strength of the positive finding reported in the study.

Without a consensus position regarding the use of HBO for CO poisoning, there are no pure, evidence-based guidelines to assist clinical decision making. While suggestions regarding the use of HBO therapy are not difficult to find,[46,48,110,111] probably the most widely cited is the Maryland Institute of Emergency Medical Services Systems indications for HBO:[48,112,113] coma, neurological impairment as evidenced by neuropsychiatric testing or other means, cardiovascular involvement, serum carboxyhemoglobin (COHb) level >40%, or COHb level >15% in pregnancy, ischemic heart disease in association with serum COHb levels >20%, recurrent symptoms up to 3 weeks after original treatment with NBO, and symptoms that do not resolve after 6 hours of continuous 100% NBO therapy (**Table 4**). Duke University operates the Divers Alert Network, which can be reached by calling 800-648-8111. In addition to maintaining a list of available HBO chambers, this service also provides emergency consultation. The use of HBO in the setting of smoke inhalation has not been specifically studied. A few patients with smoke inhalation were included in the Cochrane analysis, although burn victims were specifically excluded in one of the reports. In the double-blind, randomized study by Weaver, patients with smoke inhalation were not excluded, but 98% of patients in the HBO group and 88% in the NBO group were exposed to

Table 5. Factors That Suggest an Increased Risk of Smoke Inhalation Injury.
Closed space exposure
Loss of consciousness
Entrapment
CNS depression
Carbonaceous sputum
Edema of the posterior pharynx
Face or neck burns
Hoarseness
Singed nasal hairs
Stridor
Respiratory distress
Including wheezing, shortness of breath

Source: Goldfrank LR, Flomenbaum NE, Lewin NA, Weisman R, Howland MA, Hoffman R. Goldfrank's Toxicologic Emergencies. 6th ed. Stamford: Appleton & Lange; 1998.

CO by sources other than fires.[101] Concomitant burn injuries and multiple trauma considerations in many patients with smoke inhalation may not make HBO a feasible treatment option during the initial stabilization period. Future studies are needed to clarify this.

CUTTING EDGE

With the goal of improving the morbidity and mortality associated with smoke inhalation injury, diverse and exciting scientific efforts are ongoing. Some of the research is focused on preventing fibrin cast formation, providing exogenous surfactant, and targeting the inflammatory response to inhalation injury.[114-117] In an attempt to reduce the number of fibrin cases that form in the bronchi, nebulized heparin has been used in animal models and has been shown to reduce complications.[118-120] Nebulized tPA (tissue plasminogen activator) has also been studied in animal models as a method of limiting fibrin composed airway material.[121] Exogenous surfactant has been investigated as a potential treatment in inhalation injury. Animal models have contributed to the understanding that there is a deficiency of surfactant in smoke inhalation

due to inactivation of surfactant and decreased production by type II pneumocytes.[122,123] Similar models have also shown an improvement in oxygenation after surfactant treatment.[124,117]

DISPOSITION

Since mortality is high for burn victims with inhalation injury, patients with suspected inhalation injury and TBSA greater than 15% should be seriously considered for transfer to a qualified burn center.[91] Intubated patients should be admitted to the ICU or transferred to a burn facility. If there is clinical suspicion of inhalation injury, patients should be evaluated with bronchoscopy, transferred to a regional burn center if bronchoscopy is not available, or admitted to a monitored unit for at least 24 hours of observation.[36,89] (**Table 5**) Asymptomatic patients with low suspicion of inhalation injury can be discharged after a 4–6 hour observation in the ED. In stable patients, transfer decisions can be made without bronchoscopy. (**Table 6**) Physicians should strongly consider intubating symptomatic patients before they are transferred to another facility.[23,4]

Table 6. Criteria for Transfer to a Burn Center
• Injury
• Suspected inhalation injury with >15% TBSA burns
• Symptoms related to smoke inhalation with preexisting cardiovascular or pulmonary disease
• Moderate symptoms (wheezing, hoarseness, sputum production, CO level >10%)

Source: McAuliffe, P. Inhalation Injury and Ventilator Management. Problems in General Surgery 2003:20(1):97-105.

SUMMARY

Smoke inhalation is a major cause of morbidity in burn patients. Awareness of the pathophysiology of smoke inhalation injury can assist clinicians who care for these patients. Even without major external evidence of burns, patients can still suffer from airway injury. Patients should be treated aggressively and early, including early intubation for airway protection when indicated. Carbon monoxide and cyanide toxicity should always be considered. Bronchoscopy is an important adjunct in the assessment of inhalation injury.

REFERENCES

Evidence-based medicine requires a critical appraisal of the literature based upon study methodology and number of subjects. Not all references are equally robust. The findings of a large, prospective-1, randomized, and blinded trial should carry more weight than a case report.

1. Gill JR, Goldfeder LB, Stjic M. The Happy Land homicides: 87 deaths due to smoke inhalation. *J Forensic Sci* 2003 Jan;48(1):161-163. **(Retrospective, 87 patients)**

2. Dacey MJ. Tragedy and reponse -the Rhode Island nightclub fire. *N Engl J Med* 2003 Nov 20;349(21):1990-1992. **(Essay)**

3. Saffle JR. The 1942 Fire at Boston's Cocoanut Grove Nightclub. Am J Surg 1993 Dec;166(6):581-591. **(Retrospective)**

4. American Burn Association. Inhalation injury: diagnosis. *J Am Coll Surg* 2003 Feb;196(2):307-312. **(Review)**

5. American Burn Association. Practice Guidelines for Burn Care. *J Burn Care Rehabil* 2001 May/June Supplement;22(6):19s-26s. **(Review)**

6. Park MS, Cancio LC, Jordan BS, Brinkley WW, Rivera VR, Dubick MA. Assessment of oxidative stress in lungs from sheep after inhalation of wood smoke. *Toxicology* 2004 Feb 15;195(2-3):97-112. **(Animal study)**

7. Qi S, Sun W. The effects of inhaled nitric oxide on cardiac pathology and energy metabolism in a canine model of smoke inhalation injury. *Burns* 2004 Feb;30(1):65-71 **(Animal study)**

8. Park MS, Cancio LC, Batchinsky AI, et al. Assessment of severity of ovine smoke inhalation injury by analysis of computed tomographic scans. *J Trauma* 2003 Sep;55(3):417-427; discussion 427-429. **(Animal study)**

9. Enkhbaatar P, Murakami K, Shimoda K, et al. Ketorolac attenuates cardiopulmonary derangements in sheep with combined burn and smoke inhalation injury. *Clin Sci* 2003 Nov;105(5):621-628. **(Animal study)**

10. American Burn Association. Burn incidence and treatment in the US: 2000 fact sheet. Available at: http://www.ameriburn. org/pub/BurnIncidenceFactSheet.htm. Accessed November 16, 2004.

11. Sobel JB, Goldfarb IW, Slater H, Hammell EJ. Inhalation injury: a decade without progress. *J Burn Care Rehabil* 1992 Sep-Oct;13(5):573-575. **(Retrospective study)**

12. Tredget EE, Shankowsky HA, Taerum TV, et al. The Role of Inhalation Injury in Burn Trauma: A Canadian Experience. *Ann Surg* 1990 Dec;212(6):720-727. **(Retrospective; 1705 patients)**

13. Ryan CM, Schoenfeld DA, Thorpe WP, Sheridan RL, Cassem EH, Tompkins RG. Objective estimates of the probability of death from burn injuries. *N Engl J Med* 1998 Feb;338(6):362-366. **(Retrospective; 1665 patients)**

14. Smith DL, Cairns BA, Ramadan F, et al. Effect of inhalation injury, burn size and age on mortatlity: A study of 1447 consecutive burn patients. *J Trauma* 1994 Oct;37(4):655-659. **(Prospective; 1447 patients)**

15. Levine MS, Radford EP. Fire victims: Medical outcomes and demographic characteristics. *Am J Public Health* 1977 Nov;67(11):1077-1080. **(Retrospective)**

16. Ward EC, Uriarte M, Sppath B, Conroy AL, Sppatht B. Duration of dysphagic symptoms and swallowing outcomes after thermal burn injury. *J Burn Care Rehabil* 2001 Nov/Dec;22(6):441-453. **(Retrospective; 30 patients)**

17. Casper JR, Clark WR, Kelley RT, Colton, RH. Laryngeal and phonatory status after burn/inhalation injury: a long term follow-up study. *J Burn Care Rehabil* 2002 Jul/Aug;23(4):235-243. **(Retrospective, 10 patients)**

18. Park G, Park JW, Jeong DH, Jeong SH. Prolonged Airway and systemic inflammatory reactions after smoke inhalation. *Chest* 2003 Feb;123(2):475-480. **(Prospective case control, 9 case patients, 5 control patients)**

19. Tasaka S, Kanazawa M, Mori M, et al. Long-term course of bronchiectasis and bronchiolitis obliterans as a late complication of smoke inhalation. *Respiration* 1995;62:40-42. **(Case study)**

20. Bourbeau J, Lacasse Y, Rouleau M, Boucher S. Combined smoke inhalation and body surface burns injury does not necessarily imply long-term respiratory health consequences. *Eur Respir J* 1996 Jul;9(7):1470-1474. **(Retrospective, 23 patients)**

21. DiVincenti FC, Pruitt BA, Reckler JM. Inhalation injuries. *J Trauma* 1971 Feb;11(2):109-117. **(Retrospective, 66 patients)**

22. Barrow RE, Spies M, Barrow LN, Herndon, DN. Influence of demographics and inhalation injury on burn mortality in children. *Burns* 2004 Feb;30(1): 72-77. **(Retrospective, 1246 patients)**

23. Herndon DN, Traber DL, Niehaus GD, Linares HA, Traber LD. The pathophysiology of smoke inhalation injury in a sheep model. *J Trauma* 1984 Dec;24(12):1044-1051. **(Prospective, randomized, controlled; 35 sheep)**

24. Alpard SK, Zwischenberger JB, Tao W, Deyo DJ, Traber DL, Bidani A. New clinically relevant model of severe respiratory failure secondary to combined smoke inhalation/cutaneous flame burn injury. *Crit Care Med* 2000 May;28(5):1469-1476. **(Prospective, 22 sheep)**

25. Cox RA, Soejima K, Burke AS, et al. Enhanced pulmonary expression of endothelin-1 in an ovine model of smoke inhalation injury. *J Burn Care Rehabil* 2001 Nov/Dec;22(6):375-383. **(Prospective, 15 sheep)**

26. Tasaki O, Dubick MA, Goodwin CW, Pruitt BA. Effects of *Burns* on Inhalation Injury in sheep: a 5-day study. *J Trauma* 2002 Feb;52(2):351-358. **(Prospective, 13 sheep)**

27. Murakami K, Bjertnaes LJ, Schmalstieg FC, et al. A novel animal model of sepsis after acute lung injury in sheep. *Crit Care Med* 2002 Sep;30(9):2083-2090. **(Prospective, 21 sheep)**

28. Dries D. More than smoke with fire. *Crit Care Med* 2002 Sep;30(9):2159-2160. **(Editorial)**

29. Quinn DA, Moufarrej R, Volokhov A, Syrkina O, Hales CA. Combined smoke inhalation and scald burn in the rat. *J Burn Care Rehabil* 2003 Jul/Aug;24 (4):208-216. **(Prospective, total number of rat subjects unspecified)**

30. Cetin C, Ozyimaz M, Bayci C, et al. Effects of rolling inhibition on smoke inhalation injury. *Burns* 2003 Jun;29(4):307-314 **(Animal study)**

31. Nieman GF, Clark WR, Paskanik A, Feldbaum D. Segmental pulmonary vascular resistance following wood smoke inhalation. *Crit Care Med* 1995 Jul;23(7):1264-1271. **(Prospective, randomized control, animal study)**

32. Rabinowitz PM. Acute inhalation injury. Clin *Chest* Med 2002 Dec;23(4): 707-715. **(Review)**

33. Masanes MJ, Legendre C, Lioret N, Maillard D, Saizy R, Lebeau B. Fiberoptic bronchoscopy for the early diagnosis of subglottal inhalation injury: Comparative value in the assessment of prognosis. *J Trauma* 1994 Jan;36(1):59-67. **(Prospective, 130 patients)**

34. Heimbach DM, Waeckerle JF. Inhalation injuries. *Ann Emerg Med* 1988 Dec;17(12):1316-1320. **(Review)**

35. Cahalane M, Demling RH. Early respiratory abnormalities from smoke inhalation. *JAMA* 1984 Feb;251(6):771-773.

36. Miller K, Chang A. Acute inhalation injury. *Emerg Med Clin North Am* 2003 May;21(2):533-557. **(Review)**

37. Goldfrank LR, Flomenbaum NE, Lewin NA, Weisman R, Howland MA, Hoffman R. *Goldfrank's Toxicologic Emergencies*. 6th ed. Stamford: Appleton & Lange; 1998:1539-1549. **(Textbook)**

38. Prien T, Traber DL. Toxic smoke compounds and inhalation injury. *Burns* Incl Therm Inj 1988 Dec:14(6);451-460. **(Review)**

39. Hantson P, Butera R, Clemessy JL, Michel A, Baud FJ. Early complications and value of initial clinical and paraclinical observations in victims of smoke inhalation without burns. *Chest* 1997 Mar;111(3):671-675. **(Retrospective, 64 patients)**

40. Dyer RF, Esch VH. Polyvinyl chloride toxicity in fires. Hydrogen chloride toxicity in fire fighters. *JAMA* 1976 Jan;235(4):393-397. **(Prospective)**

41. Markowitz JS, Gutterman EM, Schwartz S, Link B, Gorman SM. Acute health effects among firefighters exposed to a polyvinyl chloride (PVC) fire. Am J Epidemiol 1989 May;129(5):1023-1031. **(Retrospective)**

42. Borak J, Diller WF. Phosgene exposure: mechanisms of injury and treatment strategies. *Occup Environ Med* 2001 Feb;43(2):110-119. **(Review)**

43. Cobb N, Etzel RA. Unintentional carbon monoxide–related deaths in the United States, 1979 through 1988. *JAMA* 1991 Aug;266(5):659–663. **(Retrospective, 56,133 patients)**

44. Tomaszewski C. Carbon Monoxide. In: Ford MD, ed. Clinical *Toxicology*. WB Saunders Co; 2001:657-665. **(Book chapter)**

45. Weaver LK. Carbon Monoxide Poisoning. *Crit Care Clin* 1999 Apr;15(2):298-317. **(Review)**

46. Ernst A, Zibrak JD. Carbon Monoxide Poisoning. *N Engl J Med* 1998 Nov;339(22):1603-1608. **(Review)**

47. Choi IS. Delayed Neurologicl Sequelae in Carbon Monoxide Intoxication.

Arch Neurol 1983 Jul;40(7):433-435. **(Retrospective, 2360 patients)**

48. Seger D, Welch L. Carbon Monoxide Controversies: Neuropsychologic Testing, Mechanism of Toxicity, and Hyperbaric Oxygen. *Ann Emerg Med* 1994 Feb; 24(2):242-248. **(Review)**

49. Jones J, McMullen MJ, Dougherty J. Toxic smoke inhalation: Cyanide poisoning in fire victims. *Am J Emerg Med* 1987 Jul;5(4):318–321. **(Review)**

50. Holland MA, Kozlowski LM. Clinical features and management of cyanide poisoning. *Clin Pharm* 1986 Sep;5(9):737-741. **(Review)**

51. Baud FJ, Barriot P, Toffis V, et al: Elevated blood cyanide concentrations in victims of smoke inhalation. *N Engl J Med* 1991 Dec; 325(25):1761–1766. **(Prospective control, 109 patients)**

52. Barillo DJ, Goode R, Esch V. Cyanide poisoning in victims of fire: analysis of 364 cases and review of the literature. *J Burn Care Rehabil* 1994 Jan-Feb;15(1):46-57. **(Review)**

53. Yen D,Tsai J, Wang LM, et al. The clinical experience of acute cyanide poisoning. *Am J Emerg Med* 1995 Sep;13(5):524-528. **(Retrospective review, 21 patients)**

54. Clark WR Jr. Smoke inhalation: diagnosis and treatment. *World J Surg* 1992 Jan-Feb;16(1):24-29. **(Review)**

55. Orzel RA. Toxicologic aspects of firesmoke: polymer pyrolysis and Combustion. *Occup Med* 1993 Jul-Sep;8(3):414-429. **(Review)**

56. Alarie Y. Toxicity of Fire Smoke. *Crit Rev Toxicol* 2002 Jul;32(4):259-289. **(Review)**

57. Sheridan, R. Airway Management and Respiratory Care of the Burn Patient. *Int Anesthesiol Clin* 2000;38(3):129-145. **(Review)**

58. MacLennan N, Heimbach DM, Cullen BF. Anesthesia for Major Thermal Injury. *Anesthesiology* 1998 Sep;89(3):749-770. **(Review)**

59. Theirbach A. Airway Management in Trauma Patients. *Anesthesiol Clin North America* 1999 Mar;17(1):63-81. **(Review)**

60. Harwood-Nuss A, Wolfson AB, Linden CH, Shepherd SM, Stenklyft PH, eds. *The Clinical Practice of Emergency Medicine.* 3rd ed. Philadelphia, Pa: Lippincott Williams & Wilkins; 2001:1690-1694. **(Textbook)**

61. Barlett RH, Niccole M, Tavis MJ, Allyn PA, Furnas DW. Acute management of the upper airway in facial burns. *Arch Surg* 1976 Jul;111(7):744-749. **(Retrospective, 740 patients)**

62. Haponik EF, Summer WR. Respiratory Complications in burn patients: Diagnosis and management of inhalation injury. J Crit Care 1987 Jun;2(2):121. **(Review)**

63. Pruitt BA Jr, Cioffi WG, Shimazu T, Ikeuchi H, Mason AD Jr. Evaluation and management of patients with inhalation injury. *J Trauma* 1990 Dec;30(12 Suppl):S63-S68. **(Review)**

64. Moylan JA Jr, Wilmore DW, Mouton DE, Pruitt BA Jr. Early Diagnosis of inhalation injury using xenon lung scan. *Ann Surg* 1972 Oct;176(4):477-484. **(Prospective, 50 patients)**

65. Schall GL, McDonald HD, Carr LB, Capozzi A. Xenon ventilation-perfusion lung scans. The early diagnosis of inhalation injury. *JAMA* 1978 Nov;240(22):2441-2445. **(Prospective, 64 patients)**

66. Clark WR, Bonaventura M, Myers W. Smoke inhalation and airway management at a regional burn unit: 1974-1983. *J Burn Care Rehabil* 1989 Jan;10(1):52-62. **(Retrospective review, 108 patients)**

67. Touger M. Relationship between venous and arterial carboxyhemoglobin levels in patients with suspected carbon monoxide poisoning. *Ann Emerg Med* 1995 Apr;25(4):481-483. **(Prospective, 61 patients)**

68. Brown DL, Archer SB, Greenhalgh DG, Washam MA, James LE, Warden GD. Inhalation injury severity scoring system: a quantitative method. *J Burn Care Rehabil* 1996 Nov-Dec;17(6):552-557. **(Retrospective, 120 patients)**

69. Hampson NB. Pulse oximetry in severe carbon monoxide poisoning. *Chest* 1998 Oct;114(4):1036-1041. **(Retrospective, 30 patients)**

70. Putman CE, Loke J, Matthay RA, Ravin CE. Radiographic manifestations of acute smoke inhalation. *Am J Roentgenol* 1977 Nov;129(5):865-870. **(Retrospective, 21 patients)**

71. Wittram C, Kenny JB. The admission chest radiograph after acute inhalation injury and burns. *Br J Radiol* 1994 Aug;67(800):751-754. **(Prospective, 30 patients)**

72. Lee MJ, O'Connell DJ. The plain chest radiograph after acute smoke inhalation. *Clin Radiol* 1988 Jan;39(1):33-37. **(Retrospective, 45 patients)**

73. Teixidor HS, Rubin E, Novick GS, Alonso DR. Smoke inhalation: radiologic manifestations. *Radiology* 1983 Nov;149(2):383-387. **(Retrospective, 62 patients)**

74. Stewart R, Baretta ED, Platte LR, et al. Carboxyhemoglobin levels in American blood donors. *JAMA* 1974 Aug; 229(9):1187–1195.

75. Levasseur L, Galliot-Guilley M, Richter F, Baud FJ. Effects of mode of

inhalation of carbon monoxide and of normobaric oxygen administration on carbon monoxide elimination from the blood. *Hum Exp Toxicol* 1996 Nov;15(11):898–903. **(Retrospective, 45 patients)**

76. Bozeman WP, Myers RA, Barish RA. Confirmation of the pulse oximetry gap in carbon monoxide poisoning. *Ann Emerg Med* 1997 Nov;30(5):608-611. **(Retropective, 124 patients)**

77. Kirk MA, Gerace R, Kulig KW. Cyanide and methemoglobin kinetics in smoke inhalation victims treated with the cyanide antidote kit. *Ann Emerg Med* 1993 Sep;22(9):1413-1418. **(Prospective, 7 patients)**

78. Levin BC, Rechani PR, Gurman JL, et al. Analysis of carboxyhemoglobin and cyanide in blood from victims of the Dupont Plaza Hotel fire in Puerto Rico. *J Forensic Sci* 1990 Jan;35(1):151-168 **(Retrospective, 97 patients)**

79. Lundquist P, Rammer L, Sorbo B. The Role of Hydrogen Cyanide and Carbon Monoxide in Fire Casualties: A Prospective Study. Forensic Sci Int 1989 Sep;43(1):9-14. **(Prospective, 18 patients)**

80. Barillo J, Goode R, Rush BF Jr, Lin RL, Freda A, Anderson EJ Jr. Lack of correlation between carboxyhemoglobin and cyanide in smoke inhalation injury. *Curr Surg* 1986 Sep-Oct;43(5):421-423.

81. Benaissa ML, Megarbane B, Borron SW, Baud FJ. Is elevated plasma lactate a useful marker in the evaluation of pure carbon monoxide poisoning? Intensive Care Med 2003 Aug;29(8):1372-1375. **(Prospective, 145 patients)**

82. McCabe MJ, Weston CF, Fraser AG. Acute myocardial infarction related to smoke inhalation and myocardial bridging. *Postgrad Med J* 1992 Sep;68(803):758-761. **(Case Report)**

83. Koren G, Sharav T, Pastuszak A, et al. A multicenter, prospective study of fetal outcome following accidental carbon monoxide poisoning in pregnancy. *Reprod Toxicol* 1991;5(5):397. **(Prospective, 31 patients)**

84. Bingham HG, Gallagher TJ, Powell MD. Early bronchosopy as a predictor of ventilatory support for burned patients. *J Trauma* 1987 Nov;27(11):1286-1289. **(Prospective, 27 patients)**

85. Robinson NB, Hudson LD, Riem M, et al. Steroid therapy following isolated smoke inhalation injury. *J Trauma* 1982 Oct;22(10):876-879. **(Randomized control trial)**

86. Lin WY, Kao CH, Wang SJ. Detection of acute inhalation injury in fire victims by means of technetium-99m DTPA radioaerosol inhalation lung scintigraphy. *Eur J Nucl Med* 1997 Feb;24(2): 125-129. **(Prospective, 10 control and 17 experimental)**

87. Rue, LW, Cioffi WG. Improved Survival of Burned Patients with Inhalation Injury. 1993 Jul;128(7):772-780. **(Retrospective review)**

88. Martyn J, Goldhill DR, Goudsouzian NG. Clinical pharmacology of muscle relaxants in patients with burns. *J Clin Pharmaology* 1986 Nov-Dec;26 (8):680-5. **(Review)**

89. Fitzpatrick JC, Cioffi WG. In: Herndon D, ed. *Total Burn Care.* 2nd ed. Philadelphia, Pa: WB Saunders; 2002:221-253. **(Textbook chapter)**

90. Park GY, Park JW, Jeong DH, Jeong SH. Prolonged airway and systemic inflammatory reactions after smoke inhalation. *Chest* 2003 Feb;123(2):475-480. **(Cross-sectional study, 9 patients)**

91. McAuliffe, P. Inhalation Injury and Ventilator Management. Problems in General Surgery 2003:20(1):97-105. **(Review)** 92. Reper P, Wibaux O, Van Laeke P, Vandeenen D, Duinslaeger L, Vanderkelen A. High frequency percussive ventilation and conventional ventilation after smoke inhalation. *Burns* 2002 Aug;28(5):503-508. **(Prospective, 35 patients)**

93. Cioffi WG Jr, Rue LW 3rd, Graves TA, McManus WF, Mason AD Jr, Pruitt BA Jr. Prophylactic use of high frequency percussive ventilation in patients with inhalation injury. *Ann Surg* 1991 Jun;213(6):575-580. **(Prospective, 54 patients)**

94. Cioffi W, Graves TA, McManus WF, Pruitt BA Jr. High Frequency percussive ventilation in patients with inhalation injury. *J Trauma* 1989 Mar;29(3):350-354. **(Retropective)**

95. Jackson MP, Philp B, Murdoch LJ, Powell BW. High frequency oscillatory ventilation successfully used to treat a severe paediatric inhalation injury. *Burns* 2002 Aug;28(5):509-511. **(Case study)**

96. Cortiella J, MIcak R, Herndon D. High frequency percussive ventilation in pediatric patients with inhalation injury. *J Burn Care Rehabil* 1999 May-Jun;20(3):232-235. **(Retrospective, 13 patients)**

97. Smailes ST. Noninvasive Positive Pressure Ventilation in burns. *Burns* 2002 Dec;28(8):795-801. **(Retrospective, 30 patients)**

98. Inoue T, Okabayashi K, Ohtani M, Yamanoue T, Wada S, Iida K. Effect of smoke inhalation injury on fluid requirement in burn resuscitation. *Hiroshima J Med Sci* 2002 Mar;51(1):1-5. **(Retrospective, 131 patients)**

99. Hughes KR, Armstrong RF, Brough MD, Parkhouse N. Fluid Requirements of patients with burns and inhalation injuries in an intensive care unit. Intensive Care Med 1989;15(7):464-466. **(Retrospective, 9 patients)**

100. Navar PD, Saffle JR, Warden GD. Effect of inhalation injury on fluid resusci-

tation requirements after thermal injury. *Am J Surg* 1985 Dec;150(6):716-720. **(Retrospective, 171 patients)**

101. Weaver LK, Hopkins RO, Chan KJ, et al. Hyperbaric oxygen for acute carbon monoxide poisoning. *N Engl J Med* 2002 Oct;347(14):1057-1067. **(Randomized Control Trial; 152 patients)**

102. Saincher A, Swirsky N, Tenenbein M. Cyanide overdose: survival with fatal blood concentration without antidotal therapy. *J Emerg Med* 1994 Jul-Aug;12(4):555-557. **(Case study)**

103. Kulig K. Cyanide antidotes and fire toxicology. *N Engl J Med* 1991 Dec;325(25):1801–1802. **(Comment)**

104. Houeto P, Hoffman JR, Imbert M, Levillain P, Baud FJ. Relation of blood cyanide to plasma cyanocobalamin concentration after a fixed-dose of hydroxocobalamin in cyanide poisoning. *Lancet* 1995 Sep;346(8975):605-608. **(Prospective, 12 patients)**

105. Mokhlesi B. Adult toxicology in critical care: Part II: specific poisonings. *Chest* 2003 Mar;123(3):897-922. **(Review)**

106. Sauer S, Keim M. Hydroxocobalamin: Improved public health readiness for cyanide disasters. *Ann Emerg Med* 2001 Jun;37(6):635-641. **(Comment)**

107. Levine B, Petroff PA, Slade L, Pruitt BA Jr. Prospective Trials of Dexamethasone and Aerosolized Gentamicin in the Treatment of Inhalation Injury in the Burned Patient. *J Trauma* 1978 Mar;18(3):188-193. **(Prospective cohort with 60 patients)**

108. Neiman GF, Clark WR. Methyprednisolone does not protect the lung from inhalation injury. *Burns* 1991 Oct;17(5):384-390. **(Animal Study)**

109. Juurlink DN, Stanbrook MB. McGuigan MA. Hyperbaric Oxygen for Carbon Monoxide Poisoning. *Cochrane Database Syst Rev* 2000(2):CD002041. **(Cochrane review)**

110. Hampson NB, Dunford RG, Kramer CC, Norkool DM. Selection Criteria Utilized for Hyperbaric Oxygen Treatment of Carbon Monoxide Poisoning. *J Emerg Med* 1995 Mar; 3(2):227-231. **(Survey)**

111. Tibbles PM, Edelsberg JS. Hyperbaric-Oxygen Therapy. *N Engl J Med* 1996 Jun;334(25):1642-1648. **(Review)**

112. Minogue MF. Hyperbaric Oxygen Therapy and Carbon Monoxide Toxicity. *Clin Toxicol Rev* 1998 Aug;20(11). **(Review)**

113. Erikson TB, Neylan VD. Carbon Monoxide Poisoning. In: Haddad L, ed. *Clinical Management of Poisoning and Drug Overdose.* 3rd ed. Philadelphia, Pa: WB Saunders; 1998:272. **(Textbook chapter)**

114. Murakami K, McGuire R, Cox RA, et al. Recombinant antithrombin attenuates pulmonary inflammation following smoke inhalation and pneumonia in sheep. *Crit Care Med* 2003 Feb;31(2):577-583. **(Animal Study)**

115. Park GY, Park JW, Jeong DH, Jeong SH., Prolonged airway and systemic inflammatory reactions after smoke inhalation. *Chest* 2003 Feb;123(2):475-480. **(Prospective, 9 patients)**

116. Dubick MA, Carden SC, Jordan BS, Langlinais PC, Mozingo DW. Indices of antioxidant status in rats subjected to wood smoke inhalation and/or ther-mal injury. *Toxicology* 2002 Jul1;176(1-2):145-157. **(Animal study)**

117. Nieman GF, Paskanik AM, Fluck RR. Comparison of exogenous surfactant in the treatment of smoke inhalation. Am J Respir *Crit Care Med* 1995 Aug;152(2):597. **(Animal study)**

118. Tasaki O, Mozingo DW, Dubick MA, Goodwin CW, Yantis LD, Pruitt BA Jr. Effects of heparin and lisofylline on pulmonary function after smoke inhalation injury in an ovine model. *Crit Care Med* 2002 Mar;30(3):637–643. **(Animal study)**

119. Cox CS Jr, Zwischenberger JB, Traber DL, Traber LD, Haque AK, Herndon DN. Heparin improves oxygenation and minimizes barotrauma after severe smoke inhalation in an ovine model. *Surg Gynecol Obstet* 1993 Apr;176(4):339–349. **(Animal study)**

120. Desai MH, MIcak R, Richardson J, Nichols R, Herndon DN. Reduction in mortality in pediatric patients with inhalation injury with aerosolized heparin/acetylcystine therapy. *J Burn Care Rehabil* 1999 Jan-Feb;19 (3):210–212. **(Retrospective, 90 patients)**

121. Enkhbaatar P, Murakami K, Cox R, et al. Aersolized Tissue Plasminogen Inhibitor Improves Pulmonary Function in Sheep with Burn and Smoke Inhalation. *Shock* 2004 Jul;22(1):70-75. **(Animal study)**

122. Nieman GF, Clark WR Jr. Effects of wood and cotton smoke on the surface properties of pulmonary surfactant. *Respir Physiol* 1994 Jun;97(1):1-12. **(Animal study)**

123. Oulton MR, Janigan DT, MacDonald JM, Faulkner GT, Scott JE. Effects of smoke inhalation on alveolar surfactant subtypes in mice. *Am J Pathol* 1994 Oct;145(4):941-950. **(Animal study)**

124. Jeng MJ, Kou YR, Sheu CC, Hwang B. Effects of exogenous surfactant supplementation and partial liquid ventilation on acute lung injury induced by wood smoke inhalation in newborn piglets. *Crit Care Med* 2003 Apr;31(4):1166-1174. **(Animal study)**

Meghal Mehta, MD, Department of Emergency Medicine, Brown University— Providence, RI.

Laura McPeake, MD, Department of Emergency Medicine, Brown University— Providence, RI.

Daren Girard, MD, Clinical Instructor in Emergency Medicine, Department of Emergency Medicine, Brown University School of Medicine, Providence, RI.

(Peer reviewers: Stephen Wolf, MD, Attending Physician, Department of Emergency Medicine, Denver Health Medical Center, Denver, CO; Andy Jagoda, MD, FACEP, Vice-Chair of Academic Affairs, Department of Emergency Medicine; Residency Program Director, Mount Sinai School of Medicine, New York, NY)

Source: Emergency Medicine Practice: *An Evidence-Based Approach to Emergency Medicine. Volume 6, Number 11. November 2004, pages 1-17. www.empractice.net. Reprinted with permission from EB Practice, LLC.*

PART SEVEN

MEDICAL MANAGEMENT IN AN EXPLOSIVE ATTACK

EXPLOSIONS AND BLAST INJURIES

A PRIMER FOR CLINICIANS

KEY CONCEPTS

- Bombs and explosions can cause unique patterns of injury seldom seen outside combat.
- The predominant post explosion injuries among survivors involve standard penetrating and blunt trauma. Blast lung is the most common fatal injury among initial survivors.
- Explosions in confined spaces (mines, buildings, or large vehicles) and/or structural collapse are associated with greater morbidity and mortality.
- Half of all initial casualties will seek medical care over a one-hour period. This can be useful to predict demand for care and resource needs.
- Expect an "upside-down" triage—the most severely injured arrive after the less injured, who bypass EMS triage and go directly to the closest hospitals.

BACKGROUND

Explosions can produce unique patterns of injury seldom seen outside combat. When they do occur, they have the potential to inflict multisystem life-threatening injuries on many persons simultaneously. The injury patterns following such events are a product of the composition and amount of the materials involved, the surrounding environment, delivery method (if a bomb), the distance between the victim and the blast, and any intervening protective barriers or environmental hazards. Because explosions are relatively infrequent, blast-related injuries can present unique triage, diagnostic, and management challenges to providers of emergency care.

Few U.S. health professionals have experience with explosive-related injuries. Vietnam-era physicians are retiring, other armed conflicts have been short-lived, and until this past decade, the U.S. was largely spared of the scourge of mega-terrorist attacks. This primer introduces information relevant to the care of casualties from explosives and blast injuries. As the risk of terrorist attacks increases in the U.S., disaster response personnel must understand the unique pathophysiology of injuries associated with explosions and must be prepared to assess and treat the people injured by them.

CLASSIFICATION OF EXPLOSIVES

Explosives are categorized as **high-order explosives** (HE) or **low-order explosives** (LE).

HE produce a defining supersonic over-pressurization shock wave. Examples of HE include TNT, C-4, Semtex, nitroglycerin, dynamite, and ammonium nitrate fuel oil (ANFO). LE create a subsonic explosion and lack HE's over-pressurization wave. Examples of LE include pipe bombs, gunpowder, and most pure petroleum-based bombs such as Molotov cocktails or aircraft improvised as guided missiles. HE and LE cause different injury patterns.

Explosive and incendiary (fire) bombs are further characterized based on their source. "Manufactured" implies standard military-issued, mass produced, and quality-tested weapons. "Improvised" describes weapons produced in small quantities, or use of a device outside its intended purpose, such as converting a commercial aircraft into a guided missile. Manufactured (military) explosive weapons are exclusively HE-based. Terrorists will use whatever is available–illegally obtained manufactured weapons or improvised explosive devices (also known as "IEDs") that may be composed of HE, LE, or both. Manufactured and improvised bombs cause markedly different injuries.

BLAST INJURIES

The four basic mechanisms of blast injury are termed as primary, secondary, tertiary, and quaternary (**Table 1**). "Blast Wave" (primary) refers to the intense over-pressurization impulse created by a detonated HE. Blast injuries are characterized by anatomical and physiological changes from the direct or reflective over-pressurization force impacting the body's surface. The HE "blast wave" (over-pressure component) should be distinguished from "blast wind" (forced super-heated air flow). The latter may be encountered with both HE and LE.

LE are classified differently because they lack the self-defining HE over-pressurization wave.

Table 1. Mechanisms of Blast Injury

Category	Characteristics	Body Part Affected	Types of Injuries
Primary	Unique to HE, results from the impact of the overpressurization wave with body surfaces.	Gas filled structures are most susceptible • lungs, GI tract, and middle ear	• Blast lung (pulmonary barotrauma) • TM rupture and middle ear damage • Abdominal hemorrhage and perforation • Globe (eye) rupture • Concussion (TBI without physical signs of head injury)
Secondary	Results from flying debris and bomb fragments	Any body part may be affected	• Penetrating ballistic (fragmentation) or blunt injuries • Eye penetration (can be occult)
Tertiary	Results from individuals being thrown by the blast wind	Any body part may be affected	• Fracture and traumatic amputation • Closed and open brain injury
Quaternary	• All explosion-related injuries, illnesses, or diseases not due to primary, secondary, or tertiary mechanisms. • Includes exacerbation or complications of existing conditions.	Any body part may be affected	• Burns (flash, partial, and full thickness) • Crush injuries • Closed and open brain injury • Asthma, COPD, or other breathing problems from dust, smoke, or toxic fumes • Angina • Hyperglycemia, hypertension

LE's mechanisms of injuries are characterized as due from ballistics (fragmentation), blast wind (not blast wave), and thermal. There is some overlap between LE descriptive mechanisms and HE's secondary, tertiary, and quaternary mechanisms.

Note: Up to 10% of all blast survivors have significant eye injuries. These injuries involve perforations from high-velocity projectiles, can occur with minimal initial discomfort, and present for care days, weeks, or months after the event. Symptoms include eye pain or irritation, foreign body sensation, altered vision, periorbital swelling or contusions. Findings can include decreased visual acuity, hyphema, globe perforation, subconjunctival hemorrhage, foreign body, or lid lacerations. Liberal referral for ophthalmologic screening is encouraged.

SELECTED BLAST INJURIES

LUNG INJURY

"Blast lung" is a direct consequence of the HE over-pressurization wave. It is the most common fatal primary blast injury among initial survivors. Signs of blast lung are usually present at the time of initial evaluation, but they have been reported as late as 48 hours after the explosion. Blast lung is characterized by the clinical triad of apnea, bradycardia, and hypotension. Pulmonary injuries vary from scattered petechae to confluent hemorrhages. Blast lung should be suspected for anyone with dyspnea, cough, hemoptysis, or chest pain following blast exposure. Blast lung produces a characteristic "butterfly" pattern on chest X-ray. A chest X-ray is recommended for all exposed persons and a prophylactic chest tube (thoracostomy) is recommended before general anesthesia or air transport is indicated if blast lung is suspected.

EAR INJURY

Primary blast injuries of the auditory system cause significant morbidity, but are easily overlooked. Injury is dependent on the orientation of the ear to the blast. TM perforation is the most common

Table 2. Overview of Explosive-Related Injuries

System	Injury or Condition
Auditory	TM rupture, ossicular disruption, cochlear damage, foreign body
Eye, Orbit, Face	Perforated globe, foreign body, air embolism, fractures
Respiratory	Blast lung, hemothorax, pneumothorax, pulmonary contusion and hemorrhage, A-V fistulas (source of air embolism), airway epithelial damage, aspiration pneumonitis, sepsis
Digestive	Bowel perforation, hemorrhage, ruptured liver or spleen, sepsis, mesenteric ischemia from air embolism
Circulatory	Cardiac contusion, myocardial infarction from air embolism, shock, vasovagal hypotension, peripheral vascular injury, air embolism-induced injury
CNS Injury	Concussion, closed and open brain injury, stroke, spinal cord injury, air embolism-induced injury
Renal Injury	Renal contusion, laceration, acute renal failure due to rhabdomyolysis, hypotension, and hypovolemia
Extremity Injury	Traumatic amputation, fractures, crush injuries, compartment syndrome, burns, cuts, lacerations, acute arterial occlusion, air embolism-induced injury

injury to the middle ear. Signs of ear injury are usually present at time of initial evaluation and should be suspected for anyone presenting with hearing loss, tinnitus, otalgia, vertigo, bleeding from the external canal, TM rupture, or mucopurulent otorrhea. All patients exposed to blast should have an otologic assessment and audiometry.

ABDOMINAL INJURY

Gas-containing sections of the GI tract are most vulnerable to primary blast effect. This can cause immediate bowel perforation, hemorrhage (ranging from small petechiae to large hematomas), mesenteric shear injuries, solid organ lacerations, and testicular rupture. Blast abdominal injury should be suspected in anyone exposed to an explosion with abdominal pain, nausea, vomiting, hematemesis, rectal pain, tenesmus, testicular pain, unexplained hypovolemia, or any findings suggestive of an acute abdomen. Clinical findings may be absent until the onset of complications.

BRAIN INJURY

Primary blast waves can cause concussions or mild traumatic brain injury (MTBI) without a direct blow to the head. Consider the proximity of the victim to the blast particularly when given complaints of

headache, fatigue, poor concentration, lethargy, depression, anxiety, insomnia, or other constitutional symptoms. The symptoms of concussion and post traumatic stress disorder can be similar.

EMERGENCY MANAGEMENT OPTIONS

- Follow your hospital's and regional disaster system's plan.
- Expect an "upside-down" triage—the most severely injured arrive after the less injured, who bypass EMS triage and go directly to the closest hospitals.
- Double the first hour's casualties for a rough prediction of total "first wave" of casualties.
- Obtain and record details about the nature of the explosion, potential toxic exposures and environmental hazards, and casualty location from police, fire, EMS, ICS Commander, regional EMA, health department, and reliable news sources.
- If structural collapse occurs, expect increased severity and delayed arrival of casualties.

MEDICAL MANAGEMENT OPTIONS

- Blast injuries are not confined to the battlefield. They should be considered for any victim exposed to an explosive force.

- Clinical signs of blast-related abdominal injuries can be initially silent until signs of acute abdomen or sepsis are advanced.
- Standard penetrating and blunt trauma to any body surface is the most common injury seen among survivors. Primary blast lung and blast abdomen are associated with a high mortality rate. "Blast Lung" is the most common fatal injury among initial survivors.
- Blast lung presents soon after exposure. It can be confirmed by finding a "butterfly" pattern on chest X-ray. Prophylactic chest tubes (thoracostomy) are recommended prior to general anesthesia and/or air transport.
- Auditory system injuries and concussions are easily overlooked. The symptoms of mild TBI and posttraumatic stress disorder can be identical.
- Isolated TM rupture is not a marker of morbidity; however, traumatic amputation of any limb is a marker for multisystem injuries.
- Air embolism is common, and can present as stroke, MI, acute abdomen, blindness, deafness, spinal cord injury, or claudication. Hyperbaric oxygen therapy may be effective in some cases.
- Compartment syndrome, rhabdomyolysis, and acute renal failure are associated with structural collapse, prolonged extrication, severe burns, and some poisonings.
- Consider the possibility of exposure to inhaled toxins and poisonings (eg, CO, CN, MetHgb) in both industrial and criminal explosions.
- Wounds can be grossly contaminated. Consider delayed primary closure and assess tetanus status. Ensure close follow-up of wounds, head injuries, eye, ear, and stress-related complaints.
- Communications and instructions may need to be written because of tinnitus and sudden temporary or permanent deafness.

SELECTED READINGS

Auf der Heide E. Disaster Response: Principles of Preparation and Coordination Disaster Response: Principles of Preparation and Coordination http://216.202.128.19/dr/flash.htm

Quenemoen LE, Davis, YM, Malilay J, Sinks T, Noji EK, and Klitzman S. The World Trade Center bombing: injury prevention strategies for high-rise building fires. *Disasters* 1996;20:125–132.

Wightman JM and Gladish SL. Explosions and blast injuries. *Ann Emerg Med;* June 2001; 37(6): 664-p678.

Stein M and Hirshberg A. Trauma Care in the New Millinium: Medical Consequences of Terrorism, the Conventional Weapon Threat. *Surg Clin North America.* Dec 1999; Vol 79 (6).

Phillips YY. Primary Blast Injuries. *Ann Emerg Med;* 1986, Dec; 106 (15); 1446-50.

Hogan D, et al. Emergency Department Impact of the Oklahoma City Terrorist Bombing. *Ann Emerg Med;* August 1999; 34 (2)

Mallonee S, et al. Physical Injuries and Fatalities Resulting From the Oklahoma City Bombing. *JAMA;* August 7, 1996; 276 (5); 382-387.

Leibovici D, et al. Blast injuries: bus versus open-air bombings—a comparative study of injuries in survivors of open-air versus confined-space explosions. *J Trauma;* 1996, Dec; 41 (6): 1030-1035.

Katz E, et al. Primary blast injury after a bomb explosion in a civilian bus. *Ann Surg;* 1989 Apr; 209 (4): 484-8.

Hill JF. Blast injury with particular reference to recent terrorists bombing incidents. *Ann Royal Coll Surg Engl* 1979;61:411.

Landesman LY, Malilay J, Bissell RA, Becker SM, Roberts L, Ascher MS. Roles and responsibilities of public health in disaster preparedness and response. In: Novick LF, Mays GP, editors. *Public Health Administration: Principles for Population-based Management.* Gaithersburg (MD): Aspen Publishers; 2001.

BLAST LUNG INJURY: WHAT CLINICIANS NEED TO KNOW

Blast lung injury (BLI) presents unique triage, diagnostic, and management challenges and is a direct consequence of the blast wave from high explosive detonations upon the body. BLI is a major cause of morbidity and mortality for blast victims both at the scene and among initial survivors. The blast wave's impact upon the lung results in tearing, hemorrhage, contusion, and edema with resultant ventilation-perfusion mismatch. BLI is a clinical diagnosis and is characterized by respiratory difficulty and hypoxia, which may occur without obvious external injury to the chest.

Current patterns in worldwide terrorist activity have increased the potential for casualties related to explosions, yet few civilian health care providers in the United States have experience treating patients with explosion-related injuries. Emergency care providers are urged to learn more about the physics of explosions and other types of injuries that can result. Basic clinical information is provided here to inform practitioners of the presentation, evaluation, management, and outcomes of BLIs. Please see the reference list below for more information about how to treat injuries from explosions.

CLINICAL PRESENTATION

- Symptoms may include dyspnea, hemoptysis, cough, and chest pain.
- Signs may include tachypnea, hypoxia, cyanosis, apnea, wheezing, decreased breath sounds, and hemodynamic instability.
- Associated pathology may include bronchopleural fistula, air emboli, and hemothoraces or pneumothoraces.
- Other injuries may be present.

DIAGNOSTIC EVALUATION

- Chest radiography is necessary for anyone who is exposed to a blast.
- A characteristic "butterfly" pattern may be revealed upon x-ray.

- Arterial blood gases, computerized tomography, and doppler technology may be used.
- Most laboratory and diagnostic testing can be conducted per resuscitation protocols and further directed based upon the nature of the explosion (eg, confined space, fire, prolonged entrapment or extrication, suspected chemical or biologic event, etc.).

MANAGEMENT

- Initial triage, trauma resuscitation, treatment, and transfer should follow standard protocols; however some diagnostic or therapeutic options may be limited in a disaster or mass casualty situation.
- In general, managing BLI is similar to caring for pulmonary contusion, which requires judicious fluid use and administration ensuring tissue perfusion without volume overload.
- Clinical interventions
  - All patients with suspected or confirmed BLI should receive supplemental high-flow oxygen sufficient to prevent hypoxemia (delivery may include non-rebreather masks, continuous positive airway pressure, or endotracheal intubation).
  - Impending airway compromise, secondary edema, injury, or massive hemoptysis requires immediate intervention to secure the airway. Patients with massive hemoptysis or significant air leaks may benefit from selective bronchus intubation.
  - Clinical evidence of or suspicion for a hemothorax or pneumothorax warrants prompt decompression.
  - If ventilatory failure is imminent or occurs, patients should be intubated; however, caution should be used in the decision to intubate patients, as mechanical ventilation and positive end pressure may increase the risk of alveolar rupture and air embolism.
  - High-flow oxygen should be administered if air embolism is suspected, and the patient should

be placed in prone, semi-left lateral, or left lateral positions. Patients treated for air emboli should be transferred to a hyperbaric chamber.

DISPOSITION AND OUTCOME

- There are no definitive guidelines for observation, admission, or discharge following emergency department evaluation for patients with possible BLI following an explosion.
- Patients diagnosed with BLI may require complex management and should be admitted to an intensive care unit. Patients with any complaints or findings suspicious for BLI should be observed in the hospital.
- Discharge decisions will also depend upon associated injuries, and other issues related to the event, including the patient's current social situation.
- In general, patients with normal chest radiographs and ABGs, who have no complaints that would suggest BLI, can be considered for discharge after 4-6 hours of observation.
- Data on the short-and long-term outcomes of patients with BLI is currently limited. However, in one study conducted on survivors one year post injury, no patients had pulmonary complaints, all had normal physical examinations and chest radiographs, and most had normal lung function tests.

REFERENCES AND READINGS

1. Patterns of global terrorism 2001. United States Department of State. May 2002. United States Department of State website. Available at: http://www.state.gov/documents/organization/10319.pdf. Accessed 4 February 2005.
2. Patterns of global terrorism 2002. United States Department of State. April 2003. United States Department of State website. Available at: http://www.state.gov/documents/organization/20177.pdf. Accessed 4 February 2005.
3. Patterns of Global Terrorism 2003. United States Department of State. April 2004. United States Department of State website. Available at: http://www.state.gov/documents/organization/31912.pdf. Accessed 4 February 2005.
4. Terrorism 2000/2001. United States Department of Justice, Federal Bureau of Investigation, Counterterrorism Division. Publication #0308. Federal Bureau of Investigation website. Available at: http://www.fbi.gov/publications/terror/terror2000_2001.htm. Accessed 4 February 2005. 5. Gadson LO, Michael ML, Walsh N (eds). FBI Bomb Data Center: 1998 Bombing Incidents, General Information Bulletin 98-1. US Department of Justice, Federal Bureau of Investigation. 1998.
6. Wightman JM, Gladish SL. Explosions and blast injuries. *Ann Emerg Med.* 2001; 37(6):664-678.
7. Horrocks CL Blast Injuries: Biophysics, pathophysiology, and management principles. *J R Army Med Corps* 2001;147:28-40.
8. Cullis, IG. Blast waves and how they interact with structures. *J R Army Med Corps* 2001;147:16-26.
9. Langworthy MJ, Sabra J, Gould M. Terrorism and blast phenomena: lessons learned from the attack on the USS Cole (DDG67). *Clinic Orthop.* 2004;422: 82-87.
10. Elsayed NM. Toxicology of Blast Overpressure. *Toxicology.* 1997; 121: 1-15.
11. Yetiser S and Ustun T. Concussive blast-type aural trauma, eardrum perforations, and their effects on hearing levels: an update on military experience in Izmir, Turkey. *Mil Med.* 1993; 158 (12):803-806.
12. Mayorga MA. The pathology of primary blast overpressure injury. *Toxicology.* 1997; 121:17-28.
13. Kluger Y. Bomb explosions in acts of terrorism-detonation, wound ballistics, triage, and medical concerns. *Isr Med Assoc J.* 2003; 5:235-240.
14. Sasser SM. Blast injuries. Turkish *J Emerg Med.* 2001; 1(1): 97-98.
15. Shaham, D, Sella T, Makori A, et al. The role of radiology in terror injuries. *Isr Med Assoc J.* 2002; 4(7): 564-567.
16. Knapp JF, Sharp RJ, Beatty R, et al. Blast trauma in a child. *Pediatric Emerg Care.* 1990; 6(2): 122-6.
17. Phillips YY. Primary blast injuries. *Ann Emerg Med.* 1986; 15:1446-1450.
18. Cooper GH, Maynard RL, Cross NL, et al. Casualties from terrorist bombings. *J Trauma.* 1983; 23(11): 955-967.
19. Stein M, Hirshberg A. Trauma care in the new millennium. *Surg Clin North Am.* 1999; 79 (6): 1537-1552.
20. Hadden WA, Rutherford WH, Merrett JD. The injuries of terrorist bombing: a study of 1532 consecutive patients. *Br J Surg.* 1978: 65(8):525-531.
21. Frykberg ER, Tepas JJ. Terrorist bombings: lessons learned from Belfast to Beirut. *Ann Surg.* 208: 569-576.
22. Mellor SG. The relationship of blast loading to death and injury from explosion. *World J Surg.* 1992; 16: 893-898.
23. Katz E, Ofek B, Adler J, et al. Primary blast injury after a bomb explosion on a civilian bus. *Ann Surg.* 1989; 209 (4): 484-488.
24. de Ceballos JPG, Turegano-Fuentes F, Perez-Diaz D, et al. 11 March 2004: The terrorist bomb explosions in Madrid, Spain-an analysis of the logistics, injuries sustained and clinical management of casualties treated at the closest hospital. *Crit Care Med.* 2005 Jan;33(1):s107-112.
25. Pizov, R, Oppenheim-Eden A, Matot I, et al. Blast lung injury from an explosion on a civilian bus. *Chest.* 1999; 115 (1): 165-172
26. Tsokos M, Paulsen F, Petri S, Burkhard M, et al. Histological, immunohistochemical, and ultra-structural findings in human blast lung injury. *Am J Respir Crit Care Med.* 2003; 168: 549-555.
27. Leibovici D, Gofrit ON, Stein M, et al. Blast injuries: bus versus open-air bombings-a comparative study of injuries in survivors of open-air versus confinedspace explosions. *J Trauma.* 1996; 41: 1030-1035.
28. Hirshberg B, Oppenheim-Eden A, Pizov R, et al. Recovery from Blast Lung Injury: One-Year Follow-up. *Chest.* 1999; 116(6): 1683-1688.
29. Frykberg ER, Tepas JJ, Alexander RH. The 1983 Beirut airport terrorist bombing: injury patterns and implications for disaster management. *Am Surg.* 1989; 55: 134-141.
30. Irwin RJ, Lerner MR, Bealer JF, Mantor PC, et al. Shock after blast wave injury is caused by a vagally mediated reflex. *J Trauma.* 1999; 47(1): 105-110.
31. Frykberg, ER. Medical management of disasters and mass casualties from terrorist bombings: how can we cope? *J Trauma.* 2002; 53:201-212.
32. Stuhmiller JH, Ho KHH, Vander Vorst MJ, et al. A model of blast overpressure injury to the lung. *J Biomech.* 1996; 29(2):227-234.
33. Stuhmiller JH. Biological response to blast overpressure: a summary of modeling. *Toxicology.* 1997; 121: 91-103.
34. Zhang J, Wang Z, Leng J, Yang Z. Studies on lung injuries caused by blast underpressure. *J Trauma.* 1996; 40 (3 supplement): s77-s80.
35. Elsayed NM, Gorbunov NV. Interplay between high energy impulse noise (blast) and antioxidants in the lung. *Toxicology.* 2003; 189(1-2):63-74.
36. Argyros, GJ. Management of Primary Blast Injury. *Toxicology.* 1997; 121: 105-115.
37. Leibovici D, Gofrit ON, Shapira SC. Eardrum perforation in explosion survivors: is it a marker of pulmonary blast injury?. *Ann Emerg Med.* 1999; 34(2): 168-172
38. Sorkine P, Szold O, Kluger Y, et al. Permissive hypercapnia ventilation in patients with severe pulmonary blast injury. *J Trauma.* 1998; 45(1): 35-38.
39. Irwin RJ, Lerner MR, Bealer JF, et al. Cardiopulmonary physiology of primary blast injury. *J Trauma.* 1997; 43 (4): 650-655.
40. Karmy-Jones R, Kissinger D, Golcovsky M. Bomb-related injuries. *Mil Med.* 1994; 159: 536-539.
41. Cohn SM. Pulmonary Contusion: review of the clinical entity. *J Trauma.* 1997 May;42(5):973-79.
42. Elsayed NM, Gorbunov NV, Kagan VE. A proposed biochemical mechanism involving hemoglobin for blast over-pressure induced injury. *Toxicology.* 1997; 121: 81-90.
43. Lavonis E. Blast injuries. Emedicine website. Available at: http://www.emedicine.com/emerg/topic63.htm. Accessed 4 February 2005.
44. Gorbunov NV, McFaul SJ, Van Albert S, et al. Assessment of inflammatory response and sequestration of blood iron transferrin complexes in a rat model of lung injury resulting from exposure to low-frequency shock waves. *Crit Care Med.* 2004 Apr; 32(4): 1028-34.
45. DePalma RG, Burris DG, Champion HR, Hodgson MJ. Blast Injuries. *N Engl J Med* 2005;352:1335-42.

SUICIDE BOMBING ATTACKS

UPDATE AND MODIFICATIONS TO THE PROTOCOL

Gidon Almogy, MD,* Howard Belzberg, MD,†
Yoaz Mintz, MD,* Alon K. Pikarsky, MD,*
Gideon Zamir, MD,* and Avraham I. Rivkind, MD*

Objective: To review the experience of a large-volume trauma center in managing and treating casualties of suicide bombing attacks.

Summary Background Data: The threat of suicide bombing attacks has escalated worldwide. The ability of the suicide bomber to deliver a relatively large explosive load accompanied by heavy shrapnel to the proximity of his or her victims has caused devastating effects.

Methods: The authors reviewed and analyzed the experience obtained in treating victims of suicide bombings at the level I trauma center of the Hadassah University Hospital in Jerusalem, Israel from 2000 to 2003.

Results: Evacuation is usually rapid due to the urban setting of these attacks. Numerous casualties are brought into the emergency department over a short period. The setting in which the device is detonated has implications on the type of injuries sustained by survivors. The injuries sustained by victims of suicide bombing attacks in semi-confined spaces are characterized by the degree and extent of widespread tissue damage and include multiple penetrating wounds of varying severity and location, blast injury, and burns.

Conclusions: The approach to victims of suicide bombings is based on the guidelines for trauma management. Attention is given to the moderately injured, as these patients may harbor immediate life-threatening injuries. The concept of damage control can be modified to include rapid packing of multiple soft-tissue entry sites. Optimal utilization of manpower and resources is achieved by recruiting all available personnel, adopting a predetermined plan, and a centrally coordinated approach. Suicide bombing attacks seriously challenge the most experienced medical facilities. (*Ann Surg* 2004;239:295–303)

The number and extent of worldwide suicide attacks has risen sharply in recent years.[1–3] Popularized by militant Islamic organizations to terrorize buses in Israel, the utilization of suicide bombers has been adopted by other groups. Suicide bombing attacks illustrate the ability of suicide attackers to mingle within a crowd and detonate an explosive device in the vicinity of their victims. The injuries sustained by survivors of these well-planned attacks combine the lethal effects of penetrating trauma, blast injury, and burns.[4–10]

Between November 2000 and May 2003, 71 suicide bombing attacks were carried out in Israel. Three settings were predominantly targeted: (A) open spaces (OS), such as pedestrian malls, open markets, and bus stops; (B) buses; and (C) semi-confined spaces (SCS), such as restaurants and cafe's (**Table 1**). Attacks in OS usually involve 1 or 2 attackers. The energy of the blast dissipates inversely with the distance to the second power, and injury is limited to victims in close proximity to the explosive device. The effects of blast injury when a bomb is detonated inside a confined space such as a bus have been described previously.[6] Victims usually sustain severe primary blast lung injury (BLI) and the fatality/casualty ratio is high (**Table 1**).[8] Attacks inside semiconfined, crowded spaces are characterized by the large number of casualties and fatalities, and by the severity and scope of penetrating injuries (**Figs. 1** and **2**). We describe the attack on the Sbarro pizzeria, which is representative of such attacks. The unique circumstances associated with suicide bombing attacks are discussed and our experience with the management of victims is analyzed.

From the *Trauma Unit and Department of Surgery, Hadassah University Hospital, Jerusalem, Israel; and the †Department of Surgery, Los Angeles County-University of Southern California Medical Center, Los Angeles, California.

Table 1. Classification of Suicide Bombing Attacks in Israel, November 2000–May 2003

Setting of Attack	Open Space	Bus	Semi-confined Space
Number of attacks	52	13	6
Number of victims injured/attack	28 (4.75–60)	40 (22–50)	70[†] (54.25–118.75)
Number of fatalities/attack	1 (0–3)	9* (7–15)	15* (12–15.75)
Number of casualties/attack	29 (5.75–62.25)	55 (30–64)	82.5[†] (66.5–132.25)
Ratio of fatalities/casualties (%)	4.8	21.9*	17.0*

Data shown as median (interquartile range).
*P   0.01 vs. open space (Mann-Whitney U test).
[†]P   0.02 vs. open space and bus (Mann-Whitney U test).

THE SBARRO ATTACK

On August 9, 2001 just before 2 p.m., a suicide bomber detonated an explosive device inside a crowded Sbarro pizza restaurant in Jerusalem. The device contained 8–10 kg of high-grade explosive material accompanied by a large amount of ball bearings, bolts, and nuts. The suicide bombing attack in the Sbarro restaurant generated 146 casualties, of which 14 were immediate deaths.

THE PROTOCOL

The only chance for victims who develop severe respiratory distress or severe hemorrhagic shock in the field is the availability of early advanced life support. Emergency medical services (EMS) crews are therefore instructed to follow the scoop-and-run approach in these circumstances. Needle thoracostomy and tracheal intubation are the only procedures performed in the field. Victims with amputated body parts who are not showing signs of movement and those who are pulseless with dilated pupils are considered dead. No further efforts are spent on these victims and attention is directed to evacuating the remaining victims.

There are 4 emergency departments (ED) in Jerusalem, and the Ein Kerem Campus ED is located furthest from the Sbarro restaurant (9.5 km, 6 mi). Regardless of the distance, EMS crews are instructed to evacuate the most severely injured victims to the Ein Kerem Campus, the only level I trauma center in Jerusalem, with more experience in recognizing and treating complex injuries. The Ein Kerem ED is divided into a designated trauma room and a general admitting area. The trauma room is equipped with respirators, monitoring devices, built-in plain film arms, and portable sonograms and has the capacity to treat 4 severely injured patients simultaneously. Surgeons have the capability to perform surgical procedures ranging from venous cut-down to ED thoracotomy.

The initial EMS report described scores of casualties with an unknown number of fatalities inside a crowded restaurant. A detailed protocol, specifically designed for such circumstances, was initiated. All patients in the ED were transferred to the floors and all nonurgent activity was halted. Elective diagnostic procedures such as plain film, sonogram, computed tomography (CT), and angiogram were deferred. Operating room (OR) administration was alerted and 7 procedures scheduled for that afternoon were postponed. Operations in process were allowed to proceed unaltered. Available OR personnel prepared an additional OR, which is dedicated to trauma patients.

The attack occurred when the majority of personnel were available almost immediately. In other circumstances, physicians, nurses, and OR personnel are contacted, irrespective of call schedules, by telephone via a structured list. In most instances this was unnecessary as hospital personnel were already alerted of the attack either by relatives or friends, the media, the Internet, or by simply hearing the blast. Surgical personnel arrived at the ED and were organized into predetermined teams. General surgery teams and subspecialty teams were led by an attending physician and included 2 surgical residents. Each team was assigned to 1 bed in the trauma room or 3–4 beds in the admitting area. An anesthesiologist was integrated into the general surgery teams assigned to the trauma room.

The most experienced trauma surgeon available was designated as surgeon-in-charge (SIC). The

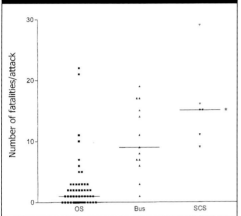

FIGURE 1. The number of fatalities per suicide bombing attack according to the different setting. OS: open space; SCS: semi-confined space. *$P=0.0003$ versus OS (Mann-Whitney U test).

FIGURE 2. The number of victims injured per suicide bombing attack according to the different setting. OS: open space; SCS: semi-confined space. *$P<0.02$ versus OS and bus (Mann-Whitney U test).

SIC received incoming EMS crews and triaged the victims into either the trauma room or the admitting area according to the presence of immediate life-threatening injuries. The SIC accompanied the most severely injured victims into the trauma room and orally communicated his findings to the treating teams. The SIC determined OR priority and did not participate in surgical procedures in the preliminary phases of triage and evaluation. Teams of general surgeons examined all the patients initially. These teams determined the need for further examination by subspecialty teams such as orthopedics, plastic surgery, and neurosurgery. Due to the high incidence of tympanic membrane trauma following blast injury, all patients were examined by teams from ear, nose, and throat (ENT).[11]

During the initial 6–8 hours, the SIC conducted repeated reassessments on all patients. These bedside reassessments were conducted following initial evaluation by the designated teams and consisted of repeated physical examination and review of the laboratory and imaging findings. Prioritization of treatment was determined by the SIC according to the presence and severity of life- and limb-threatening injuries, the degree of respiratory compromise, and the availability of operating rooms.

THE INJURIES

Within 6 minutes 18 patients were brought to the ED. Four patients were brought to the trauma room and 14 patients were directed to the admitting area. A 17-year-old male with severe brain injury was pulseless and underwent ED thoracotomy. Resuscitative efforts failed, he was pronounced dead, and transferred to the admitting area. Following initial evaluation, 1 patient with an injury severity score (ISS) of 22 was transferred from the admitting area to the trauma room and 1 patient from the trauma room with an ISS of 5 was transferred to the admitting area (**Fig. 3**). Fifty-seven minutes later a fifth patient with head injury was transferred to the trauma room from another hospital. Ten patients with minor injuries were discharged from the ED and were excluded from the analysis. The condition of the 8 survivors, the teams that participated in their evaluation and treatment, and the initial diagnostic work up are shown in **Tables 2, 3** and **4**. The pattern of injuries sustained by the 3 patients who were taken to the OR within the initial 4 hours is shown in **Table 5**.

ANALYSIS

The Circumstances

There are several factors to consider in understanding the bodily damage caused by the recent wave of suicide bombing attacks in Israel: (A) the high-grade explosive material used by the attackers; (B) the ability of the

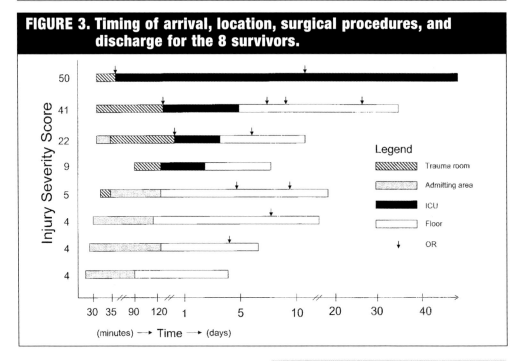

FIGURE 3. Timing of arrival, location, surgical procedures, and discharge for the 8 survivors.

attackers to detonate the explosive device in proximity to the victims by concealing the explosive device and mingling within a crowd; (C) the ability of the attacker to precisely time the explosion at his or her discretion; and (D) the large load of heavy shrapnel that accompany the explosive material. All the above factors are combined by the attackers to increase the number of casualties and the severity of their injuries. The injuries sustained by the victim depend on the proximity of the victim to the explosive device, the angle at which the victim stands in relation to the center of the explosion, and the height of the explosive device in relation to the victim. The circumstances associated with these attacks also influence management and decision-making. The uncertainty as to the arrival of additional victims, the mayhem associated with the arrival of anxious family members, the florid scenes associated with these injuries, the often young age of the victims, the possibility that family members of hospital personnel are among the victims, and the risk of second-hit explosions, intensify the chaotic atmosphere that already exists in the ED. These factors underline the importance of forming a plan at the hospital level designed to deal with these circumstances.

HOSPITAL RESPONSE

The demand on hospitals dealing with trauma victims varies according to the number of casualties and the severity of their injuries. Everyday resources are used in delivering treatment to one seriously injured patient. Conversely, in a scenario of mass casualties, medical resources are overwhelmed. It has been recently proposed that the circumstances associated with terrorist attacks, ie, the massive influx of casualties over a short time-span, inhibit the ability of medical crews to deliver efficient treatment to all the victims.[12] This view is based on mass casualty scenarios in which large numbers of casualties overwhelmed existing medical resources.[13] Thus, in dealing with mass casualty scenarios such as the bombing of the Murrah Federal Building in Oklahoma City in 1995, a selective approach is encouraged: one in which overtriage is discouraged; the treatment of moderately injured patients is prioritized over severely injured patients; and imaging studies are restricted or avoided. This approach seems justified in mass casualty scenarios. The Israeli experience with treating victims of suicide bombing attacks likely represents an intermediate situation, one in which the number of casualties is limited

Table 2. Clinical Characteristics of the 8 Survivors

	ISS ≤ 8 (n = 4)	ISS > 8 (n = 4)
Female: Male	3:1	3:1
Age*	49.5 (24–65)	17 (15–31)
ISS*	4 (4–5)	31.5 (9–50)
ICU stay*	0 (0–0)	4 (2–48)
Intubated upon arrival	0/4	3/4
Blast lung injury	1/4	4/4

ISS, injury severity score; ICU, intensive care unit.
*Data shown as median (range).

Table 3. The Teams Participating in the Evaluation and Treatment of the 8 Survivors

Teams	Number of Patients
General surgery	8/8
ENT	8/8
Plastic surgery	7/8
Orthopedic surgery	6/8
Neurosurgery	4/8
Maxillo-facial surgery	3/8
Cardiothoracic surgery	1/8

ENT, Ear, nose and throat.

Table 4. Imaging Studies Performed During the Initial 4 Hours for the 8 Survivors

Imaging study	Number of Patients
Chest x-ray	7/8
Other plain films	6/8
FAST	7/8
Head CT	6/8
Chest CT	3/8
Abdominal CT	3/8

FAST, Focused abdominal sonogram for trauma; CT, computerized tomography.

by the capacity of the target, ie, bus or restaurant. In these circumstances, ordinary hospital resources are heavily burdened, yet delivery of efficient medical treatment is possible by recruitment of all available personnel and resources.

It is difficult to predict the number of casualties based on the setting and on initial EMS reports. The number of casualties generated by attacks in OS depends on the density of victims at the scene, the number of attackers, and the explosive load. Premature detonation of devices in isolated OS, such as occurred when security personnel confronted the attackers, results in fewer casualties. In these situations EMS reports are reliable and the number of casualties is predictable. When these attacks involve crowded OS, SCS,

Table 5. Injuries Sustained by the 3 Patients Who Were Taken to the OR Within the Initial 4 Hours

	Patients		
Age (years)	15	15	31
Sex	Female	Female	Female
ISS	22	41	50
Injuries	Blast lung injury	Blast lung injury	Blast lung injury
	Penetrating rectal wound	Splenic laceration	Cardiac tear
	Open fracture left tibia	Open fracture left femur	FB to head, chest and trunk
	15% BSA second degree burns	20% BSA second degree burns	
	FB to head, face and limbs	FB to head, face, trunk and limbs	
Procedures	Laparotomy, colostomy	Laparotomy, splenectomy	ED thoracotomy
	Fixation of fracture	Fixation of fracture	Thoracotomy, repair of cardiac tear
	Debridement of burns	Debridement of burns	Laparotomy
	Removal of FB	Removal of FB	Tracheostomy*
Participating teams	General Surgery	General Surgery	Cardiothoracic surgery
	Orthopedics	Orthopedics	General Surgery
	Plastic Surgery	Plastic Surgery	ENT*
	ENT	Neurosurgery	
Time to OR (minutes)	235	185	20
Time in OR (minutes)	200	280	195
ICU time (days)	3	5	48

ISS, Injury severity score; OR, Operating room; ICU, Intensive care unit; ENT, Ear, nose and throat; FB, Foreign body; BSA, Body surface area.
*Performed on day 12.

and buses, initial EMS reports are confused and often contradictory. We have therefore adopted a universal response to attacks in crowded places. Evacuation of the ER, a halt to scheduled OR activity, and mobilization of personnel is routinely performed. Partial normalization of activity may follow confirmation of the magnitude of the attack.

TRIAGE

After an attack, many victims are brought to the admitting area over a period of minutes either by qualified prehospital personnel or many times by by-standers. Triage is of utmost importance in these scenarios.[14–15] A trauma-qualified, general surgeon is designated as SIC and waits at the ambulance unloading point to perform triage. The attack on the Sbarro restaurant occurred at 2 p.m. and this was therefore possible. In other circumstances, the most experienced trauma surgeon available is designated as SIC. Attention is focused on signs of severe respiratory distress and hemodynamic instability. Evaluation and treatment of the severely injured is initiated in a trauma room setting. The short evacuation times secondary to the proximity of suicide attacks to the urban setting and the usually young age of the victims favor an aggressive approach in the majority of

cases.[16] In retrospect, of the 2 patients without signs of life who underwent ED thoracotomy, 1 had severe brain injury and was obviously unsalvageable. The second patient had penetrating cardiac injury and was potentially salvageable,[17] but developed hypoxic brain damage secondary to prolonged hypotension. Terminating resuscitative efforts in these chaotic circumstances where little is known regarding prehospital status is extremely difficult. Nonetheless, performing these procedures on unsalvageable victims such as those without any signs of life or those with severe brain injury, may compromise delivery of efficient care to salvageable victims.

INITIAL EVALUATION

We consider undertriage unavoidable in these chaotic situations, and the importance of repeated surveys cannot be over-emphasized. Attention is initially given to identifying patients with signs of BLI such as shortness of breath, tachycardia, and confusion, and those with multiple entry sites and extensive tissue damage, which are markers of more severe trauma. These patients require immediate transfer to a higher-level care environment or to the OR. This is illustrated by the course of events of an 18-year-old male who was injured in the attack on the number 32 bus in Jerusalem, on

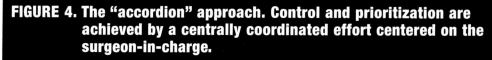

FIGURE 4. The "accordion" approach. Control and prioritization are achieved by a centrally coordinated effort centered on the surgeon-in-charge.

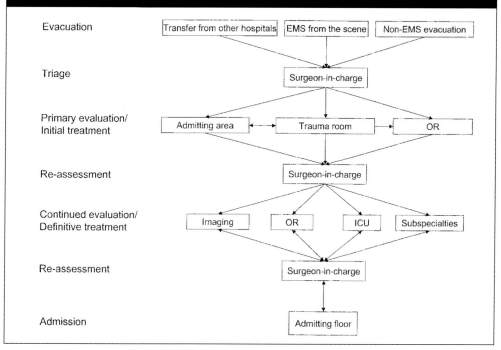

June 18, 2002. He was diagnosed with burns, and triaged to the admitting area. Within minutes he developed acute respiratory distress caused by BLI. He was immediately transferred to the trauma room where he was ventilated and bilateral chest drains were inserted.

The majority of victims of penetrating trauma sustain injuries to isolated parts of the body such as the head, chest, abdomen, or limbs. Blunt trauma is more commonly a multisite injury, the severity of which depends on the mechanism of injury. The injuries sustained by victims of suicide bombing attacks share the worst of both worlds. The multitude of heavy particles causes damage to a large surface area of the victim, much like blunt trauma. Each particle causes extensive tissue damage at the site of entry, much like penetrating trauma. Survivors typically suffer a combination of wounds of varying severity and location, and the diagnostic work up is focused on determining the extent of damage caused by each missile.

CONTROL

Control and coordination are achieved by the "accordion" approach. According to this approach, patient evaluation and management proceed through repeated cycles consisting of a dispersal phase and a convergence phase (**Fig. 4**). Activity is coordinated and controlled by the SIC who is aware of the overall situation and has the oversight to prioritize evaluation and treatment. Chaos is gradually managed once the number of patients requiring further work up is reduced. Patients undergoing surgery, often simultaneously by different teams, are reassessed by the SIC in the OR with the treating teams. The overall condition of the patient, the sequence of therapy, the need for further imaging studies, and the need for intensive care unit (ICU) admission are discussed and finalized.

In analyzing this approach we must consider the following: (A) many hours and sometimes days are required for the situation to stabilize and eventually normalize (**Fig. 3**); (B) treating teams are physically and emotionally exhausted from the continuous workload, especially when repeat attacks occur within days; and (C) repeated reassessment by the treating teams and SIC to ascertain that all patients receive optimal care is fundamental. In these circumstances, a strong personal commitment by the treating teams and SIC is pivotal to success. Depending on the magnitude of the attack, this commitment may last from several hours to several days. During this period, other professional and personal commitments are sacrificed.

TREATMENT

The basic rules of trauma, the ABC, and the concepts of trauma management such as the abbreviated laparotomy and damage control, are applied universally.[18–22] Their application may be modified in different situations. As in all trauma cases, airway control and acute breathing problems are prioritized. Hypotensive victims of penetrating abdominal or thoracic trauma are taken to the operating room to perform laparotomy and/or thoracotomy. This approach stems from our understanding that the mechanism of hypotension is major intra-abdominal and/or intrathoracic bleeding.

Hypotensive victims of suicide bombing attacks with abdominal and/or thoracic injuries believed to contribute significantly to their instability are also taken to the OR. The approach in the OR to victims of suicide attacks may be slightly modified in these cases. Multiple shrapnel entry sites are common in survivors and it is impossible to determine which of the numerous entry sites is the cause of hypotension. The degree of soft-tissue damage associated with these injuries is also difficult to quantitate. Since the attackers usually approach the victims from behind, the majority of entry sites are located on the backsides. Positioning the patient in the supine position and performing routine abbreviated laparotomy may actually postpone treatment of these potentially more serious injuries. We propose a modification to the concept of damage control in these cases. Up to 10 to 15 entry sites, ranging in size from 2–6 cm in diameter and up to 5–8 cm deep, are packed by 2 to 3 teams in a swift manner with the patient in the left or right lateral decubitus positions. Rapid hemostasis should be achieved within 2–3 minutes.

Hypothermia, a leading cause of coagulopathy in trauma patients, may also be diminished by covering these wounds.[23] The patient is then positioned in the supine position and laparotomy and/or thoracotomy initiated. This modification may attenuate the degree of soft-tissue damage, lessen hypothermia, achieve better overall hemostasis, and improve survival.

Recombinant activated factor VIIa (rFVIIa) has been successfully used to treat bleeding patients with various coagulopathies. When bound to tissue factor, which is exposed at sites of vessel injury, circulating FVIIa is activated. This complex initiates the coagulation cascade on activated platelet surfaces, which adhere to the site of injury, resulting in the formation of a fibrin clot at the site of injury only.[24] Animal studies have shown a significant improvement in mean prothrombin time, mean arterial blood pressure, and mean blood loss in hypothermic, coagulopathic pigs after administration of rFVIIa.[25] Noncontrolled reports in trauma patients have suggested that administration of rFVIIa results in improvement of prothrombin time and blood requirement.[24] We have used rFVIIa in 3 cases. After the Zion Square attack, a 14-year-old girl sustained multiple shrapnel wounds to her lower extremities with extensive soft-tissue damage. Her injuries included bilateral multiple open fractures of the femur and tibia, and bilateral obstruction of the posterior tibial artery. The fractures were nailed, but because she developed hypothermia and coagulopathy, the vascular injuries were not repaired and she was transferred to the ICU. She continued to bleed profusely from multiple entry sites and received 57 units of red blood cells, 39 units of FFP, 14 units of platelets, and 19 units of cryoprecipitate. Twenty-two hours after admission, she received 100 microgram/kilogram of rFVIIa with an immediate improvement of her INR from 2.11 to 0.64. More importantly, the bleeding stopped and over the following 24 hours she received 1 unit of red blood cells. Since then, we have successfully treated 2 additional penetrating trauma patients with rFVIIa. These are anecdotal reports. However, in light of recent publications and our experience, we encourage the use of rFVIIa in exsanguinating trauma patients as an adjunct to surgical hemostasis, with or without participation in ongoing randomized trials.

COMMUNICATION WITH FAMILIES

Family members injured in suicide bombing attacks have been brought to different hospitals because of different patterns of injuries and confusion at the scene. Families are unaware of the condition and location of their relatives. A crisis information center staffed by psychologists, social workers, nurses, hospital spokesperson, and police, is set up and efforts are made to identify and locate the victims and to retrieve information regarding their condition. Identification of victims is facilitated by using Polaroid™ and digital photos. The center is accessible by telephone, and the numbers are shown in the media and on the internet.

During the early hours following an attack, the treating teams do not have the opportunity to communicate directly with the families. We have therefore adopted the role of a nurse coordinator to contact the families and inform them of the condition and progress of their loved ones. The nurse has access to the ED, trauma room, OR, and crisis center and is updated by the surgeons. Once the situation stabilizes, the surgeons join the coordinator and update the families.

AFTERMATH

Debriefings are conducted regularly following partial normalization, usually within 12–18 hours of the attack. The SIC, department chairmen, treating teams, nurses, nurse coordinators, hospital administration, hospital spokesperson, and EMS representatives participate in the discussion. The event is reviewed and analyzed beginning with the correlation between initial EMS reports and the number and condition of casualties, the number and makeup of teams participating in the event, the number of patients requiring surgery and timing of their surgery, the requirement for additional ICU beds, and the need to cancel nonurgent procedures. Some of the recommendations that we have implemented include: recruitment of personnel via telephone lines and not pagers or cellular phones that crash due to overload, placement of a portable sonogram in the trauma room, transformation of recovery room beds into temporary ICU beds, regulation of

physicians' leave, and creation of the roles of SIC and nurse coordinator.

The days following such attacks are not normal. After the attack on the Sbarro restaurant and as a result of the overload on the ICU, 2 major surgical procedures scheduled for the next morning were postponed. The Israeli Center for Organ Donation was alerted and organ donations were transferred to other centers. Other factors such as physical and emotional burden are more difficult to quantify. Physicians and hospital administration are aware of the difficulties, and nonurgent activity is reduced for several days.

CONCLUSIONS

In summary, the approach to victims of suicide bombing attacks leans on the guidelines for trauma victims in general. Specific considerations include the large number of victims, the combined effects of penetrating trauma, blast injury and burns, and the numerous penetrating wounds sustained by each victim. Attention is given to the moderately injured, as these seemingly stable patients may harbor immediate life-threatening injuries. Repeated reassessments can prevent late diagnosis of potentially life- and limb-threatening injuries. Modifications to the damage control concept in the severely injured hemodynamically unstable patient may include packing of multiple entry sites prior to abbreviated laparotomy. A predetermined plan and a coordinated approach, centered on the SIC, are essential to optimize utilization of manpower and resources. Hospital personnel and resources are heavily burdened in these circumstances.

REFERENCES

1. Eiseman B. Combat casualty management for tomorrow's battlefield: urban terrorism. *J Trauma.* 2001;51:821–823.
2. Karmy-Jones R, Kissinger D, Golocovsky M, et al. Bomb-related injuries. *Mil Med.* 1994;159:536–539.
3. Slater MS, Trunkey DD. Terrorism in America: an evolving threat. *Arch Surg.* 1997;132:1059–1066.
4. Philips YY. Primary blast injuries. *Ann Emerg Med.* 1986;15:1446–1450.
5. Wightman JM, Gladish SL. Explosions and blast injuries. *Ann Emerg Med.* 2001;37:664–678.
6. Leibovici D, Gofrit ON, Stein M, et al. Blast injuries in a bus versus open air bombings: a comparative study of injuries in survivors of open air versus confined space explosions. *J Trauma.* 1996;41:1030–1035.
7. Cooper GJ, Maynard RL, Cross NL, et al. Casualties from terrorist bombings. *J Trauma.* 1983;23:955–967.
8. Pizov R, Oppenheim-Eden A, Matot I, et al. Blast lung injury from an explosion on a civilian bus. *Chest.* 1999;115:165–172.
9. Katz E, Ofek B, Adler J, et al. Primary blast injury after a bomb explosion in a civilian bus. *Ann Surg.* 1989;209:484–488.

10. Almogy G, Makori A, Zamir O, et al. Rectal penetrating injuries from blast trauma. *Isr Med Assoc J*. 2002;4:557–558.
11. Leibovici D, Gofrit ON, Shapira SC. Eardrum perforation in explosion survivors: is it a marker of pulmonary blast injury? *Ann Emerg Med*. 1999;34:168–172.
12. Frykberg ER. Medical management of disasters and mass casualties from terrorist bombings: how can we cope? J Trauma. 2002;53:201– 212.
13. Caro D. Major disasters. *Lancet*. 1974;2:1309–1310.
14. Stein M, Hirshberg A. Medical consequences of terrorism. The conventional weapon threat. *Surg Clin North Am*. 1999;79:1537–1552.
15. Stein M, Hirshberg A. Limited mass casualties due to conventional weapons-the daily reality of a level I trauma center. In: Shemer J, Shoenfeld Y, eds. *Terror and Medicine: Medical Aspects of Biological, Chemical and Radiological Terrorism*. Lengerich: Pabst Science Publishers; 2003:378–393.
16. Kluger Y. Bomb explosions in acts of terrorism-detonation, wound ballistics, triage and medical concerns. *Isr Med Assoc J*. 2003;5:235–240.
17. Rhee PM, Acosta J, Bridgeman A, et al. Survival after emergency department thoracotomy: review of published data from the past 25 years. *J Am Coll Surg*. 2000;190:288–298.

18. Hirshberg A, Walden R. Damage control for abdominal trauma. *Surg Clin North Am*. 1997;77:813–820.
19. Moore EE, Burch JM, Franciose RJ, et al. Staged physiologic restoration and damage control surgery. *World J Surg*. 1998;22:1184–1190.
20. Mattox KL. Introduction, background, and future projections of damage control surgery. *Surg Clin North Am*. 1997;77:753–759.
21. Moore EE. Staged laparotomy for the hypothermia, acidosis and coagulopathy syndrome. *Am J Surg*. 1996;172:405–410.
22. Rotondo MF, Schwab CW, McGonigal MD, et al. "Damage control": an approach for improved survival in exsanguinating penetrating abdominal injury. *J Trauma*. 1993;35:375–383.
23. Jurkovich GJ, Greiser WB, Luterman A, et al. Hypothermia in trauma victims: an ominous predictor of survival. *J Trauma*. 1987;27:1019–1024.
24. Martinowitz U, Kenet G, Segal E, et al. Recombinant activated factor VII for adjunctive hemorrhage control in trauma. *J Trauma*. 2001;51:4319.
25. Shreiber MA, Holcomb JB, Hedner U, et al. The effect of recombinant factor VIIa on coagulopathic pigs with grade V liver injuries. *J Trauma* 2002;53:252–257.

Source: *Annals of Surgery*, Vol.239, No.3, March 2004. Reprinted with permission.

PART EIGHT

MEDICAL MANAGEMENT IN A NUCLEAR/RADIATION ATTACK

INTERIM GUIDELINES FOR HOSPITAL RESPONSE TO MASS CASUALTIES FROM A RADIOLOGICAL INCIDENT

James M. Smith, PhD
Marie A. Spano, MS

BACKGROUND

A variety of potential terrorist incidents involving radiation could result in mass casualties that could present at hospitals in the area near the incident. The following are meant to be examples of possible radiological scenarios and are sorted in ascending order of potential health effects:

- **Radiation Dispersal Device.** For example, a conventional explosion has scattered radioactive material ("dirty bomb"), or saboteurs blow up a truck carrying radioactive material, or an aerosol containing radioactive material has been spread over a large area. There may be tens to hundreds of injured people and many hundreds of contaminated or exposed people. However, the radiation levels are not sufficient to cause acute radiation sickness in anyone; however, there *are* immediate psychological effects and an additional risk of long-term health effects.
- **Major event at or near a nuclear facility.** For example, an airplane crashes into a nuclear power plant or into a spent nuclear fuel pool. Significant amounts of radioactive material might then be released. It is likely there would be dozens of injured people at the facility, many experiencing symptoms related to acute radiation syndrome, as well as thousands of contaminated or exposed people in the surrounding area who would have an increased probability of long-term health effects.
- **Nuclear detonation.** The immediate physical devastation could rival that of the World Trade

Center following the events of September 11, 2001. However, the dust and debris from this event would be highly radioactive. Thousands of people would be both contaminated and injured at the scene. In addition, there would be thousands of people with serious radiation exposures in a large area potentially extending many miles outward from the initial point of attack, although they might initially have no obvious physical injury or contamination. Radioactive fallout with potential for long-term health effects would extend over a large region far from ground zero. Many people would probably experience symptoms related to acute radiation syndrome.

HEALTH EFFECTS OF RADIATION EXPOSURE

Exposure to radiation can cause two kinds of health effects:

- **Deterministic effects** are observable health effects that occur soon after receipt of large doses. These may include hair loss, skin burns, nausea, or death.
- **Stochastic effects** are long-term effects, such as cancer. The radiation dose determines the severity of a deterministic effect and the probability of a stochastic effect.

The object of any radiation control program is to prevent any deterministic effects and minimize the risk for stochastic effects. When a person inhales or ingests a radionuclide (*an unstable and therefore radioactive form of a nuclide*), the body will absorb different amounts of that radionuclide in different organs, so each organ will receive a different **organ dose**.

The dose conversion factor for each organ is the number of rem (*roentgen equivalent—rem relates*

Division of Environmental Hazards and Health Effects, National Center for Environmental Health, Centers for Disease Control and Prevention, Department of Health and Human Services, December 2003.

the absorbed dose in human tissue to the effective biological damage of the radiation) delivered to that organ by each curie *(37 billion disintegrations per second—the number of disintegrations per second in 1 gram of pure radium)* or becquerel *(one disintegration per second)* of intake of a specific radioisotope.

EXTERNAL, INTERNAL, AND ABSORBED DOSES

A person can receive an **external dose** by standing near a gamma or high-energy beta-emitting source. A person can receive an **internal dose** by ingesting or inhaling radioactive material. The external exposure stops when the person leaves the area of the source. The internal exposure continues until the radioactive material is flushed from the body by natural processes or decay.

A person who has ingested a radioactive material receives an internal dose to several different organs. The absorbed dose to each organ is different, and the sensitivity of each organ to radiation is different.

The Environmental Protection Agency (EPA) assigns a different weighting factor to each organ. To determine a person's risk for cancer, multiply each organ's dose by its weighting factor and add the results. The sum is the **effective dose equivalent**—"effective" because it is not really the dose to the whole body but a sum of the relative risks to each organ, and "equivalent" because it is presented in rem or sieverts (*a unit used to derive a dose equivalent; one sievert—or Sv—equals 100 rem*) instead of rads or gray.

COMMITTED AND TOTAL EFFECTIVE DOSE EQUIVALENTS

When a person inhales or ingests a radionuclide, that radionuclide is distributed to different organs and stays there for days, months, or years until it decays or is excreted. The radionuclide will deliver a radiation dose over a period of time. The dose that a person receives from the time the radionuclide enters the body until it is gone is the **committed dose**.

The EPA calculates doses over a 50-year period and presents the **committed dose equivalent** for each organ plus the **committed effective dose equivalent** (CEDE).

A person can receive both an internal dose and an external dose. The sum of the CEDE and the external dose is called the **total effective dose equivalent** (TEDE).

TRIAGE

PLANNING FOR TRIAGE

- In most mass casualty incidents:
  - A large majority of people will self-triage and go directly to the closest and most familiar hospitals; they will probably bypass field triage and treatment whether contaminated or not. Therefore, hospitals often have little, if any, advance notification of incoming patients.
  - Most of the individuals who come to the hospital are ambulatory and either minimally injured or concerned about potential contamination.
  - The general medical needs of the community must continue to be met despite the occurrence of a disaster.
- Hospitals should have plans in place to transfer patients (if conditions allow) to other hospitals or other medical facilities during disasters according to pre-arranged formal agreements. Hospitals are protected from having to transfer unstable patients under the provisions of the Emergency Medical Treatment and Active Labor Act (EMTALA).
- Every individual involved in the response to a mass casualty incident, especially the fire and police, should be familiar with the triage process and know how to determine who should be sent to the hospital.
- The triage plan should include a process for establishment of an assessment center, separate from the emergency department. The assessment center can be used to rapidly screen victims for injury and contamination, as well as to serve as a location removed from the emergency department where decontamination of victims can take place. The assessment center should also be used for observation, limited treatment and evaluation, and reuniting with family members where possible.
- Consideration should be given to setting up a temporary *primary* assessment center that

would be located on the hospital campus, removed from the emergency department, or, depending on logistics and the magnitude of the event, a temporary *secondary* assessment center located within the community but removed from the hospital. If practical, any outside assessment center should be set-up upwind from the patient arrival area.

- Hospitals must ensure that the triage process has an efficient record-keeping process to be sure injured persons are not missed.
- Hospitals need to take into consideration that corpses from a radiological event may be contaminated with radioactive material.

THE TRIAGE PROCESS

- The hospital triage plan should be based on and coordinated with the community plan. It should focus on training and exercises.
- Triage will be conducted at the scene and at the hospital, but communities and responders should attempt to do as much as possible at the scene.
- After a mass casualty or hazardous materials (hazmat) incident, hospitals should "lock down," providing only two entrances:
  - A site for triage and patients
  - A site for personnel, staff, press, officials, etc.
    - ✔ This site will require community support and local law enforcement to assist in the lock down, as the hospital is an important disaster response asset.
  - Casualty distribution to participating health care facilities should be based on and coordinated with the community plan.
  - Hospital space must be reserved for the most critically injured or ill.
- The assessment center should be used for observation, decontamination, limited treatment and evaluation, and reuniting with family members where possible.
- Under the triage process for patients with life-threatening conditions, emergency department staff should stabilize and treat physical symptoms according to standard procedures. The threat of contamination should not preclude patient treatment.
- Under the triage process for patients with non-life-threatening conditions:

- When possible, trained staff should survey all patients for radioactive contamination.
  - ✔ If contamination is detected or suspected, remove the patient's clothing, give the patient a shower, then treat physical symptoms according to standard procedures.
  - ✔ Localized contamination can be rinsed off with premoistened wipes or washed with soap and water, as opposed to showering the individual.
  - ✔ If radiation is still detected after washing, admit the patient if medically warranted and arrange for further evaluation and decontamination.

KEY PRINCIPLES OF CONTAMINATION CONTAINMENT

- Hospitals should use contamination containment processes with which the staff are familiar and should apply universal precautions and isolation techniques. Staff should use universal precautions when making direct contact with contaminated patients.
- Staff should double bag, tie, seal, and label any contaminated material in plastic bags to be stored in a predetermined, secure storage area (labeling should include appropriate identifying information—e.g., patient name, hospital number, date, and time of day). The bagged items should be removed from the patient treatment area as soon as possible to eliminate any further contamination.
- In a mass-casualty emergency, staff should dispose of the water used to decontaminate patients via the sewer system. (It is unlikely hospitals will have an effective water-holding system for any mass casualty event.) The EPA has issued the following guideline: "Contaminated runoff should be avoided whenever possible, but should not impede necessary and appropriate actions to protect human life and health. Once the victims are removed and safe from further harm and the site is secured and stable, the first responders should be doing everything reasonable to prevent further migration of contamination into the environment."
- Hospitals should prepare personnel to rapidly identify and notify pre-identified resources who can provide assistance.

- Hospitals should use appropriately trained staff with properly maintained and tested radiation survey meters to determine contamination.
- Hospitals should consider purchasing personal dosimeters for rapid response teams or others who might be subject to contact with contaminated patients or materials. Personal dosimeter data for hospital staff provide exposure documentation after the fact.
- Hospital staff should remember that it may take time before a disaster is recognized as a *radiological* incident and assume contamination is present; however, the first time radioactive contamination is clearly identified, all staff and first responders must be notified as soon as possible.

KEY PRINCIPLES OF CONTROL

- Hospitals should designate a central point where patients are funneled into the hospital (ensure that it is within walking distance from the hospital).
- Hospitals should clearly identify demarcation points (use control points, pylons, or tape) where people will be monitored when coming in and going out of the hospital. The hospital should provide survey monitors at both points. This also includes the restricting staff movement.
  - Designate separate "clean" versus "contaminated" areas in the hospital.
  - Segregate contaminated and noncontaminated patients and arrange a location where contaminated patients can be observed with limited staff contact.
- Hospitals should plan to contact local law enforcement and to augment hospital security staff to control facility ingress and egress (including the parking lot).
  - Hospital security staff must also control entrance of vehicles.
  - Hospital security staff will also work with EMS to determine how to address contaminated EMS vehicles.

PATIENT MANAGEMENT

- The management of patients following suspected or confirmed radiological events involving mass casualties must be well-organized and well-rehearsed.

- Patient management includes:
  - Determining the signs and symptoms of acute radiation exposure
  - Determining the extent the patient may be contaminated
  - Providing for decontamination, when necessary
  - Treating specific injuries
  - Collecting specimens for laboratory testing
  - Providing care for special populations (eg, pregnant women)
  - Providing discharge information
  - Follow-up care
  - Post-mortem procedures
  - Addressing the psychological effects of patients and their mental health concerns
- The psychological trauma in a radiological incident may be as varied in severity and type as physical trauma and will require special skills and training to adequately meet the needs of those affected.

HOW DO YOU KNOW IF SOMEONE IS CONTAMINATED?

- Radiological contamination cannot be detected without specialized equipment. (For information on this equipment, see **Appendix A** at the end of this article.)
- When conducting a radiation survey of the patient, the technician should initially conduct a scan of the face, hands, and feet using a standard radiation survey instrument. If the meter results are positive, then the technician should conduct a thorough survey (five to eight minutes per person). The speed of the survey should not exceed two inches per second, and the distance between the probe and the patient should be approximately one inch. Staff should consider covering the survey probe in plastic to prevent contamination of the instrument.
- Ensure that data recorded from radiation detection instrumentation is understandable to clinical practitioners.
- The provider should arrange for bioassays if internal contamination is suspected. Body fluids used for laboratory analysis include blood, urine, feces, nasal and saliva swabs, sputum, vomitus, and wound secretions.

DECONTAMINATION

- Radiation decontamination should not interfere with medical care of patients with life-threatening injuries or illness.
- If possible, staff should screen and survey for levels of contamination before moving a patient into the facility; this will minimize staff and equipment exposure. As a control, staff should attempt a background reading of the facility before surveying the patient.
- Only properly trained personnel should use radiation survey equipment.
  - Most things needed for decontamination are already available in a hospital. The only additional recommended equipment is radiation survey equipment to measure beta and gamma rays. Radiation survey equipment to detect contamination includes a Geiger counter to detect beta and gamma radiation. Although not specifically designed to quantify alpha radiation, pancake probes that are available for Geiger counters will detect the presence of most alpha radiation sources, as well as beta and gamma radiation (see **Appendix A**). Many hospitals have at least one survey instrument in-house. Make certain that trained personnel are always on duty and know how to use survey instruments properly.
- Hospitals should ensure that personnel have proper personal protection equipment. Universal precautions as practiced with any other mass-casualty incidents (trauma, chemical, biological, etc.) are generally sufficient for protection from radioactive contamination.
  - Under standard precautions, surgical masks are used to reduce the possibility of blood splashes to the mouth and nose and hand-oral contamination. Surgical masks do not protect against inhaling all respiratory hazards.
  - A higher level of protection is provided by fitted particulate respirators such as N95 or higher. These respirators should be available in hospitals, as they already are recommended for health care worker protection against SARS, tuberculosis, and certain other infectious diseases. However, these respirators must be used in an OSHA-compliant respiratory protection program that includes medical clearance, training, and fit testing.

- Experience in human decontamination indicates that careful procedures for removing clothing and decontaminating patients prevents aerosolization of radioactive particles, and dosimetry of health care workers using surgical masks has not found evidence of contamination. This suggests that if N95 respirators are not available, surgical masks should provide adequate protection if other precautions are observed.
- Responders should attempt as much decontamination as possible either at the designated assessment center or outside the hospital. Minimize the amount of contamination that actually enters the emergency department or the hospital. Decontamination areas should be separated from the hospital.
- Removing the clothing from the patient should remove 70% to 90% of the contamination. Staff or responders should bag and tag clothing, dressings, etc., for future evaluation and potential use as criminal evidence.
- Small personal belongings (jewelry, wallet, etc.) should be surveyed for contamination. If personal belongings are not contaminated, they can be returned to the patient. Otherwise, steps must be taken to decontaminate the items before returning them. If the patient is medically able to remove his own clothing and wash, then he should be allowed to do so. However, providers should maintain communication during the process.
- Staff should address privacy concerns of patients who are undressing. Disposable dressing gowns should be provided for patients concerned about modesty and to ensure that the environment is appropriate to remove clothing (e.g., not too cold).
- The patient should be washed with water and soap, taking care not to abrade or irritate the skin. Water is the most important ally in this setting. Ambulatory patients can easily be washed; however, nonambulatory patients must be on gurneys that can be washed.
- Staff trained in using survey instrumentation should resurvey the patient after washing. The patient should be rewashed until no further reduction in contamination is detected or a set threshold is attained, generally considered less than two or three times background. After

washing, providers should isolate and cover with a plastic bag or wrap any area of the skin that is still positive.

- Care should be taken with the washing procedure, ensuring that radioactive materials are not incorporated into a wound.
- If a patient has both wounds and very high, localized levels of internal contamination, this may indicate that the patient contains a radioactive fragment or fragments internally. The physician—in consultation with the hospital radiation safety officer, if possible—should consider surgically removing the fragment(s) using forceps to avoid potential local radiation injury to his own hands.
- To ensure best use of the health care providers' time and resources, hospitals should consider having other personnel perform the decontamination process. But these other personnel should be appropriately trained to prevent injury to the patient and to minimize the possibility of contaminating themselves during decontamination of the patient.
- Hospitals should decontaminate the facility and staff who had contact with contaminated patients to prevent the spread of contamination. Staff should consult their radiation safety officer for step-by-step procedures.
- If the patient does not show any signs of contamination or meet hospital admittance criteria, providers should nevertheless recommend that the patient take a thorough shower as soon as possible as a safety precaution.

PATIENT TREATMENT

- Staff must not allow the threat of contamination to impede the delivery of medical assistance. When an individual who is contaminated and has a life-threatening condition appears in the emergency department, that person should be admitted to the emergency department for immediate care.
- It is crucial to educate staff on the realities and history of a patient's contamination to provide appropriate patient treatment. Staff who work in an emergency department expose themselves to certain risks, including ordinary hospital radiation sources, as part of the job.
- Initially, hospitals should obtain as much patient and situation history as possible, noting circum-

stances surrounding the patient and the situation that might indicate exposure. This also includes looking for corroborating evidence.

- Emergency department staff can measure complete blood counts (CBCs) with differential to serve as an initial baseline measurement. CBCs taken over the next several days can then be compared to the baseline measurements and used to assess the radiation dose received. These data are of key importance in evaluating patients for acute radiation syndrome. (For further details, see "Acute radiation syndrome: A fact sheet for physicians" in this section.)
- When internal contamination is suspected, body excreta may contain radioactive substances. Collection of urine and feces should be considered for those patients. Also, swabs from body orifices should be taken for survey or analysis for radionuclides. Although state and federal assistance may be made available for receiving and analyzing these samples, during their emergency planning, hospitals should identify which agencies or laboratories the samples should go to for analysis.
- In the first 48 hours, physicians should conduct standard patient assessment, take care of immediately life-threatening problems, and attend to all other problems that require immediate attention. Emergency department staff should:
  - Treat symptoms according to ordinary patient treatment practices and procedures.
  - Treat wounds by irrigating, debriding, and covering as well as possible.
  - Look for the symptoms of acute radiation syndrome. Have a trained technician perform a radiation survey if symptoms, patient history, and situation history indicate the possibility of contamination.
  - Supplies and medications to stock in large quantities include IVs, fluid support, anti-diarrhea medications, anti-emetic medications, and potassium iodide tablets.
  - Keeping supply of potassium iodide in particular is worth considering. Potassium iodide helps reduce the risk of thyroid cancer from radioactive iodine exposure. Such exposures may arise from a nuclear power plant incident or in radioactive fallout from a terrorism event involving the detonation of a nuclear device.

Table 1. FDA Recommendations for the Administration of Potassium Iodide (KI)

Threshold thyroid radioactive exposures and recommended doses of KI for different risk groups

	Predicted radiation dose to thyroid (cGy¹ or rad)	KI dose (mg)	Number of 130 mg tablets	Number of 65 mg tablets
Adults over 40 years	≥500	130	1	2
Adults over 18 through 40 years	≥ 10	130	1	2
Pregnant or lactating women	≥ 5	130	1	2
Adolescents over 12 through 18 years	≥ 5	65	1/2	1
Children over 3 through 12 years	≥ 5	65	1/2	1
Over 1 month through 3 years	≥ 5	32	1/4	1/2
Birth through 1 month	≥ 5	16	1/8	1/4

¹1 Gy = 100 rad; 1 centigray (cGy) = 1 rad
²Adolescents approaching adult size (≥70 kg) should receive the full adult dose (130 mg)

- Hospitals should adhere to FDA recommendations for the administration of potassium iodide, which are summarized in **Table 1**.
- Potassium iodide supplementation is less effective for patients over 40 years. As such, it is recommended that these individuals receive potassium iodide supplementation only if their exposure seems significant enough to potentially destroy the thyroid gland, leading to hypothyroidism.
- Potassium iodide should be taken immediately, although it may still have a significant impact if taken even three to four hours after exposure. It should be available to those in a radioactive fallout area.
- States with a population within the 10-mile emergency planning zone of a commercial nuclear power plant are required by the Nuclear Regulatory Commission to consider maintaining a store of potassium iodide as a public protective measure to supplement sheltering and evacuation in the event of a severe nuclear power plant incident. Check to see whether your state maintains such a store of potassium iodide.
- Hospital staff should also note that an FDA "Guidance" document recommends "that persons with known iodine sensitivity should avoid potassium iodide, as should individuals with dermatitis herpetiformis and hypocomplementemic vasculitis, extremely rare conditions associated with an increased risk of iodine hypersensitivity."

- Individuals with multinodular goiter, Graves' disease, and autoimmune thyroiditis should be treated with caution—especially if dosing extends beyond a few days. Unless other protective measures are not available, repeat dosing for pregnant females and neonates is *not* recommended because of the potential for potassium iodide to suppress thyroid function in the fetus and neonate.
- Hospital staff should not leave patients and the community with the impression that potassium iodide prevents adverse health effects from radiation exposure in general, although offering patients potassium iodide may help address some of their psychological concerns.

CARE OF SPECIAL POPULATIONS

- Special populations—immunocompromised patients, equipment-dependent patients (especially those requiring ventilators), disabled people requiring wheelchairs or other mechanisms of assistance, nursing home residents, mentally ill people, elderly people, and so on—do not generally require special treatment, although pregnant women may need extra reassurance and communication.
- If radioactive iodine exposure has occurred, consider giving children potassium iodide tablets in the doses listed in **Table 1**.

PATIENT DISCHARGE AND FOLLOW-UP

- If the incident is thought to be of criminal intent, the discharge staff should explain the need for reporting to and cooperation with law enforcement.
- Along with discharge sheets, hospitals should provide Q&A sheets and fact sheets. Fact sheets should include expert contacts, phone numbers, and reliable sources of information.
- Patients may be overwhelmed by too much information. Printed materials should be brief and easy to understand. The Centers for Disease Control and Prevention offer comprehensive information to the general public on every aspect of radiation emergencies. It is available at: *www.bt.cdc.gov/radiation/#public*.
- Hospital staffers should avoid generic discussions about radiation with patients or the general public, which could promote unwarranted concern. Information that is tailored to an individual's unique circumstances is the most helpful.

LABORATORY ISSUES

- In the management of mass casualties, basic precepts of medicine should take hold with regard to testing: Minimize the amount of testing and only perform those tests that can affect the immediate care of the patient.
- In a mass casualty incident, hundreds to thousands of patients may flood hospitals, a situation in which they cannot practically take a blood count on every patient. Anyone who has or might exhibit prodromal effects would need to be considered for a CBC with differential to test for acute radiation syndrome. If possible, this should be repeated every six hours for about 72 hours.
- Other laboratory tests to consider, if warranted, include cytogenetic analysis (ie, collecting blood for dosimetry). All samples must be placed in separate, labeled containers that specify patient name, date, and time of sampling. In the planning process, hospitals should consider how to manage the shipping and transportation of samples to qualified laboratories.
- Preparation steps that hospitals can take to address laboratory capacity include:
  - Ensure that mutual aid agreements with area laboratories are in place.
  - Determine whether it is possible to transfer noncritical patients to other local facilities.
  - Keep a stockpile of CBC tubes (use purple-top tubes* for CBCs).
- Hospitals should keep in mind that while they are treating casualties, other local, state, and federal organizations are dealing with the scene. Hospitals need to know how to communicate with these responding organizations to get such needed information as radionuclide data and radiation dose assessment.
- A lesson learned from past incidents is that health care providers should have heightened awareness of significant political pressure to use the most accurate tests available and avoid reliance on random testing of individuals.

PATIENT MENTAL HEALTH CONCERNS

- A mass casualty event involving radiation has the potential to yield a large number of psychological casualties.
  - Most casualties will not have severe psychiatric conditions that result from the incident. The initial reaction of many people will be shock, immobilization, and fear. Most people will exhibit understandably higher levels of anxiety rather than psychotic behavior; however, some will also experience posttraumatic stress disorder (PTSD).
  - In addition, many people with a mental illness even in noncatastrophic times, such as those suffering from schizophrenia, major depression, or bipolar disorder, will be likely to come to the hospital because they fear losing access to their mental health medications.
  - Family members are apt come to the hospital in an attempt to gain information on loved ones who have sought medical attention for heightened anxiety. Hospitals should dedicate space in their facilities to accommodate these people, and—if possible—a phone number to keep them informed about the

---

* Tubes for blood collection and testing are standardized by the color of the rubber stopper placed in each. The different stopper colors refer to the additives placed in each tube--additives that are necessary to preserve the appropriate blood product for different blood tests. A purple-top tube contains (K3) EDTA as a preservative for whole blood.

health status of loved ones who are patients.

- Long-term psychological effects, which could arise from 48 to 72 hours after the incident and from then on for several months, include anxiety disorders, PTSD, depression, traumatic neurosis, insomnia, and acute stress disorder.
- It is important to distinguish between people who are merely concerned about potential exposure and people who have a genuine, nonincident-based psychological dysfunction.
- Since a radiological event is a frightening event, hospitals should be proactive in communicating with the community, and in offering reassurance, to reduce intensity of psychological issues and the number of people who experience them. To this end:
  - Dispense timely and accurate information to the public, including an accurate description of the incident and its location. This will allow people to take appropriate action before they come to the hospital.
  - Counsel patients on both acute and potential long-term physical and psychological effects. Include this information in patient discharge sheets.
- Hospitals also should ensure that trained counselors are on site, and screen for people who may be at higher risk for PTSD (i.e., people who have been previously traumatized or have been in other disasters). These individuals will require follow-up.
  - Dedicate a lead person responsible for the counselor.
  - Provide radiological education/training for the staff performing the psychological evaluations and counseling. Staff who cannot function in times of high stress should not be assigned to these duties.

HEALTH CARE PROVIDER PROTECTION

While patient care is a top hospital priority, it is vital that hospital personnel be protected from injury and disease while doing their jobs. During a mass-casualty radiological event it is likely that hospital personnel will be concerned about radia-

tion contamination. To alleviate their concern, hospital personnel should be educated about the potential health effects resulting from radiation exposure, learn what personal protection equipment they will need for precautionary measures, and be trained so they can respond effectively to a radiological incident. In addition, hospitals must prepare for potential psychological effects among their own staffers resulting from such a stressful event.

PHYSICAL PROTECTION OF HOSPITAL EMPLOYEES

- Proactive protection of hospital employees starts with obtaining as much patient and incident site information as is feasible from first responders.
- It is also important to establish an assessment center removed from the emergency department to rapidly screen victims for injury and contamination and to decontaminate those who need it.
- Radiation control zones, where potential radioactive contamination may exist, should be established within the hospital. Hospital administrators should ensure that someone is in charge of access to/from these control zones, and that law enforcement officer is present to control entry and egress.
- Personnel protection equipment that facilitates the ease of clean-up includes:
  - Universal precautions clothing (facemask, goggles, gowns, and double gloves with the inner glove taped and the outer glove removed after each contact).
  - Plastic wrap (eg, disposable trash bags, Saran™ Wrap, Ziploc® storage bags, etc.) to cover and protect instruments and equipment.
  - Disposable shoe coverings.
  - Butcher paper or the equivalent to cover floors.
  - If possible, personal dosimeters (see **Appendix A**) for staff members who might have frequent contact with contaminated patients.
- Hospitals should purchase and maintain radiation survey meters for detection procedures.
  - Each hospital should have at least three

actively working and maintained radiation survey meters, one each at point of egress and ingress and the third in circulation.
- Large hospitals might consider a portal monitor for 24/7 monitoring and protection (see **Appendix A**).
- Hospitals should ensure that designated personnel are properly trained in the use of the survey meters, and that the meters are maintained and calibrated according to the manufacturer's instructions.

• Protective clothing does not always reduce the risk of exposure, since penetrating beta and gamma radiation may go through it. However, such clothing does prevent personal contamination of radioactive substances and limits the spread of contamination.

• Hospitals should take extra precautions to –protect special populations, especially pregnant employees.

• Hospitals should provide employees with immediate and accurate communication, including public announcements, media packets, information packets for the emergency department waiting area, and website updates.

• Issues to consider in funding or obtaining needed equipment include:
- Consider a billable patient surcharge for disaster preparedness. Federal or state government grants may be available for personal protection equipment and radiation detection devices.
- Consider other community resources that may have survey meters and equipment that can be borrowed for disaster preparedness exercises or during an actual emergency.

• When there is a probability of a radiological mass casualty event, hospitals should immediately implement the radiological component of their emergency response plan to best protect their employees.

• In a radiological emergency, employees should remember to apply time, distance, and shielding principles—limit the time spent near contamination, keep as much distance as is practicable from the contaminated area, and shield yourself with any available material.

APPENDIX A:
RADIATION DETECTION AND DECONTAMINATION MONITORING EQUIPMENT

RADIATION DETECTION AND MEASUREMENT INSTRUMENTATION

Note: In the descriptions below, the term "radiation" in the context of radiation detection refers to beta/gamma radiation unless noted otherwise. The detection of alpha radiation, or even low-energy beta or gamma radiation (like that emitted from tritium), requires special probes or devices and is generally not included in the instruments discussed, unless specifically mentioned.

Thermoluminescent dosimeters (TLD) — TLDs are devices that store radiation readings, which can later be measured using an electronic reader. They are rugged and can be stockpiled and rapidly issued. They are usually housed in cards that can color code for different technical specialties or be used as ID cards. TLDs do not have readouts that can be read by those wearing them, so they cannot be used as early warning devices or as indicators that radiation exposure limits have been reached. Once a TLD is read, its reading is cleared, so it can be reused many times. The TLD reader must be regularly calibrated and operated by a qualified and knowledgeable person. TLDs are appropriate for people involved in reentry and cleanup, but should not be used alone by first responders entering high-radiation areas. In the latter case, real-time detection instrumentation should also be carried by the first responders.

Self-reading dosimeters (SRD) — This type of dosimeter, a small tube about the size of a ballpoint pen, is easy to use and does not require an expensive training program or a skilled technician. The wearer can look through the tube and get a reading of total absorbed dose in real time, so an SRD can be used as an aid in controlling the amount of time spent in the radiation area. However, SRDs are fragile and tend to lurch to a maximum reading when dropped, leading to lost data. SRDs can be initialized by electronic chargers and reused many times. SRDs could be used by emergency responders, but because of their sensitivity to mechanical shock and environmental conditions, dosimeter cards are preferred.

Dosimeter cards — These devices, about the size of a credit card, can be carried in a pocket. Successive dots on the card change color as levels of radiation exposure are exceeded. A dosimeter card can only be used once, and then must be thrown away, but at $5 per card, the cost is minimal. The reading can be instantly understood. Dosimeter cards are recommended for immediate issue to emergency responders. Because their readings are only approximate and because they can be used only once, they are not recommended for reentry and cleanup personnel.

MONITORING DEVICES FOR DECONTAMINATION STATIONS

Decontamination stations should be established as soon as possible after the event. People without serious injuries should be directed to these stations instead of to hospital emergency departments. Decontamination stations require instruments that can read radiation levels below-normal background, but such instruments do not need a very high range. Accurate readings of high radiation levels have no practical value; if a person is contaminated, he or she should be immediately decontaminated.

Geiger-Mueller (GM) counter — GM counters are sensitive radiation-detection devices capable of measuring alpha, beta, and gamma radiation. The GM counter, or Geiger counter, has a probe that can be aimed at the area of interest, producing readout measurements in mR/hr (milliroentgens per hour) or counts/minute. A special probe, generally referred to as a "pancake" probe, is required for detecting alpha radiation. GM counters also offer an audio option that allows the user to hear clicking sounds of varying intensity proportional to the radiation level. Because they are directional and can give erroneous readings in extremely high radiation fields, GM counters are not recommended for general area readings by the teams entering intense radiation areas to save

lives or to map the areas. The devices are easy to use but require periodic recalibration, which a service provider can perform. Organizations using Geiger counters should have access to a qualified technician who can train the team members in use of the device.

Pancake probe — A pancake probe is a Geiger-Mueller counter with a wide, flat probe capable of detecting alpha, beta, or gamma radiation. The wide sensitive area of the probe allows for a more rapid search of an area, and the shield on the back of the probe helps prevent radiation from some other source from interfering with the readings on the area of interest. The detector should be able to read levels below-normal background. Because such devices are directional and can give erroneous readings in extremely high radiation fields, pancake probes are not recommended for general area readings by the teams entering intense radiation areas to save lives or to map the areas. They are easy to use but require periodic recalibration, which a service provider can perform. Organizations using pancake probes should have access to a qualified technician who can train the team members in use of the device.

Alpha detectors — An alpha detector must be very close to the alpha source to detect that source. It should be noted that the measurement of alpha radiation can be confounded by the presence of beta/gamma radiation. Alpha emitters are internal hazards, not external hazards. However, if there is any concern about the former, first responders who enter a building or room with respiratory protection need not worry about the presence of the alpha-emitting material. Decontamination station personnel can determine whether radioactive material is present using a pancake probe. Alpha detectors are only useful in the reentry and cleanup phase of the incident.

Portable spectrometer — Portable spectrometers are used to determine the specific radioisotopes present. Since the presence or absence of radiation, and its magnitude, are all that emergency responders entering an area to save lives need to be aware of, knowing the specific radioisotope involved would not be immediately helpful. Therefore, portable spectrometers are not recommended for first responders. However, personnel making protective-action recommendations need to know which radioisotopes are present, specifically to guide the treatment of internal contamination; as such, they need the capability of performing isotopic identification.

Area monitor — These monitors are stationary devices set up to continuously detect radiation over a wide area. One type of device, the gate monitor, is an omnidirectional probe and meter mounted in a fixed location to check incoming or outgoing material for radiation. An area monitor should be capable of reading below-normal background, and it would be worthwhile to connect it to a computer or data-logging device. Logged data would then enable the reconstruction of the extent of possible contamination or staff exposure, especially when emergency department or relocation center staff miss an alarm or choose to ignore it to care for a gravely injured patient.

Portal monitor — A portal monitor is a doorway-type device that allows people to walk through to detect the presence of radiation. A portal monitor can be used to check large numbers of people more rapidly than a technician with a handheld meter, so such devices are useful at decontamination stations established for screening mobile but possibly contaminated people. Many types of portal monitors are not wide enough to accommodate wheelchairs or gurneys, and all such devices require periodic recalibration and testing. Some portal monitors can be expanded to allow vehicles to pass through, but most are designed only to monitor to people.

Air monitor/Air sampler — These terms sometimes create confusion. An air *monitor* is technically an omnidirectional probe mounted in an area of concern, which can record or transmit dose rates in units such as rad per hour. An air *sampler* is a calibrated vacuum cleaner-type device that collects particles from the air in a filter for later analysis. Some hybrid devices pull air through a moving paper tape, after which particles are then counted by a detector, usually called an *air particle detector*. An air monitor is useful where there is concern about airborne radiation posing an immediate health risk. An air sampler is more sensitive than an air monitor, but it does not provide real-time information. Samples can be analyzed in a laboratory for total counts or for specific isotopes.

For assistance in selecting a particular instrument or set of instruments, contact your state's Radiation Control Program Director. You can find the name and telephone number by contacting the Conference of Radiation Control Program Directors in Frankfort, KY, at (502) 227-4543 (8 am to 4:30 pm EST) or on the Internet at *http://www.crcpd.org/Map/map.asp.*

ACUTE RADIATION SYNDROME:
A FACT SHEET FOR PHYSICIANS

Acute Radiation Syndrome (ARS) (sometimes known as radiation toxicity or radiation sickness) is an acute illness caused by irradiation of the entire body (or most of the body) by a high dose of penetrating radiation in a very short period of time (usually a matter of minutes). The major cause of this syndrome is depletion of immature parenchymal stem cells in specific tissues. Examples of people who suffered from ARS are the survivors of the Hiroshima and Nagasaki atomic bombs, the firefighters that first responded after the Chernobyl Nuclear Power Plant event in 1986, and some unintentional exposures to sterilization irradiators.

THE REQUIRED CONDITIONS FOR ARS ARE:

- **The radiation dose must be large** (i.e., greater than 0.7 Gray (Gy)*† or 70 rads).
  - Mild symptoms may be observed with doses as low as 0.3 Gy or 30 rads.
- **The dose usually must be external** (i.e., the source of radiation is outside of the patient's body).
  - Radioactive materials deposited inside the body have produced some ARS effects only in extremely rare cases.
- **The radiation must be penetrating** (i.e., able to reach the internal organs).
  - High energy X-rays, gamma rays, and neutrons are penetrating radiations.
- **The entire body** (or a significant portion of it) must have received the dose.‡

---

* The Gray (Gy) is a unit of absorbed dose and reflects an amount of energy deposited into a mass of tissue (1 Gy = 100 rads). In this document, the referenced absorbed dose is that dose inside the patient's body (i.e., the dose that is normally measured with personal dosimeters).

† The referenced absorbed dose levels in this document are assumed to be from beta, gamma, or x radiation. Neutron or proton radiation produces many of the health effects described herein at lower absorbed dose levels.

‡ The dose may not be uniform, but a large portion of the body must have received more than 0.7 Gy (70 rads).

§ Note: Although the dose ranges provided in this document apply to most healthy adult members of the public, a great deal of variability of radiosensitivity among individuals exists, depending upon the age and condition of health of the individual at the time of exposure. Children and infants are especially sensitive.

- Most radiation injuries are local, frequently involving the hands, and these local injuries seldom cause classical signs of ARS.
- **The dose must have been delivered in a short time** (usually a matter of minutes).
  - Fractionated doses are often used in radiation therapy. These large total doses are delivered in small daily amounts over a period of time. Fractionated doses are less effective at inducing ARS than a single dose of the same magnitude.

THE THREE CLASSIC SYNDROMES ASSOCIATED WITH ARS ARE:

- **Bone marrow syndrome** (sometimes referred to as hematopoietic syndrome): The full syndrome will usually occur with a dose greater than approximately 0.7 Gy (70 rads) although mild symptoms may occur as low as 0.3 Gy or 30 rads.§
  - The survival rate of patients with this syndrome decreases with increasing dose. The primary cause of death is the destruction of the bone marrow, resulting in infection and hemorrhage.
- **Gastrointestinal (GI) syndrome:** The full syndrome will usually occur with a dose greater than approximately 10 Gy (1,000 rads) although some symptoms may occur as low as 6 Gy or 600 rads.
  - Survival is extremely unlikely with this syndrome. Destructive and irreparable changes in the GI tract and bone marrow usually cause infection, dehydration, and electrolyte imbalance. Death usually occurs within two weeks.
- **Cardiovascular (CV)/central nervous system (CNS) syndrome:** The full syndrome will usually occur with a dose greater than approximately 50 Gy (5000 rads), although some symptoms may occur as low as 20 Gy or 2000 rads.
  - Death occurs within three days. Death likely is due to collapse of the circulatory system as well as increased pressure in the confining

cranial vault as the result of increased fluid content caused by edema, vasculitis, and meningitis.

THE FOUR STAGES OF ARS ARE:

- **Prodromal stage (N-V-D stage):** The classic symptoms for this stage are nausea and vomiting, as well as anorexia and possibly diarrhea (depending on the dose), which occur from minutes to days following exposure. The symptoms may last (episodically) for minutes up to several days.
- **Latent stage:** In this stage, the patient looks and feels generally healthy for a few hours or even up to a few weeks.
- **Manifest illness stage:** In this stage, the symptoms depend on the specific syndrome (see **Table 1**) and last from hours up to several months.
- **Recovery or death:** Most patients who do not recover will die within several months of exposure. The recovery process lasts from several weeks up to two years.

These stages are described in more detail in **Table 1.**

CUTANEOUS RADIATION SYNDROME

The concept of cutaneous radiation syndrome (CRS) was introduced in recent years to describe the complex pathological syndrome that results from acute radiation exposure to the skin.

ARS usually will be accompanied by some skin damage. It is also possible to receive a damaging dose to the skin without symptoms of ARS, especially with acute exposures to beta radiation or X-rays. Sometimes this occurs when radioactive materials contaminate a patient's skin or clothes.

When the basal cell layer of the skin is damaged by radiation, inflammation, erythema, and dry or moist desquamation can occur. Also, hair follicles may be damaged, causing epilation. Within a few hours after irradiation, a transient and inconsistent erythema (associated with itching) can occur. Then a latent phase may occur and last from a few days up to several weeks, when intense reddening, blistering, and ulceration of the irradiated site are visible.

In most cases, healing occurs by regenerative means; however, very large skin doses can cause permanent hair loss, damaged sebaceous and sweat glands, atrophy, fibrosis, decreased or increased skin pigmentation, and ulceration or necrosis of the exposed tissue.

For more on CRS, see "Cutaneous radiation syndrome: A fact sheet for physicians" in this section.

PATIENT MANAGEMENT

TRIAGE

If radiation exposure is suspected:

- Secure ABCs (airway, breathing, circulation) and physiologic monitoring (blood pressure, blood gases, electrolytes, and urine output) as appropriate.
- Treat major trauma, burns, and respiratory injury, if evident.
- In addition to the blood samples required to address the trauma, obtain blood samples for CBC (complete blood count), with attention to lymphocyte count, and HLA (human leukocyte antigen) typing prior to any initial transfusion and at periodic intervals following transfusion.
- Treat contamination as needed.
- If exposure occurred within eight to 12 hours, repeat CBC, with attention to lymphocyte count, two or three more times (approximately every two to three hours) to assess lymphocyte depletion.

DIAGNOSIS

The diagnosis of ARS can be difficult to make because ARS causes no unique disease. Also, depending on the dose, the prodromal stage may not occur for hours or days after exposure, or the patient may already be in the latent stage by the time they receive treatment, in which case the patient may appear and feel well when first assessed.

If a patient received more than 0.05 Gy (5 rads) and three or four CBCs are taken within eight to 12 hours of the exposure, a quick estimate of the dose can be made. If these initial blood counts are not taken, the dose can still be estimated by using CBC results over the first few days. It would

Table 1: Acute Radiation Syndromes

Syndrome	Dose*	Prodromal stage	Latent stage	Manifest illness stage	Recovery
Hematopoietic (bone marrow)	0.7 Gy (>70 rads)-- mild symptoms may occur as low as 0.3 Gy or 30 rads.	•Symptoms are anorexia, nausea, and vomiting •Onset occurs 1 hour to 2 days after exposure. •Stage lasts for minutes to days	•Stem cells in bone marrow are dying, although patient may appear and feel well. •Stage lasts one to six weeks.	•Symptoms are anorexia, fever, and malaise. Drop in all blood cell counts occurs for several weeks. •Primary cause of death is infection and hemorrhage •Survival decreases with increasing dose. •Most deaths occur within a few months after exposure.	•In most cases, bone barrow cells will begin to repopulate the marrow. •There should be full recovery for a large percentage of individuals from a few weeks up to two years after exposure. •Death may occur in some individuals at 1.2 Gy (120 rads). •The $LD_{50/60}$[†] is about 2.5 to 5 Gy (250 to 500 rads).
Gastrointestinal (GI)	>10 Gy (1,000 rads) some symptoms may occur as low as 6 Gy or 600 rads	•Symptoms are anorexia, severe nausea, vomiting, cramps, and diarrhea. •Onset occurs within a few hours after exposure. •Stage lasts about two days.	•Stem cells in bone marrow and cells lining the GI tract are dying, although patient may appear and fell well. •Stage lasts less than one week.	•Symptoms are malaise, anorexia, severe diarrhea, fever dehydration, and electrolyte imbalance. •Death is due to infection, dehydration, and electrolyte imbalance. •Death occurs within two weeks of exposure.	The LD_{100}[‡] is about 10 Gy (1,000 rads).
Cardiovascular (CV)/Central Nervous System (CNS)	>50 Gy (5,000 rads) some symptoms may occur as low as 20 Gy or 2,000 rads.	•Symptoms are extreme nervousness and confusion; severe nausea, vomiting, and watery diarrhea; loss of consciousness; and burning sensations of the skin. •Onset occurs within minutes of exposure. •Stage lasts for minutes to hours.	•Patients may return to partial functionality. •Stage may last for hours but often is less.	•Symptoms are the return of watery diarrhea, convulsions, and coma. •Onset occurs five to six hours after exposure. •Death occurs within three days of exposure	No recovery is expected.

* The absorbed doses quoted here are "gamma equivalent" values. Neutrons or protons generally produce the same effects as gamma, beta, or x-rays but at lower doses. If the patient has been exposed to neutrons or protons, consult radiation experts on how to interpret the dose.

† The $LD_{50/60}$ is the dose necessary to kill 50% of the exposed population in 60 days.

‡ The LD_{100} is the dose necessary to kill 100% of the exposed population.

Figure 1. Andrews Lymphocyte Nomogram.

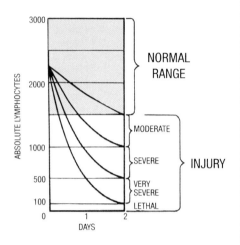

From Andrews GA, Auxier JA, Lushbaugh CC. *The Importance of Dosimetry to the Medical Management of Persons Exposed to High Levels of Radiation.* In *Personal Dosimetry for Radiation Accidents.* Vienna, Austria: International Atomic Energy Agency; 1965.

be best to have radiation dosimetrists conduct the dose assessment, if possible.

If a patient is known to have been or suspected of having been exposed to a large radiation dose, draw blood for CBC analysis—with special attention to the lymphocyte count—every two to three hours during the first eight hours after exposure (and every four to six hours for the next two days). Observe the patient during this time for symptoms, and consult with radiation experts before ruling out ARS.

If no radiation exposure is initially suspected, you may consider ARS in the differential diagnosis if a history exists of nausea and vomiting that is unexplained by other causes. Other indications are bleeding, epilation, or white blood count (WBC) and platelet counts abnormally low a few days or weeks after unexplained nausea and vomiting. Again, consider CBC and chromosome analysis and consultation with radiation experts to confirm the diagnosis.

INITIAL TREATMENT AND DIAGNOSTIC EVALUATION

- Treat vomiting (collect vomitus in the first few days for later analysis)
- Repeat CBC analysis with special attention to the lymphocyte count every two to three hours for

the first eight to 12 hours after exposure (and every four to six hours for the following two or three days). Sequential changes in absolute lymphocyte counts over time are demonstrated in the Andrews Lymphocyte Nomogram (see **Figure 1**).

- Precisely record all clinical symptoms, particularly nausea, vomiting, diarrhea, and itching, reddening or blistering of the skin. Be sure to include time of onset.
- Note and record areas of erythema. If possible, take color photographs of suspected radiation skin damage.
- Consider tissue, blood typing, and initiating viral prophylaxis.
- Promptly consult with radiation, hematology, and radiotherapy experts about dosimetry, prognosis, and treatment options. Call the Radiation Emergency Assistance Center/Training Site (REAC/TS) at (865) 576-3131 (M-F, 8 am to 4:30 pm EST) or (865) 576-1005 (after hours) to record the incident in the Radiation Accident Registry System.

After consultation, begin the following treatment (as indicated):

- Supportive care in a clean environment (if available, the use of a burn unit may be quite effective)
- Prevention and treatment of infections
- Stimulation of hematopoiesis by use of growth factors
- Stem cell transfusions or platelet transfusions (if platelet count is too low)
- Psychological support
- Careful observation for erythema (document locations), hair loss, skin injury, mucositis, parotitis, weight loss, or fever
- Confirmation of initial dose estimate using chromosome aberration cytogenetic bioassay when possible. Although resource intensive, this is the best method of dose assessment following acute exposures
- Consultation with experts in radiation accident management

FOR MORE ASSISTANCE

Technical assistance can be obtained from the Radiation Emergency Assistance Center/Training

Site (REAC/TS) at (865) 576-3131 (M-F, 8 am to 4:30 pm EST) or (865) 576-1005 (after hours) or on their web site at *www.orau.gov/reacts*, and from the Medical Radiobiology Advisory Team (MRAT) at (301) 295-0316.

Also, more information can be obtained from the CDC Health Alert Network at (800) 311-3435 or *http://www.bt.cdc.gov/radiation*.

Source: *Centers of Disease Control and Prevention, Department of Health and Human Services, March 2005.*

CUTANEOUS RADIATION INJURY: FACT SHEET FOR PHYSICIANS

Injury to the skin and underlying tissues from acute exposure to a large external dose of radiation is referred to as cutaneous radiation injury (CRI). Acute radiation syndrome (ARS)* will usually be accompanied by some skin damage; however, CRI can occur without symptoms of ARS. This is especially true with acute exposures to beta radiation or low-energy x-rays, because beta radiation and low-energy x-rays are less penetrating and less likely to damage internal organs than gamma radiation is. CRI can occur with radiation doses as low as 2 Gray (Gy) or 200 rads† and the severity of CRI symptoms will increase with increasing doses.

Most cases of CRI have occurred when people inadvertently came in contact with unsecured radiation sources from food irradiators, radiotherapy equipment, or well depth gauges. In addition, cases of CRI have occurred in people who were overexposed to x-radiation from fluoroscopy units.

Early signs and symptoms of CRI are itching, tingling, or a transient erythema or edema without a history of exposure to heat or caustic chemicals. Exposure to radiation can damage the basal cell layer of the skin and result in inflammation, erythema, and dry or moist desquamation. In addition, radiation damage to hair follicles can cause epilation. Transient and inconsistent erythema (associated with itching) can occur within a few hours of exposure and be followed by a latent, symptom-free phase lasting from a few days to several weeks.

After the latent phase, intense reddening, blistering, and ulceration of the irradiated site are visible. Depending on the radiation dose, a third and even fourth wave of erythema are possible over the ensuing months or possibly years. In most cases, healing occurs by regenerative means;

however, large radiation doses to the skin can cause permanent hair loss, damaged sebaceous and sweat glands, atrophy, fibrosis, decreased or increased skin pigmentation, and ulceration or necrosis of the exposed tissue. With CRI, it is important to keep the following things in mind:

- The visible skin effects depend on the magnitude of the dose as well as the depth of penetration of the radiation.
- Unlike the skin lesions caused by chemical or thermal damage, the lesions caused by radiation exposures do not appear for hours to days following exposure, and burns and other skin effects tend to appear in cycles.
- The key treatment issues with CRI are infection and pain management.

STAGES AND GRADES OF CRI

CRI will progress over time in stages and can be categorized by grade, with characteristics of the stages varying by grade of injury, as shown in **Table 1**. For a detailed description of the various skin responses to radiation, see **Appendix A**.

Prodromal stage (within hours of exposure)—This stage is characterized by early erythema (first wave of erythema), heat sensations, and itching that define the exposure area. The duration of this stage is from one to two days.

Latent stage (one to two days postexposure)—No injury is evident. Depending on the body part, the larger dose, the shorter this period will last. The skin of the face, chest, and neck will have a shorter latent stage than will the skin of the palms of the hands or the soles of the feet.

Manifest illness stage (days to weeks postexposure)—The basal layer is repopulated through proliferation of surviving clonogenic cells. This stage begins with main erythema (second

---

* See "Acute Radiation Syndrome: A Fact Sheet for Physicians," *Centers of Disease Control and Prevention, Department of Health and Human Services*

† Both the Gray (Gy) and the rad are units of absorbed dose and reflect the amount of energy deposited in a mass of tissue (1 Gy = 100 rads). In this document, the absorbed dose refers to that dose received by at least 10 cm² of the basal cell layer of the skin. The referenced absorbed dose levels in this document are assumed to be from beta, gamma, or x-radiation. Neutron or proton radiation produces many of the health effects described herein at lower absorbed dose levels.

wave), a sense of heat, and slight edema, which are often accompanied by increased pigmentation. The symptoms that follow vary from dry desquamation or ulceration to necrosis, depending on the severity of the CRI (see **Table 1**).

Third wave of erythema (10-16 weeks postexposure, especially after beta exposure)— The exposed person experiences late erythema, injury to blood vessels, edema, and increasing pain. A distinct bluish color of the skin can be observed. Epilation may subside, but new ulcers, dermal necrosis, and dermal atrophy (and thinning of the dermis layer) are possible.

Late effects (months to years postexposure; threshold dose ~10 Gy or 1,000 rads)— Symptoms can vary from slight dermal atrophy (or thinning of dermis layer) to constant ulcer recurrence, dermal necrosis, and deformity.

Possible effects include occlusion of small blood vessels with subsequent disturbances in the blood supply (telangiectasia); destruction of the lymphatic network; regional lymphostasis; and increasing invasive fibrosis, keratosis, vasculitis, and subcutaneous sclerosis of the connective tissue. Pigmentary changes and pain are often present. Skin cancer is possible in subsequent years.

Recovery (months to years).

Table 1. Grades of Cutaneous Radiation Injury

Grade	Skin dose*	Prodromal stage	Latent stage	Manifest illness stage	Third wave of erythema[†]	Recovery	Late effects
I	>2 Gy (200 rads) [‡]	1-2 days postexposure or not seen	No injury evident for 2-5 weeks postexposure[§]	•2-5 weeks postexposure, lasting 20-30 days: redness of skin, slight edema, possible increased pigmentation •6-7 weeks postexposure, dry desquamation	Not seen	Complete healing expected 28-40 days after dry desquamation (3-6 months postexposure)	•Possible slight skin atrophy •Possible skin cancer decades after exposure
II	>15 Gy (1500 rads)	6-24 hours postexposure with immediate sensation of heat lasting 1-2 days	No injury evident for 1-3 weeks postexposure	•1-3 weeks postexposure: redness of skin, sense of heat, edema, skin may turn brown •5-6 weeks postexposure: edema of subcutaneous tissues and blisters with moist desquamation •Possible epithelialization later	•10-16 weeks postexposure: injury of blood edema; and increasing pain •Epilation may subside, but new ulcers and necrotic changes are possible	Healing depends on size of injury and the possibility of more cycles of erythema	•Possible skin atrophy or ulcer recurrence •Possible telangiectasia (up to 10 years postexposure) •Possible skin cancer decades after exposure

Continued on next page

Table 1. Grades of Cutaneous Radiation Injury   *continued*

Grade	Skin dose*	Prodromal stage	Latent stage	Manifest illness stage	Third wave of erythema[†]	Recovery	Late effects
III	>40 Gy (4000 rads)	4-24 hours postexposure, with immediate pain or tingling lasting 1-2 days	None or less than 2 weeks	•1-2 weeks postexposure: redness of skin, blisters, sense of heat, slight edema, possible increased pigmentation •These are followed by erosions and ulceration as well as severe pain	•10-16 weeks postexposure: injury of blood vessels, edema, new ulcers, and increasing pain •Possible necrosis	Can involve ulcers that are extremely difficult to treat and that can require months to heal fully	•Possible skin atrophy, depigmentation, constant ulcer recurrence, or deformity •Possible occlusion of small vessels with subsequent disturbances in the blood supply, destruction of the lymphatic network, regional lymphostasis, and increasing fibrosis and sclerosis of the connective tissue •Possible telangiectasia •Possible skin cancer decades after exposure
IV	>550 Gy (55,000 rads)	Occurs minutes to hours postexposure with immediate pain or tingling, accompanied by swelling	None	•1-4 days postexposure accompanied by blisters •Early ischemia (tissue turns white, then dark blue or black with substantial pain) in most severe cases •Tissue becomes necrotic within 2 weeks following exposure, accompanied by substantial pain	Does not occur due to necrosis of skin in the affected area	Recovery possible following amputation of severely affected areas and possible skin grafts	•Continued plastic surgery may be required over several years •Possible skin cancer decades after exposure

* Absorbed dose to at least 10 cm² of the basal cell layer of the skin
† Especially with beta exposure
‡ The Gray (Gy) is a unit of absorbed dose and reflects an amount of energy deposited in a mass of tissue (1 Gy=100 rads).
§ Skin of the face, chest, and neck will have a shorter latent phase than the skin of the palms of the hands and the skin of the feet.

PATIENT MANAGEMENT

DIAGNOSIS

The signs and symptoms of CRI are as follows:

- Intensely painful burn-like skin injuries (including itching, tingling, erythema, or edema) without a history of exposure to heat or caustic chemicals. (Erythema will not be seen for hours to days following exposure, and its appearance is cyclic.)

- Epilation
- A tendency to bleed
- Possible signs and symptoms of ARS

As mentioned previously, local injuries to the skin from acute radiation exposure evolve slowly over time, and symptoms may not manifest for days to weeks after exposure. Consider CRI in the differential diagnosis if the patient presents with a skin lesion without a history of chemical or thermal burn, insect bite, or skin disease or allergy. If the patient gives a history of possible radiation exposure (such as from a radiography source, x-ray device, or accelerator) or a history of finding and handling an unknown metallic object, note the presence of any of the following: erythema, blistering, dry or wet desquamation, epilation, and/or ulceration.

Regarding lesions associated with CRI be aware that:

- Days to weeks may pass before lesions appear
- Unless patients are symptomatic, they will not require emergency care
- Lesions can be debilitating and life threatening after several weeks

Medical follow-up is essential, and victims should be cautioned to avoid trauma to the involved areas.

INITIAL TREATMENT

Localized injuries should be treated symptomatically as they occur, and radiation injury experts should be consulted for detailed information. Such information can be obtained from the Radiation Emergency Assistance Center/Training Site (*www.orau.gov/reacts* or call and ask for REAC/TS (865) 576-1005).

As with ARS, if the patient also has other trauma, wounds should be closed, burns covered, fractures reduced, surgical stabilization performed, and definitive treatment given within the first 48 hours after injury. After 48 hours, surgical interventions should be delayed until hematopoietic recovery has occurred.

A baseline CBC and differential should be taken and repeated in 24 hours. Because cutaneous radiation injury is cyclic, areas of early erythema should be noted and recorded. These areas should also be sketched and photographed, if possible, ensuring that the date and time are recorded. The following should be initiated as indicated:

- Supportive care in a clean environment (a burn unit if one is available)
- Prevention and treatment of infections
- Use of the following:
  - Medications to reduce inflammation, inhibit protealysis, relieve pain, stimulate regeneration, and improve circulation
  - Anticoagulant agents for widespread and deep injury
- Pain management
- Psychological support

RECOMMENDATIONS FOR TREATMENT BY STAGE

The following recommendations for treatment by stage of the illness are authoritative but do not represent official recommendations of the CDC.

Prodromal Stage—Use antihistamines and topical antipruriginous preparations, which act against itch and also might prevent or attenuate initiation of the cycle that leads to the manifestation stage. Anti-inflammatory medications such as corticosteroids and topical creams, as well as slight sedatives, may prove useful.

Latent Stage—Continue anti-inflammatory medications and sedatives. At midstage, use proteolysis inhibitors, such as Gordox®.

Manifestation Stage—Use repeated swabs, antibiotic prophylaxis, and anti-inflammatory medications, such as Lioxasol®, to reduce bacterial, fungal, and viral infections

- Apply topical ointments containing cortico-steroids along with locally acting antibiotics and vitamins.
- Stimulate regeneration of DNA by using Lioxasol® and later, when regeneration has started, biogenic drugs, such as Actovegin® and Solcoseril®.
- Stimulate blood supply in third or fourth week using Pentoxifylline® (contraindicated for patients with atherosclerotic heart disease).
- Puncture blisters if they are sterile, but do not remove them as long as they are intact.
- Stay alert for wound infection. Antibiotic therapy should be considered according to the individual patient's condition.
- Treat pain according to the individual patient's condition. Pain relief is very difficult and is the most demanding part of the therapeutic process.
- Debride areas of necrosis thoroughly but cautiously.

TREATMENT OF LATE EFFECTS

After immediate treatment of radiation injury, an often long and painful process of healing will ensue. The most important concerns are the following:

- Pain management
- Fibrosis or late ulcers (Use of medication to stimulate vascularization, inhibit infection, and reduce fibrosis may be effective. Examples include Pentoxifylline®, vitamin E, and interferon gamma. Otherwise, surgery may be required.)
- Necrosis
- Plastic/reconstructive surgery (Surgical treatment is common. It is most effective if performed early in the treatment process. Full-thickness graft and microsurgery) techniques usually provide the best results.
- Psychological effects, such as post-traumatic stress disorder
- Possibility of increased risk of skin cancer later in life

FOR MORE ASSISTANCE

Technical assistance can be obtained from the Radiation Emergency Assistance Center/Training Site (REAC/TS) at (865) 576-3131 (Mon.-Fri., 8 am to 4:30 pm EST) or (865) 576-1005 (after hours), and from the Medical Radiobiology Advisory Team (MRAT) at (301) 295-0316.

Also, more information can be obtained from the CDC Health Alert Network at *www.bt.cdc.gov/radiation* or call (800)-311-3435. For emergency response, call (800) 232-4636.

APPENDIX A: RESPONSES OF THE SKIN TO RADIATION

Acute epidermal necrosis (time of onset: <10 days postexposure; threshold dose: ~550 Gy or 55,000 rads)—Interphase death of postmitotic keratinocytes in the upper visible layers of the epidermis (may occur with high-dose, low-energy beta irradiation)

Acute ulceration (time of onset: <14 days postexposure; threshold dose: ~20 Gy or 2000 rads)—Early loss of the epidermis (and, to a varying degree, deeper dermal tissue) that results from the death of fibroblasts and endothelial cells in interphase

Dermal atrophy (time of onset: >26 weeks postexposure; threshold dose: ~10 Gy or 1000 rads)—Thinning of the dermal tissues associated with the contraction of the previously irradiated area

Dermal necrosis (time of onset >10 weeks postexposure; threshold dose: ~20 Gy or 2000 rads)—Necrosis of the dermal tissues as a consequence of vascular insufficiency

Dry desquamation (time of onset: 3-6 weeks postexposure; threshold dose: ~8 Gy or 800 rads)—Atypical keratinization of the skin caused by the reduction in the number of clonogenic cells within the basal layer of the epidermis

Early transient erythema (time of onset: within hours of exposure; threshold dose: ~2 Gray [Gy] or 200 rads)—Inflammation of the skin caused by activation of a proteolytic enzyme that increases the permeability of the capillaries

Epilation (time of onset: 14–21 days; threshold dose: ~3 Gy or 300 rads)—Hair loss caused by the depletion of matrix cells in the hair follicles

Late erythema (time of onset: 8–20 weeks postexposure; threshold dose: ~20 Gy or 2000 rads)—Inflammation of the skin caused by injury of blood vessels. Edema and impaired lymphatic clearance precede a measured reduction in blood flow.

Invasive fibrosis (time of onset: months to years postexposure; threshold dose: ~20 Gy or 2000 rads)—Method of healing associated with acute ulceration, secondary ulceration, and dermal necrosis that leads to scar tissue formation

Main erythema (time of onset: days to weeks postexposure; threshold dose: ~3 Gy or 300 rads)—Inflammation of the skin caused by hyperemia of the basal cells and subsequent epidermal hypoplasia

Moist desquamation (time of onset: 4-6 weeks postexposure; threshold dose: ~15 Gy or 1500 rads)—Loss of the epidermis caused by sterilization of a high proportion of clonogenic cells within the basal layer of the epidermis

Secondary ulceration (time of onset: >6 weeks postexposure; threshold dose: ~15 Gy or 1500 rads)—Secondary damage to the dermis as a consequence of dehydration and infection when moist desquamation is severe, and protracted because of reproductive sterilization of the vast majority of the clonogenic cells in the irradiated area

Telangiectasia (time of onset: >52 weeks postexposure; threshold dose for moderate severity at 5 years: ~40 Gy or 4000 rads)— Atypical dilation of the superficial dermal capillaries

Source: *Centers of Disease Control and Prevention, Department of Health and Human Services*

DRUGS FOR TERRORISM RESPONSE

ANTHRAX (BACILLUS ANTHRACIS) TREATMENT

ANTHRAX VACCINE ADSORBED
Biothrax *(Bioport)*
HOW SUPPLIED: Inj: 5mL
THERAPEUTIC CLASS: Vaccine
INDICATION: Active immunization against *Bacillus anthracis* in individuals who come in contact with animal products (eg, hides, hairs, bones) that come from anthrax endemic areas and that may be contaminated with spores. Also for individuals at high risk of exposure to these spores (eg, veterinarians, laboratory workers).
DOSAGE: *Adults:* 18-65 yrs: 0.5mL SQ for 3 doses given 2 weeks apart, followed by 3 additional doses of 0.5mL given at 6, 12, 18 months. Booster injections of 0.5mL recommended at 1-year intervals.
CONTRAINDICATIONS: History of anaphylactic or anaphylactic-like reaction following a previous dose of anthrax vaccine adsorbed, or any of the vaccine components.
WARNINGS/PRECAUTIONS: May cause birth defects if given during pregnancy. Review history for vaccine sensitivities. Avoid with history of Guillain-Barré syndrome. Increased risk of local adverse reaction with history of anthrax disease. Possible inadequate immunization with impaired immune responsiveness (eg, congenital/acquired immunodeficiency). Postpone vaccination with moderate to severe illness. Caution with latex sensitivity.
PREGNANCY: Category D, safety in nursing not known.
INTERACTIONS: Possible inadequate immunization with immunosuppressives. Chemotherapy, high-dose corticosteroid therapy >2 week duration, or radiation therapy may cause suboptimal vaccine response; defer vaccination until 3 months after completion of therapy.
ADVERSE REACTIONS: (Local) tenderness, erythema, SQ nodule, induration, warmth, pruritus, arm motion limitation. (Systemic) headache, respiratory difficulty, fever, malaise, myalgia, fever, anorexia, nausea, vomiting.

CHLORAMPHENICOL
Chloramphenicol *(Various)*

> Aplastic anemia, hypoplastic anemia, thrombocytopenia, and granulocytopenia may occur. Also reported is aplastic anemia terminating in leukemia. Blood dyscrasias occurred after both short-term and prolonged therapy. Do not use when less potentially dangerous drugs are effective. Not to be used for trivial infections, prophylaxis of bacterial infections, or to treat colds, flu, or throat infections. Perform adequate blood studies during treatment.

HOW SUPPLIED: Cap: 250mg; Inj: 100mg/mL
THERAPEUTIC CLASS: Bacteriostatic antibiotic
INDICATION: Alternative treatment of anthrax.[†]
DOSAGE: *Adults:* 50-100mg/kg/day divided every 6 hours.[†]
Pediatrics: 50-75mg/kg/day divided every 6 hours.[†]
CONTRAINDICATIONS: Hypersensitivity to chloramphenicol; pregnancy, especially near term and during labor. Avoid with other drugs that may depress bone marrow.
WARNINGS/PRECAUTIONS: Caution in patients with intermittent porphyria; G6PD deficiency; premature and full-term infants.
PREGNANCY: Category D, not for use in nursing.
INTERACTIONS: Decreased liver breakdown and increased effect of anticoagulants, barbiturates, tacrolimus, phenytoin, and oral antidiabetic agents with concomitant use. Acetaminophen increases serum levels of chloramphenicol; rifampin decreases chloramphenicol effect.
ADVERSE REACTIONS: Nausea, vomiting, diarrhea, headache, glossitis, stomatitis.

CIPROFLOXACIN
Cipro *(Schering/Bayer)*
HOW SUPPLIED: Inj: (vial) 200mg/20mL, 400mg/40mL, (flexible container) 200mg/100mL, 400mg/200mL; Sus: 250mg/5mL, 500mg/5mL [100mL]; Tab: 250mg, 500mg, 750mg
THERAPEUTIC CLASS: Fluoroquinolone
INDICATION: Post-exposure inhalational anthrax.
DOSAGE: *Adults:* Inhalational Anthrax: (PO) 500mg q12h for 60 days.

(IV) 400mg q12h for 60 days. CrCl 30-50mL/min: 250-500mg q12h. CrCl 5-29mL/min: 250-500mg q18h. Hemodialysis/Peritoneal Dialysis: 250-500mg q24h (after dialysis).
Pediatrics: <18 yrs: Inhalational Anthrax: IV: 10mg/kg q12h for 60 day. Max: 400mg/dose. PO: 15mg/kg q12h for 60 days. Max: 500mg/dose. Administer at least 2 hrs before or 6 hrs after magnesium or aluminum containing antacids, sucralfate, Videx® (didanosine) chewable/buffered tablets or pediatric powder, or other products containing calcium, iron, or zinc.
CONTRAINDICATIONS: History of hypersensitivity to ciprofloxacin or any member of the quinolone class of antimicrobial agents.
WARNINGS/PRECAUTIONS: Convulsions, increased intracranial pressure and toxic psychosis reported. Caution with CNS disorders or if predisposed to seizures. Severe, fatal hypersensitivity reactions may occur. Pseudomembranous colitis, achilles and other tendon ruptures reported. Discontinue at first sign of rash or if pain, inflammation, or ruptured tendon occurs. Maintain hydration; avoid alkaline urine. Avoid excessive sunlight and UV light. Do not give via feeding tube. Monitor renal, hepatic, and hematopoietic function with prolonged use. Dose adjustment with renal dysfunction.
PREGNANCY: Category C, not for use in nursing.
INTERACTIONS: Increases theophylline and caffeine levels and prolongs effects. Fatal reactions have occurred with theophylline. Magnesium or aluminum containing antacids, sucralfate, Videx® (didanosine) chewable/buffered tablets or pediatric powder, and products containing calcium, iron, or zinc decrease serum and urine levels; space doses at least 2 hrs before or 6 hrs after administration. Altered serum levels of phenytoin. Severe hypoglycemia with glyburide (rare). Potentiated by probenecid. Transient serum creatinine elevations with cyclosporine. Enhances oral anticoagulant effects. Monitor PT. Caution with drugs that lower seizure threshold.
ADVERSE REACTIONS: Nausea, dizziness, headache, CNS disturbances, vomiting, diarrhea, rash, abdominal pain/discomfort.

CLARITHROMYCIN
Biaxin *(Abbott)*, Biaxin XL *(Abbott)*
HOW SUPPLIED: Sus: 125mg/5mL, 250mg/5mL [50mL, 100mL]; Tab: 250mg, 500mg; Tab, Extended Release: 500mg
THERAPEUTIC CLASS: Macrolide antibiotic
INDICATION: Adjunct treatment of Anthrax (in conjunction with ciprofloxacin or doxycycline).[†]
DOSAGE: *Adults:* (Sus/Tab) 250-500mg q12h. (Tab, ER) 1000mg qd. [†]
Pediatrics: ≥6 months: Usual: 7.5mg/kg q12h for 10 days. CrCl <30mL/min: Give 50% dose or double interval.[†]
CONTRAINDICATIONS: Concomitant cisapride, pimozide, terfenadine, or other macrolide antibiotics.
WARNINGS/PRECAUTIONS: Avoid in pregnancy. Pseudomembranous colitis reported. Adjust dose with severe renal impairment.
PREGNANCY: Category C, caution in nursing.
INTERACTIONS: Increases serum levels of theophylline, digoxin, HMG-CoA reductase inhibitors, omeprazole, carbamazepine, drugs metabolized by CYP450. Decreases zidovudine plasma levels. Potentiates oral anticoagulant effects. Acute ergot toxicity with ergotamine or dihydroergotamine reported. Decreased clearance of triazolam. Avoid astemizole. Avoid ranitidine, bismuth citrate if CrCl <25mL/min or history of porphyria. Reduce dose with ritonavir if CrCl <60mL/min. Increased levels with fluconazole.
ADVERSE REACTIONS: Diarrhea, nausea, abnormal taste, dyspepsia, abdominal pain, headache, vomiting, rash.

CLINDAMYCIN
Cleocin *(Pharmacia & Upjohn)*

> Pseudomembranous colitis reported; may range in severity from mild to life threatening.

HOW SUPPLIED: Cap: (HCl) 75mg, 150mg, 300mg; Inj: (Phosphate) 150mg/mL, 300mg/50mL, 600mg/50mL, 900mg/50mL; Sus: (HCl) 75mg/5mL [100g]
THERAPEUTIC CLASS: Lincomycin derivative
INDICATION: Adjunct treatment of Anthrax (in conjunction with ciprofloxacin or doxycycline).[†]
DOSAGE: *Adults:* Serious Infection: 150-300mg PO q6h or 600-1200mg/day IM/IV given bid-qid. More Severe Infection: 300-450mg PO q6h or

[†] Not FDA-approved for this indication.

1200-2700mg/day IM/IV given bid-qid. Life-threatening Infections: Up to 4800mg/day IV. Max: 600mg per IM injection. Take oral form with full glass of water. [†]

Pediatrics: (Birth-16 yrs: Serious Infection: 8-16mg/kg/day PO. More Severe Infection: 16-20mg/kg/day PO. 1 month-16 yrs: 20-40mg/kg/day IM/IV given tid-qid; use higher dose for more severe infection. <1 month: 15-20mg/kg/day IM/IV given tid-qid. Take oral form with full glass of water. [†]

WARNINGS/PRECAUTIONS: Discontinue if diarrhea occurs. May permit overgrowth of clostridia. Not for treatment of meningitis. Caution with atopic patients, GI disease (eg, colitis), hepatic disease and the elderly. Monitor blood, hepatic and renal function with long-term use. Do not give injection undiluted as a bolus. The 75mg and 100mg capsules contain tartrazine.
PREGNANCY: Category B, not for use in nursing.
INTERACTIONS: Antagonism may occur with erythromycin. May potentiate neuromuscular blockers.
ADVERSE REACTIONS: Abdominal pain, pseudomembranous colitis, esophagitis, nausea, vomiting, diarrhea, hypersensitivity reactions, metallic taste (Inj), jaundice, blood dyscrasias, pruritus, vaginitis, superinfection (prolonged use).

DOXYCYCLINE
Doryx *(Warner Chilcott)*, Monodox *(Watson)*, Vibramycin *(Pfizer)*
HOW SUPPLIED: Doryx: Cap, Delayed-Release: (doxycycline hyclate) 75mg, 100mg. Monodox: Cap: (doxycycline monohydrate) 50mg, 100mg. Vibramycin: Cap: (doxycycline hyclate) 50mg, 100mg; Inj: (vial) 100mg, 200mg; Syrup: (doxycycline calcium) 50mg/5mL [473mL]; Sus: (doxycycline monohydrate) 25mg/5mL [60mL]; Tab: (Vibra-Tabs) 100mg
THERAPEUTIC CLASS: Tetracycline derivative
INDICATION: Inhalational anthrax (post-exposure): To reduce the incidence or progression of disease following exposure to aerosolized *Bacillus anthracis.*
DOSAGE: *Adults:* Inhalational Anthrax (post-exposure): 100mg bid for 60 days.
Pediatrics: >8 yrs: Inhalational Anthrax (post-exposure): <100lbs: 1mg/lb bid for 60 days. ≥100lbs: 100mg bid for 60 days.
CONTRAINDICATIONS: Hypersensitivity to any of the tetracyclines.
WARNINGS/PRECAUTIONS: May cause fetal harm during pregnancy. Use during tooth development (last half of pregnancy, infancy, <8 yrs) may cause permanent discoloration of the teeth or enamel hypoplasia. Photosensitivity, increased BUN, superinfection may occur. Monitor hematopoietic, renal, and hepatic values periodically with long term therapy. Bulging fontanels in infants and benign intracranial HTN in adults reported. May decrease bone growth in premature infants.
PREGNANCY: Category D, not for use in nursing.
INTERACTIONS: May require downward adjustments of anticoagulant dosage. May interfere with bactericidal action of penicillin; avoid concurrent use when possible. Avoid antacids containing aluminum, calcium, or magnesium, sodium bicarbonate, and iron-containing preparations.
ADVERSE REACTIONS: Anorexia, nausea, vomiting, diarrhea, dysphagia, enterocolitis, rash, exfoliative dermatitis, renal toxicity, hypersensitivity reactions, blood dyscrasias.

IMIPENEM/CILASTATIN
Primaxin *(Merck)*
HOW SUPPLIED: Inj: (Imipenem-Cilastatin) 250mg-250mg, 500mg-500mg
THERAPEUTIC CLASS: Thienamycin/dehydropeptidase I inhibitor
INDICATION: Adjunct treatment of Anthrax (in conjunction with ciprofloxacin or doxycycline).[†]
DOSAGE: *Adults:* Mild Infection: 250-500mg q6h. Moderate Infection: 500mg q6-8h or 1g q8h. Severe, Life Threatening Infection: 500mg-1g q6h or 1g q8h. Max dose: 50mg/kg/day or 4g/day, whichever is lower. Renal Impairment and/or <70kg: Refer to prescribing information. CrCl 6-20mL/min: 125-250mg q12h. CrCl ≤5mL/min: Administer hemodialysis within 48 hrs of dose.
Pediatrics: ≥3 months: Dose based on imipenem component. Non-CNS Infections: 15-25mg/kg q6h. Max: 2g/day if susceptible or 4g/day if moderately susceptible. May use up to 90mg/kg/day in older cystic fibrosis children. 4 weeks-3 months and ≥1500g: 25mg/kg q6h. 1-4 weeks and ≥1500g: 25mg/kg q8h. <1 week and ≥1500g: 25mg/kg q12h. Not recommended with CNS infection, and <30kg with impaired renal function. [†]
WARNINGS/PRECAUTIONS: Serious, fatal hypersensitivity reactions reported. Increased incidence of reactions with previous hypersensitivity to cephalosporins, penicillins, other beta-lactams, and other allergens. Pseudomembranous colitis reported. Prolonged use may result in overgrowth of non-susceptible organisms. CNS adverse events (eg, myoclonic activity, confusion, seizures) reported most commonly with CNS disorders and renal dysfunction.
PREGNANCY: Category C, caution in nursing.
DRUG INTERACTIONS: Seizures reported with ganciclovir; avoid concomitant use. Avoid probenecid. Do not mix or physically add to other antibiotics.

[†] Not FDA-approved for this indication.

May give concomitantly with other antibiotics.
ADVERSE REACTIONS: Phlebitis/thrombophlebitis, nausea, diarrhea, vomiting, rash, fever, hypotension, seizures, dizziness, pruritus, urticaria, somnolence.

LEVOFLOXACIN
Levaquin *(Ortho-McNeil)*
HOW SUPPLIED: Inj: (vial) 25mg/mL [20mL, 30mL] (flexible container) 5mg/mL [50mL, 100mL, 150mL]; Sol: 25mg/mL [480mL]; Tab: 250mg, 500mg, 750mg
THERAPEUTIC CLASS: Fluoroquinolone
INDICATION: Prevention of inhalational anthrax following exposure to *Bacillus anthracis.*
DOSAGE: *Adults:* Inhalational Anthrax: 500mg qd for 60 days. CrCl 20-49mL/min: 500mg, then 250mg q24h. CrCl 10-19mL/min/Hemodialysis/CAPD: 500mg, then 250mg q48h.
CONTRAINDICATIONS: History of hypersensitivity to levofloxacin or any member of the quinolone class of antimicrobial agents.
WARNINGS/PRECAUTIONS: Only administer injection via IV infusion over a period of not less than 60 or 90 minutes depending on dosage. Convulsions, toxic psychoses, increased ICP, CNS stimulation reported; DC if any of these occur. Caution with CNS disorders that may predispose to seizures/lower seizure threshold (eg, epilepsy, renal insufficiency, drug therapy). Hyper- or hypoglycemia with insulin or oral hypoglycemics. Moderate to severe phototoxicity can occur. Serious/fatal hypersensitivity reactions; discontinue at first sign of rash. Pseudomembranous colitis and torsade de pointes (rare) have been reported. May permit overgrowth of clostridia. Caution in renal insufficiency. Stop therapy if pain, inflammation, or ruptured tendon occurs.
PREGNANCY: Category C, not for use in nursing.
INTERACTIONS: Decreased levels with antacids, sucralfate, didanosine, metal cations (eg, iron), and multivitamins with zinc; separate dosing by 2 hrs. Concomitant NSAIDs may increase seizure risk and CNS stimulation. Blood glucose changes with concomitant antidiabetic agents. Monitor theophylline levels. Increases PT with warfarin; monitor closely.
ADVERSE REACTIONS: Nausea, diarrhea, headache, insomnia, constipation.

MINOCYCLINE
Dynacin *(Par)*, Minocin *(Lederle)*
HOW SUPPLIED: Dynacin: Cap: 50mg, 75mg, 100mg; Tab: 50mg, 75mg, 100mg. Minocin: Cap: 50mg, 100mg
THERAPEUTIC CLASS: Tetracycline derivative
INDICATION: Alternative drug in the treatment of anthrax due to *Bacillus anthracis.*
DOSAGE: *Adults:* Usual: 200mg initially, then 100mg q12h; alternative is 100-200mg initially, then 50mg qid.
Pediatrics: >8 yrs: 4mg/kg initially followed by 2mg/kg q12h. Take with plenty of fluids.
CONTRAINDICATIONS: Hypersensitivity to any of the tetracyclines.
WARNINGS/PRECAUTIONS: May cause fetal harm during pregnancy. Use during tooth development (last half of pregnancy, infancy, <8 yrs) may cause permanent discoloration of the teeth or enamel hypoplasia; avoid use during this period. Renal toxicity, hepatotoxicity, photosensitivity, increased BUN, superinfection, pseudotumor cerebri may occur; perform hematopoietic, renal, and hepatic monitoring. May impair mental/physical abilities. Use alternate form of contraception other than oral contraceptives. May decrease bone growth in premature infants.
PREGNANCY: Category D, not for use in nursing.
INTERACTIONS: May require downward adjustments of anticoagulant dosage. May interfere with bactericidal action of penicillin; avoid concurrent use when possible. May decrease efficacy of oral contraceptives. Impaired absorption with antacids containing aluminum, calcium, or magnesium and iron-containing products. Fatal renal toxicity with methoxyflurane has been reported.
ADVERSE REACTIONS: Anorexia, nausea, vomiting, diarrhea, dysphagia, enterocolitis, pancreatitis, increased LFTs, hepatitis, liver failure, renal toxicity, rash, exfoliative dermatitis, Stevens-Johnson syndrome, skin and mucous membrane pigmentation, blood dyscrasias, headache, tooth discoloration.

PENICILLIN G
Pfizerpen *(Pfizer)*
HOW SUPPLIED: Inj: 1MU, 5MU, 20MU
THERAPEUTIC CLASS: Penicillin
INDICATION: Therapy of severe infections caused by Penicllin G-susceptible microorganisms when rapid and high penicillin levels are required (eg, Anthrax).
DOSAGE: *Adults:* Anthrax: Minimum of 5 million units/day in divided doses until cure is effected.

CONTRAINDICATIONS: Hypersensitivity reaction to any penicillin.
WARNINGS/PRECAUTIONS: Serious, fatal anaphylactic reactions reported; increased risk with hypersensitivity to penicillins, cephalosporins, and other allergens. Avoid IV, intra-arterial administration, or injection into/near major peripheral nerves or blood vessels; may cause severe neurovascular damage. Take culture after therapy completion to determine streptococci eradication. Caution with history of significant allergies or asthma. May result in overgrowth of nonsusceptible organisms. Evaluate renal, hepatic and hematopoietic systems with prolonged therapy. Administer slowly to avoid electrolyte imbalance from potassium or sodium content; monitor electrolytes and consider dose reductions with renal, cardiac, or vascular dysfunction. Caution in newborns; evaluate organ system function frequently.
PREGNANCY: Category B, caution in nursing.
INTERACTIONS: Bacteriostatic agents (eg, tetracycline, erythromycin) may diminish effects. Prolonged levels with probenecid.
ADVERSE REACTIONS: Skin rash (eg, maculopapular eruption, exfoliative dermatitis) urticaria, chills, fever, edema, arthralgia, prostration, anaphylaxis, arrhythmias, cardiac arrest, Jarisch-Herxheimer reaction.

RIFAMPIN
Rifadin *(Aventis)*
HOW SUPPLIED: Cap: 150mg, 300mg; Inj: 600mg
THERAPEUTIC CLASS: Rifamycin derivative
INDICATION: Adjunct treatment of Anthrax (in conjunction with ciprofloxacin or doxycycline).†
DOSAGE: *Adults:* 10mg/kg PO/IV qd. Max: 600mg/day.†
Pediatrics: 10-20mg/kg PO/IV qd. Max: 600mg/day.†
CONTRAINDICATIONS: Hypersensitivity to any of the rifamycins.
WARNINGS/PRECAUTIONS: May produce liver dysfunction. May cause hyperbilirubinemia. Not for treatment of meningococcal disease. May produce reddish coloration of the urine, sweat, sputum, and tears. May permanently stain soft contact lenses.
PREGNANCY: Category C, not for use in nursing.
INTERACTIONS: May accelerate elimination of drugs metabolized by CYP450 (eg, anticonvulsants, antiarrhythmics, anticoagulants, azole antifungals, barbiturates, beta-blockers, calcium channel blockers, chloramphenicol, clarithromycin, corticosteroids, cyclosporine, cardiac glycosides, clofibrate, oral or systemic contraceptives, dapsone, diazepam, doxycycline, fluoroquinolones, haloperidol, oral hypoglycemics, levothyroxine, methadone, narcotics, nortriptyline, progestins, quinine, tacrolimus, theophylline, TCAs, and zidovudine). Give antacids at least 1 hr before rifampin. Increased hepatotoxicity with halothane or isoniazid. Increased serum levels with probenecid and cotrimoxazole. Caution with other hepatotoxic agents. Concomitant ketoconazole decreases both drug serum levels. Decreased levels of enalapril, atovaquone. Increased levels with atovaquone.
ADVERSE REACTIONS: GI distress, thrombocytopenia, visual disturbances, menstrual disturbances, edema of face and extremities, elevated BUN and serum uric acid levels.

TETRACYCLINE
Sumycin *(Par)*
HOW SUPPLIED: Sus: 125mg/5mL [473mL]; Tab: 250mg, 500mg
THERAPEUTIC CLASS: Streptomyces aureofaciens derivative
INDICATION: When penicillin is contraindicated, tetracycline HCl is an alternative drug in the treatment of anthrax due to *Bacillus anthracis*.
DOSAGE: *Adults:* Mild-Moderate: 250mg qid or 500mg bid. Severe: 500mg qid. Renal Dysfunction: Reduce dose or extend dose interval.
Pediatrics: >8 yrs: Usual: 25-50mg/kg divided bid-qid. Renal Dysfunction: Reduce dose or extend dose interval.
CONTRAINDICATIONS: Hypersensitivity to any of the tetracyclines.
WARNINGS/PRECAUTIONS: May cause fetal harm with pregnancy, permanent tooth discoloration during tooth development (last half of pregnancy and children <8 yrs). May increase BUN. Photosensitivity, enamel hypoplasia reported. Superinfection with prolonged use. Suspension contains sodium metabisulfite. Bulging fontanels in infants and benign intracranial HTN in adults reported. Monitor renal/hepatic and hematopoietic function with long-term use. Caution with history of asthma, hay fever, urticaria, and allergy.
PREGNANCY: Category D, not for use in nursing.
INTERACTIONS: May decrease PT; adjust anticoagulants. May interfere with bactericidal agents (eg, penicillin). May decrease effects of oral contraceptives. Take 1 hr before or 2 hrs after dairy products. Aluminum-, calcium-, iron- and magnesium-containing products impair absorption. Fatal renal toxicity reported with concurrent methoxyflurane.
ADVERSE REACTIONS: GI effects, photosensitivity, increased BUN, hypersensitivity reactions, blood dyscrasias, dizziness, headache.

† Not FDA-approved for this indication.

BRUCELLOSIS *(BRUCELLA SPECIES)* TREATMENT

CHLORAMPHENICOL
Chloramphenicol *(Various)*

> Aplastic anemia, hypoplastic anemia, thrombocytopenia, and granulocytopenia may occur. Also reported is aplastic anemia terminating in leukemia. Blood dyscrasias occurred after both short-term and prolonged therapy. Do not use when less potentially dangerous drugs are effective. Not to be used for trivial infections, prophylaxis of bacterial infections, or to treat colds, flu, or throat infections. Perform adequate blood studies during treatment.

HOW SUPPLIED: Cap: 250mg; Inj: 100mg/mL
THERAPEUTIC CLASS: Bacteriostatic antibiotic
INDICATION: Alternative treatment of brucellosis.†
DOSAGE: *Adults:* 50-100mg/kg/day divided every 6 hours.†
Pediatrics: 50-75mg/kg/day divided every 6 hours.†
CONTRAINDICATIONS: Hypersensitivity to chloramphenicol; pregnancy, especially near term and during labor. Avoid with other drugs that may depress bone marrow.
WARNINGS/PRECAUTIONS: Caution in patients with intermittent porphyria; G6PD deficiency; premature and full-term infants.
PREGNANCY: Category D, not for use in nursing.
INTERACTIONS: Decreased liver breakdown and increased effect of anticoagulants, barbiturates, tacrolimus, phenytoin, and oral antidiabetic agents with concomitant use. Acetaminophen increases serum levels of chloramphenicol; rifampin decreases chloramphenicol effect.
ADVERSE REACTIONS: Nausea, vomiting, diarrhea, headache, glossitis, stomatitis.

CIPROFLOXACIN
Cipro *(Schering/Bayer)*
HOW SUPPLIED: Inj: (vial) 200mg/20mL, 400mg/40mL, (flexible container) 200mg/100mL, 400mg/200mL; Sus: 250mg/5mL, 500mg/5mL [100mL]; Tab: 250mg, 500mg, 750mg
THERAPEUTIC CLASS: Fluoroquinolone
INDICATION: Alternative treatment of brucellosis.†
DOSAGE: *Adults:* 500-750 bid.†
Pediatrics: 10-20mg/kg q12h.†
Administer at least 2 hrs before or 6 hrs after magnesium or aluminum containing antacids, sucralfate, Videx® (didanosine) chewable/buffered tablets or pediatric powder, or other products containing calcium, iron, or zinc.
CONTRAINDICATIONS: History of hypersensitivity to ciprofloxacin or any member of the quinolone class of antimicrobial agents.
WARNINGS/PRECAUTIONS: Convulsions, increased intracranial pressure and toxic psychosis reported. Caution with CNS disorders or if predisposed to seizures. Severe, fatal hypersensitivity reactions may occur. Pseudomembranous colitis, achilles and other tendon ruptures reported. Discontinue at first sign of rash or if pain, inflammation, or ruptured tendon occurs. Maintain hydration; avoid alkaline urine. Avoid excessive sunlight and UV light. Do not give via feeding tube. Monitor renal, hepatic, and hematopoietic function with prolonged use. Dose adjustment with renal dysfunction.
PREGNANCY: Category C, not for use in nursing.
INTERACTIONS: Increases theophylline and caffeine levels and prolongs effects. Fatal reactions have occurred with theophylline. Magnesium or aluminum containing antacids, sucralfate, Videx® (didanosine) chewable/buffered tablets or pediatric powder, and products containing calcium, iron, or zinc decrease serum and urine levels; space doses at least 2 hrs before or 6 hrs after administration. Altered serum levels of phenytoin. Severe hypoglycemia with glyburide (rare). Potentiated by probenecid. Transient serum creatinine elevations with cyclosporine. Enhances oral anticoagulant effects. Monitor PT. Caution with drugs that lower seizure threshold.
ADVERSE REACTIONS: Nausea, dizziness, headache, CNS disturbances, vomiting, diarrhea, rash, abdominal pain/discomfort.

DOXYCYCLINE
Doryx *(Warner Chilcott)*, Monodox *(Watson)*, Vibramycin *(Pfizer)*
HOW SUPPLIED: Doryx: Cap, Delayed-Release: (doxycycline hyclate) 75mg, 100mg. Monodox: Cap: (doxycycline monohydrate) 50mg, 100mg. Vibramycin: Cap: (doxycycline hyclate) 50mg, 100mg; Inj: (vial) 100mg, 200mg; Syrup: (doxycycline calcium) 50mg/5mL [473mL]; Sus: (doxycycline monohydrate) 25mg/5mL [60mL]; Tab: (Vibra-Tabs) 100mg
THERAPEUTIC CLASS: Tetracycline derivative

INDICATION: Brucellosis due to *Brucella* species (in conjunction with streptomycin).
DOSAGE: *Adults:* Brucellosis: 100mg PO bid for 6 weeks. Complicated Brucellosis: 100mg PO bid for 8-12 weeks.
Pediatrics: >8 yrs: 1 to 2 mg/kg PO bid for 6 weeks.
CONTRAINDICATIONS: Hypersensitivity to any of the tetracyclines.
WARNINGS/PRECAUTIONS: May cause fetal harm during pregnancy. Use during tooth development (last half of pregnancy, infancy, <8 yrs) may cause permanent discoloration of the teeth or enamel hypoplasia. Photosensitivity, increased BUN, superinfection may occur. Monitor hematopoietic, renal, and hepatic values periodically with long term therapy. Bulging fontanels in infants and benign intracranial HTN in adults reported. May decrease bone growth in premature infants.
PREGNANCY: Category D, not for use in nursing.
INTERACTIONS: May require downward adjustments of anticoagulant dosage. May interfere with bactericidal action of penicillin; avoid concurrent use when possible. Avoid antacids containing aluminum, calcium, or magnesium, sodium bicarbonate, and iron-containing preparations.
ADVERSE REACTIONS: Anorexia, nausea, vomiting, diarrhea, dysphagia, enterocolitis, rash, exfoliative dermatitis, renal toxicity, hypersensitivity reactions, blood dyscrasias.

GENTAMICIN SULFATE
Gentamicin sulfate *(Various)*

Potential nephrotoxicity, neurotoxicity, ototoxicity. Risk of toxicity is greater with impaired renal function, high dosage, or prolonged therapy. Monitor serum concentrations closely. Avoid prolonged peak levels >12mcg/mL and trough levels >2mcg/mL. Monitor renal and eight cranial nerve function, urine, BUN, serum creatinine, and CrCl. Obtain serial audiograms. Advanced age and dehydration increase risk of toxicity. Adjust dose or discontinue use with evidence of ototoxicity or nephrotoxicity. May cause fetal harm during pregnancy. Avoid concurrent and/or sequential systemic or topical use of other potentially neurotoxic and/or nephrotoxic drugs, such as cisplatin, cephaloridine, kanamycin, amikacin, neomycin, polymyxin B, colistin, paromomycin, streptomycin, tobramycin, vancomycin, and viomycin. Avoid concurrent use with potent diuretics, such as ethacrynic acid or furosemide.

HOW SUPPLIED: Inj: 10mg/mL, 40mg/mL
THERAPEUTIC CLASS: Aminoglycoside
INDICATION: Treatment of Brucellosis in combination with a tetracycline.
DOSAGE: *Adults:* IM/IV: Brucellosis: 5mg/kg/day for 2-3 weeks. Complicated Brucellosis: 5mg/kg/day for 2-4 weeks. Renal Impairment: Reduced dose given q8h or usual dose given at prolonged intervals based on either CrCl or serum creatinine. Dialysis: 1-1.7mg/kg, depending on severity of infection, at end of each dialysis period. Obese Patients: Calculate dose based on estimated lean body mass.
Pediatrics: Brucellosis: 2.5mg/kg q8h for 2-3 weeks. Complicated Brucellosis: 2.5mg/kg q8h for 2-4 weeks. Renal Impairment: Reduced dose given q8h or usual dose given at prolonged intervals based on either CrCl or serum creatinine. Dialysis: 2mg/kg at end of each dialysis period. Obese Patients: Calculate dose based on estimated lean body mass.
CONTRAINDICATIONS: Hypersensitivity to aminoglycosides.
WARNINGS/PRECAUTIONS: Contains metabisulfite. Neuromuscular blockade, respiratory paralysis, ototoxicity, and nephrotoxicity may occur after local irrigation or topical application during surgical procedures. Caution with neuromuscular disorders (eg, myasthenia gravis, parkinsonism). Caution in elderly; monitor renal function. Keep patients well-hydrated during treatment. May cause fetal harm when administered to pregnant women.
PREGNANCY: Category D, safety not known in nursing.
INTERACTIONS: Increased nephrotoxicity with cephalosporins. Do not premix with other drugs; administer separately. Neuromuscular blockade and respiratory paralysis may occur in anesthetized patients or those receiving neuromuscular blockers (eg, succinylcholine, tubocurarine, decamethonium). See Black Box Warning.
ADVERSE REACTIONS: Nephrotoxicity, neurotoxicity, rash, fever, urticaria, nausea, vomiting, headache, lethargy, confusion, depression, decreased appetite, weight loss, BP changes, blood dyscrasias, elevated LFTs.

MINOCYCLINE
Dynacin *(Par)*, Minocin *(Lederle)*
HOW SUPPLIED: Dynacin: Cap: 50mg, 75mg, 100mg; Tab: 50mg, 75mg, 100mg. Minocin: Cap: 50mg, 100mg
THERAPEUTIC CLASS: Tetracycline derivative
INDICATION: Treatment of Brucellosis due to *Brucella* species (in conjunction with streptomycin).

† Not FDA-approved for this indication.

DOSAGE: *Adults:* Usual: 200mg initially, then 100mg q12h; alternative is 100-200mg initially, then 50mg qid.
Pediatrics: >8 yrs: 4mg/kg initially followed by 2mg/kg q12h. Take with plenty of fluids.
CONTRAINDICATIONS: Hypersensitivity to any of the tetracyclines.
WARNINGS/PRECAUTIONS: May cause fetal harm during pregnancy. Use during tooth development (last half of pregnancy, infancy, <8 yrs) may cause permanent discoloration of the teeth or enamel hypoplasia; avoid use during this period. Renal toxicity, hepatotoxicity, photosensitivity, increased BUN, superinfection, pseudotumor cerebri may occur; perform hematopoietic, renal, and hepatic monitoring. May impair mental/physical abilities. Use alternate form of contraception other than oral contraceptives. May decrease bone growth in premature infants.
PREGNANCY: Category D, not for use in nursing.
INTERACTIONS: May require downward adjustments of anticoagulant dosage. May interfere with bactericidal action of penicillin; avoid concurrent use when possible. May decrease efficacy of oral contraceptives. Impaired absorption with antacids containing aluminum, calcium, or magnesium and iron-containing products. Fatal renal toxicity with methoxyflurane has been reported.
ADVERSE REACTIONS: Anorexia, nausea, vomiting, diarrhea, dysphagia, enterocolitis, pancreatitis, increased LFTs, hepatitis, liver failure, renal toxicity, rash, exfoliative dermatitis, Stevens-Johnson syndrome, skin and mucous membrane pigmentation, blood dyscrasias, headache, tooth discoloration.

RIFAMPIN
Rifadin *(Aventis)*
HOW SUPPLIED: Cap: 150mg, 300mg; Inj: 600mg
THERAPEUTIC CLASS: Rifamycin derivative
INDICATION: Treatment of Brucellosis due to Brucella species (in conjunction with a tetracycline).†
DOSAGE: *Adults:* Brucellosis: 600-900mg PO qd for 6 weeks. Complicated Brucellosis: 900mg PO qd for 8-12 weeks.
Pediatrics: Brucellosis: 15-20mg/kg PO qd for 6 weeks. Max: 600mg. Complicated Brucellosis: 20mg/kg PO qd for 8-12 weeks. Max: 600mg.†
CONTRAINDICATIONS: Hypersensitivity to any of the rifamycins.
WARNINGS/PRECAUTIONS: May produce liver dysfunction. May cause hyperbilirubinemia. Not for treatment of meningococcal disease. May produce reddish coloration of the urine, sweat, sputum, and tears. May permanently stain soft contact lenses.
PREGNANCY: Category C, not for use in nursing.
INTERACTIONS: May accelerate elimination of drugs metabolized by CYP450 (eg, anticonvulsants, antiarrhythmics, anticoagulants, azole antifungals, barbiturates, beta-blockers, calcium channel blockers, chloramphenicol, clarithromycin, corticosteroids, cyclosporine, cardiac glycosides, clofibrate, oral or systemic contraceptives, dapsone, diazepam, doxycycline, fluoroquinolones, haloperidol, oral hypoglycemics, levothyroxine, methadone, narcotics, nortriptyline, progestins, quinine, tacrolimus, the-ophylline, TCAs, and zidovudine). Give antacids at least 1 hr before rifampin. Increased hepatotoxicity with halothane or isoniazid. Increased serum levels with probenecid and cotrimoxazole. Caution with other hepatotoxic agents. Concomitant ketoconazole decreases both drug serum levels. Decreased levels of enalapril, atovaquone. Increased levels with atovaquone.
ADVERSE REACTIONS: GI distress, thrombocytopenia, visual disturbances, menstrual disturbances, edema of face and extremities, elevated BUN and serum uric acid levels.

STREPTOMYCIN SULFATE
Streptomycin sulfate *(Various)*

Risk of severe neurotoxic reactions (eg, vestibular and cochlear disturbances) increased significantly with renal dysfunction or pre-renal azotemia. Optic nerve dysfunction, peripheral neuritis, arachnoiditis, and encephalopathy may occur. Monitor renal function; reduce dose with renal impairment and/or nitrogen retention. Do not exceed peak serum level of 20-25mcg/mL with kidney damage. Avoid other neurotoxic and/or nephrotoxic drugs (eg, neomycin, kanamycin, gentamicin, cephaloridine, paromomycin, viomycin, polymyxin B, colistin, tobramycin, cyclosporine). Respiratory paralysis can occur, especially if given soon after anesthesia or muscle relaxants. Reserve parenteral form when adequate lab and audiometric testing is available.

HOW SUPPLIED: Inj: 1g
THERAPEUTIC CLASS: Aminoglycoside
INDICATION: Treatment of moderate to severe infections such as Brucella (second-line agent).
DOSAGE: *Adults:* IM only. 1-2g/day in divided doses q6-12h. Max: 2g/day.

Pediatrics: 20-40mg/kg/day (8-20mg/lb/day) in divided doses q6-12h.
CONTRAINDICATIONS: Hypersensitivity to aminoglycosides.
WARNINGS/PRECAUTIONS: Vestibular and auditory dysfunction may occur. Contains sodium metabisulfite. Can cause fetal harm in pregnancy. Caution with dose selection in renal impairment. Alkalinize urine to minimize or prevent renal irritation with prolonged therapy. CNS depression (eg, stupor, flaccidity) reported in infants with higher than recommended doses. If syphilis is suspected when treating venereal infections, perform dark field exam before initiating treatment, and monthly serologic tests for at least 4 months. Overgrowth of nonsusceptible organisms may occur. Terminate therapy when toxic symptoms appear, when impending toxicity is feared, when organisms become resistant, or when full treatment effect has been obtained
PREGNANCY: Category D, not for use in nursing.
INTERACTIONS: See Black Box Warning. Increased ototoxicity with ethacrynic acid, furosemide, mannitol and possibly other diuretics.
ADVERSE REACTIONS: Vestibular ototoxicity (nausea, vomiting, vertigo), paresthesia of face, rash, fever, urticaria, angioneurotic edema, eosinophilia.

TETRACYCLINE

Sumycin *(Par)*
HOW SUPPLIED: Sus: 125mg/5mL [473mL]; Tab: 250mg, 500mg
THERAPEUTIC CLASS: Streptomyces aureofaciens derivative
INDICATION: Treatment of Brucellosis due to Brucella (in conjunction with streptomycin).
DOSAGE: *Adults:* 500mg qid for 3 weeks accompanied by streptomycin 1g IM bid for the first week, then qd the second week.
Pediatrics: >8 yrs: Usual: 25-50mg/kg divided bid-qid. Renal Dysfunction: Reduce dose or extend dose interval.
CONTRAINDICATIONS: Hypersensitivity to any of the tetracyclines.
WARNINGS/PRECAUTIONS: May cause fetal harm with pregnancy, permanent tooth discoloration during tooth development (last half of pregnancy and children <8 yrs). May increase BUN. Photosensitivity, enamel hypoplasia reported. Superinfection with prolonged use. Suspension contains sodium metabisulfite. Bulging fontanels in infants and benign intracranial HTN in adults reported. Monitor renal/hepatic and hematopoietic function with long-term use. Caution with history of asthma, hay fever, urticaria, and allergy.
PREGNANCY: Category D, not for use in nursing.
INTERACTIONS: May decrease PT; adjust anticoagulants. May interfere with bactericidal agents (eg, penicillin). May decrease effects of oral contraceptives. Take 1 hr before or 2 hrs after dairy products. Aluminum-, calcium-, iron- and magnesium-containing products impair absorption. Fatal renal toxicity reported with concurrent methoxyflurane.
ADVERSE REACTIONS: GI effects, photosensitivity, increased BUN, hypersensitivity reactions, blood dyscrasias, dizziness, headache.

TRIMETHOPRIM-SULFAMETHOXAZOLE

Bactrim *(Women First)*, Septra *(King)*, Sulfatrim Pediatric *(Alpharma)*
HOW SUPPLIED: Bactrim: (Sulfamethoxazole [SMX]-Trimethoprim [TMP]) Tab: 400mg-80mg*; Tab, DS: 800mg-160mg*. Septra: (Sulfamethoxazole [SMX]-Trimethoprim [TMP]) Inj: (Septra) 80mg-16mg/mL; Sus: (Sulfatrim Pediatric, Septra) 200mg-40mg/5mL [100mL, 473mL]; Tab: (Septra) 400mg-80mg*; Tab, DS: (Septra) 800mg-160mg* *scored
THERAPEUTIC CLASS: Sulfonamide/tetrahydrofolic acid inhibitor
INDICATION: Treatment of Brucellosis due to *Brucella* in children <8 yrs (in conjunction with rifampin or gentamicin).†
DOSAGE: *Pediatrics:* <8 yrs: Brucellosis: 10mg/kg/day PO in 2 divided doses for 6 weeks. Complicated Brucellosis: 10mg/kg/day PO in 2 divided doses for 8-12 weeks.†
CONTRAINDICATIONS: Megaloblastic anemia due to folate deficiency, pregnancy at term, nursing, infants <2 months old.
WARNINGS/PRECAUTIONS: Fatal hypersensitivity reactions (eg, Stevens-Johnson syndrome, toxic epidermal necrolysis, fulminant hepatic necrosis, agranulocytosis, aplastic anemia) may occur. Pseudomembranous colitis, cough, SOB, and pulmonary infiltrates reported. Avoid with group A beta-hemolytic streptococcal infections. Caution with hepatic/renal impairment, elderly, folate deficiency (eg, chronic alcoholics, anticonvulsants, malabsorption, malnutrition), bronchial asthma, and other allergies. In G6PD deficiency, hemolysis may occur. Increased incidence of adverse events in AIDS patients. Maintain adequate fluid intake.
PREGNANCY: Category C, contraindicated in nursing.
INTERACTIONS: Increase risk of thrombocytopenia with purpura with diuretics (especially thiazides) in the elderly. Caution with warfarin; may prolong PT. Increased effects of phenytoin, methotrexate.
ADVERSE REACTIONS: Anorexia, nausea, vomiting, rash, urticaria, cholestatic jaundice, agranulocytosis, anemia, hyperkalemia, renal failure, interstitial nephritis, hyponatremia, convulsions, arthralgia, myalgia, weakness.

† Not FDA-approved for this indication.

BZ TREATMENT

PHYSOSTIGMINE SALICYLATE

Physostigmine Salicylate *(Akorn)*
HOW SUPPLIED: Inj: 1mg/mL
THERAPEUTIC CLASS: Cholinesterase inhibitor
INDICATION: Treatment of anticholinergic drug overdose.
DOSAGE: *Adults:* 2mg IV, no faster than 1mg/min; dose may be repeated if necessary.
Pediatrics: 0.02mg/kg IV, no faster than 0.5mg/min; dose may be repeated in 20 minutes or thereafter if necessary. Max: 2mg.
CONTRAINDICATIONS: Active inflammation of the iris or ciliary body, asthma, cardiovascular disease, concomitant ester or depolarizing neuromuscular blocker use, diabetes, gangrene, mechanical obstruction of the intestine or urogenital tract, vagotonic state.
WARNINGS/PRECAUTIONS: Caution in ophthalmic surgery and retinal detachment. Atropine sulfate injection should be available to reverse toxic effects of physostigmine injection. Caution in tricyclic antidepressant overdose.
PREGNANCY: Unknown.
INTERACTIONS: Increased neuromuscular blockade with succinylcholine.
ADVERSE REACTIONS: Bradyarrhythmia, bronchospasm, cardiac arrest, cardiac dysrhythmia, dyspnea, increased cardiac output, seizure.

CHOLERA TREATMENT

CIPROFLOXACIN

Cipro *(Schering/Bayer)*
HOW SUPPLIED: Inj: (vial) 200mg/20mL, 400mg/40mL, (flexible container) 200mg/100mL, 400mg/200mL; Sus: 250mg/5mL, 500mg/5mL [100mL]; Tab: 250mg, 500mg, 750mg
THERAPEUTIC CLASS: Fluoroquinolone
INDICATION: Treatment of Cholera.†
DOSAGE: *Adults:* 250mg po qd for 3 days. †
CONTRAINDICATIONS: History of hypersensitivity to ciprofloxacin or any member of the quinolone class of antimicrobial agents.
WARNINGS/PRECAUTIONS: Convulsions, increased intracranial pressure and toxic psychosis reported. Caution with CNS disorders or if predisposed to seizures. Severe, fatal hypersensitivity reactions may occur. Pseudomembranous colitis, achilles and other tendon ruptures reported. Discontinue at first sign of rash or if pain, inflammation, or ruptured tendon occurs. Maintain hydration; avoid alkaline urine. Avoid excessive sunlight and UV light. Do not give via feeding tube. Monitor renal, hepatic, and hematopoietic function with prolonged use. Dose adjustment with renal dysfunction.
PREGNANCY: Category C, not for use in nursing.
INTERACTIONS: Increases theophylline and caffeine levels and prolongs effects. Fatal reactions have occurred with theophylline. Magnesium or aluminum containing antacids, sucralfate, Videx® (didanosine) chewable/buffered tablets or pediatric powder, and products containing calcium, iron, or zinc decrease serum and urine levels; space doses at least 2 hrs before or 6 hrs after administration. Altered serum levels of phenytoin. Severe hypoglycemia with glyburide (rare). Potentiated by probenecid. Transient serum creatinine elevations with cyclosporine. Enhances oral anticoagulant effects. Monitor PT. Caution with drugs that lower seizure threshold.
ADVERSE REACTIONS: Nausea, dizziness, headache, CNS disturbances, vomiting, diarrhea, rash, abdominal pain/discomfort.

DOXYCYCLINE

Doryx *(Warner Chilcott)*, Monodox *(Watson)*, Vibramycin *(Pfizer)*
HOW SUPPLIED: Doryx: Cap, Delayed-Release: (doxycycline hyclate) 75mg, 100mg. Monodox: Cap: (doxycycline monohydrate) 50mg, 100mg. Vibramycin: Cap: (doxycycline hyclate) 50mg, 100mg; Inj: (vial) 100mg, 200mg; Syrup: (doxycycline calcium) 50mg/5mL [473mL]; Sus: (doxycycline monohydrate) 25mg/5mL [60mL]; Tab: (Vibra-Tabs) 100mg
THERAPEUTIC CLASS: Tetracycline derivative
INDICATION: Treatment of *Vibrio cholerae*.
DOSAGE: *Adults:* Usual: 100mg q12h on day 1, then 100mg qd or 50mg q12h. Severe Infection: 100mg q12h.
Pediatrics: >8 yrs: ≤100 lbs: 1mg/lb bid on day 1, then 1mg/lb qd or 0.5mg/lb bid. Severe Infections: Maint: 2mg/lb. >100lbs: Usual: 100mg q12h on day 1, then 100mg qd or 50mg q12h. Severe Infection: 100mg q12h.
CONTRAINDICATIONS: Hypersensitivity to any of the tetracyclines.
WARNINGS/PRECAUTIONS: May cause fetal harm during pregnancy. Use during tooth development (last half of pregnancy, infancy, <8 yrs) may cause permanent discoloration of the teeth or enamel hypoplasia.

Photosensitivity, increased BUN, superinfection may occur. Monitor hematopoietic, renal, and hepatic values periodically with long term therapy. Bulging fontanels in infants and benign intracranial HTN in adults reported. May decrease bone growth in premature infants.
PREGNANCY: Category D, not for use in nursing.
INTERACTIONS: May require downward adjustments of anticoagulant dosage. May interfere with bactericidal action of penicillin; avoid concurrent use when possible. Avoid antacids containing aluminum, calcium, or magnesium, sodium bicarbonate, and iron-containing preparations.
ADVERSE REACTIONS: Anorexia, nausea, vomiting, diarrhea, dysphagia, enterocolitis, rash, exfoliative dermatitis, renal toxicity, hypersensitivity reactions, blood dyscrasias.

MINOCYCLINE
Dynacin *(Par)*, Minocin *(Lederle)*
HOW SUPPLIED: Dynacin: Cap: 50mg, 75mg, 100mg; Tab: 50mg, 75mg, 100mg. Minocin: Cap: 50mg, 100mg[†]
THERAPEUTIC CLASS: Tetracycline derivative
INDICATION: Treatment of Cholera due to *Vibrio cholerae.*
DOSAGE: *Adults:* Usual: 200mg initially, then 100mg q12h; alternative is 100-200mg initially, then 50mg qid.
Pediatrics: >8 yrs: 4mg/kg initially followed by 2mg/kg q12h.
CONTRAINDICATIONS: Hypersensitivity to any of the tetracyclines.
WARNINGS/PRECAUTIONS: May cause fetal harm during pregnancy. Use during tooth development (last half of pregnancy, infancy, <8 yrs) may cause permanent discoloration of the teeth or enamel hypoplasia; avoid use during this period. Renal toxicity, hepatotoxicity, photosensitivity, increased BUN, superinfection, pseudotumor cerebri may occur; perform hematopoietic, renal, and hepatic monitoring. May impair mental/physical abilities. Use alternate form of contraception other than oral contraceptives. May decrease bone growth in premature infants.
PREGNANCY: Category D, not for use in nursing.
INTERACTIONS: May require downward adjustments of anticoagulant dosage. May interfere with bactericidal action of penicillin; avoid concurrent use when possible. May decrease efficacy of oral contraceptives. Impaired absorption with antacids containing aluminum, calcium, or magnesium and iron-containing products. Fatal renal toxicity with methoxyflurane has been reported.
ADVERSE REACTIONS: Anorexia, nausea, vomiting, diarrhea, dysphagia, enterocolitis, pancreatitis, increased LFTs, hepatitis, liver failure, renal toxicity, rash, exfoliative dermatitis, Stevens-Johnson syndrome, skin and mucous membrane pigmentation, blood dyscrasias, headache, tooth discoloration.

TRIMETHOPRIM-SULFAMETHOXAZOLE
Bactrim *(Women First)*, Septra *(King)*, Sulfatrim Pediatric *(Alpharma)*
HOW SUPPLIED: Bactrim: (Sulfamethoxazole [SMX]-Trimethoprim [TMP]) Tab: 400mg-80mg*; Tab, DS: 800mg-160mg*. Septra: (Sulfamethoxazole [SMX]-Trimethoprim [TMP]) Inj: (Septra) 80mg-16mg(mL); Sus: (Sulfatrim Pediatric, Septra) 200mg-40mg/5mL [100mL, 473mL]; Tab: (Septra) 400mg-80mg*; Tab, DS: (Septra) 800mg-160mg* *scored
THERAPEUTIC CLASS: Sulfonamide/tetrahydrofolic acid inhibitor
INDICATION: Treatment of cholera.[†]
DOSAGE: *Adults:* 1 DS tab bid for 3 days.[†]
CONTRAINDICATIONS: Megaloblastic anemia due to folate deficiency, pregnancy at term, nursing, infants <2 months old.
WARNINGS/PRECAUTIONS: Fatal hypersensitivity reactions (eg, Stevens-Johnson syndrome, toxic epidermal necrolysis, fulminant hepatic necrosis, agranulocytosis, aplastic anemia) may occur. Pseudomembranous colitis, cough, SOB, and pulmonary infiltrates reported. Avoid with group A beta-hemolytic streptococcal infections. Caution with hepatic/renal impairment, elderly, folate deficiency (eg, chronic alcoholics, anticonvulsants, malabsorption, malnutrition), bronchial asthma, and other allergies. In G6PD deficiency, hemolysis may occur. Increased incidence of adverse events in AIDS patients. Maintain adequate fluid intake.
PREGNANCY: Category C, contraindicated in nursing.
INTERACTIONS: Increase risk of thrombocytopenia with purpura with diuretics (especially thiazides) in the elderly. Caution with warfarin; may prolong PT. Increased effects of phenytoin, methotrexate.
ADVERSE REACTIONS: Anorexia, nausea, vomiting, rash, urticaria, cholestatic jaundice, agranulocytosis, anemia, hyperkalemia, renal failure, interstitial nephritis, hyponatremia, convulsions, arthralgia, myalgia, weakness.

CRYPTOSPORIDIUM TREATMENT

NITAZOXANIDE
Alinia *(Romark)*
HOW SUPPLIED: Sus: 100mg/5mL [60mL]; Tab: 500mg [60*, 3-Day Therapy Packs, 6†]

[†] Not FDA-approved for this indication.

THERAPEUTIC CLASS: Antiprotozoal agent
INDICATION: Treatment of diarrhea caused by *Cryptosporidium parvum* and *Giardia lamblia.*
DOSAGE: *Adults:* ≥12 yrs: *G. lamblia* Diarrhea: 500mg q12h for 3 days. Take with food.
Pediatrics: *C.parvum/G.lamblia* Diarrhea: 1-3 yrs: 100mg (5mL) q12h for 3 days. 4-11yrs: 200mg (10mL) q12h for 3 days. *G.lamblia* Diarrhea: ≥12 yrs: 500mg (1 tab or 25mL) q12h for 3 days. Take with food.
WARNINGS/PRECAUTIONS: Caution with hepatic and biliary disease, renal disease. Contains 1.48g sucrose/5mL. Safety and effectiveness have not been established in HIV positive or immunodeficient patients.
PREGNANCY: Category B; caution in nursing.
INTERACTIONS: Highly protein bound; caution with other highly plasma protein-bound drugs with narrow therapeutic indices.
ADVERSE REACTIONS: Abdominal pain, diarrhea, headache, nausea.

CYANIDE POISONING TREATMENT

AMYL NITRITE/SODIUM NITRITE/ SODIUM THIOSULFATE
Cyanide Antidote Package *(Akorn)*
HOW SUPPLIED: Amyl Nitrite Inhalants: 0.3mL [12 ampoules]. Sodium Nitrite: 200mg/10mL [2 ampoules]. Sodium Thiosulfate: 12.5mg/50mL [2 vials]
THERAPEUTIC CLASS: Antidote
INDICATION: Treatment of cyanide poisoning.
DOSAGE: *Adults:* Apply 1 ampoule of Amyl Nitrite to a handkerchief and hold in front of patient's mouth for 15 seconds followed by a rest for 15 seconds. Then reapply until Sodium Nitrite can be administered. Discontinue Amyl Nitrite and give Sodium Nitrite IV 300mg at the rate of 2.5 to 5mL/minute. Immediately after inject 12.5g of Sodium Thiosulfate. If the poison was taken by mouth, gastric lavage should be performed as soon as possible. If signs of poisoning reappear repeat Sodium Nitrite and Sodium Thiosulfate at one-half of the original dose.
Pediatrics: Apply 1 ampoule of Amyl Nitrite to a handkerchief and hold in front of patient's mouth for 15 seconds followed by a rest for 15 seconds. Then reapply until Sodium Nitrite can be administered. Discontinue Amyl Nitrite and give 6-8mL/m² of Sodium Nitrite IV, max of 10mL. Immediately after inject 7g/m² of Sodium Thiosulfate, max of 12.5g. If the poison was taken by mouth, gastric lavage should be performed as soon as possible. If signs of poisoning reappear repeat Sodium Nitrite and Sodium Thiosulfate at one-half of the original dose.
CONTRAINDICATIONS: None known.
WARNINGS/PRECAUTIONS: Sodium Nitrite and Amyl Nitrite in high doses induce methemoglobinemia and can cause death.
PREGNANCY: Safety in pregnancy and nursing not known.
ADVERSE REACTIONS: None known.

SODIUM NITRITE
Sodium Nitrite *(Hope)*
HOW SUPPLIED: Inj: 30mg/mL
THERAPEUTIC CLASS: Antidote
INDICATION: Treatment of cyanide poisoning.
DOSAGE: *Adults:* 300mg (10mL of 3% solution) at rate of 2.5-5mL/minute. Immediately thereafter inject 12.5g (50mL of a 25% solution) of Sodium Thiosulfate. Monitor for 24 to 48 hours, if symptoms reappear, repeat Sodium Nitrite and Sodium Thiosulfate at half the original dose.
Pediatrics: 6-8mL/m² (0.2mL/kg) at rate of 2.5-5mL/minute. Max: 10mL. Immediately thereafter inject 7g/m² (Max: 12.5g) of Sodium Thiosulfate. Monitor for 24 to 48 hours, if symptoms reappear, repeat Sodium Nitrite and Sodium Thiosulfate at half the original dose.
CONTRAINDICATIONS: None known.
WARNINGS/PRECAUTIONS: May induce dangerous methemoglobinemia and can cause death.
PREGNANCY: Use in pregnancy and nursing unknown.
ADVERSE REACTIONS: Methemoglobinemia (blue skin and mucous membranes, vomiting, shock, coma).

SODIUM THIOSULFATE
Sodium Thiosulfate *(American Regent)*
HOW SUPPLIED: Inj: 100mg/mL, 250mg/mL
THERAPEUTIC CLASS: Antidote
INDICATION: Treatment of cyanide poisoning.
DOSAGE: *Adults:* 12.5g IV over 10 minutes. Monitor for 24-48 hours, if symptoms reappear repeat at half the original dose.
Pediatrics: 7g/m² BSA IV over 10 minutes. Max: 12.5g. Monitor for 24-48 hours, if symptoms reappear repeat at half the original dose.
CONTRAINDICATIONS: None known.

WARNINGS/PRECAUTIONS: None known.
PREGNANCY: Category C, safety in nursing not known.
ADVERSE REACTIONS: None known.

FENTANYL TREATMENT

NALOXONE

Naloxone *(Various)*, Narcan *(Endo)*
HOW SUPPLIED: Inj: 0.4mg/mL, 1mg/mL
THERAPEUTIC CLASS: Opioid antagonist
INDICATION: For complete or partial opioid depression reversal induced by natural and synthetic opioids. Diagnosis of suspected opioid tolerance or acute opioid overdose. Adjunct in management of septic shock to increase blood pressure.
DOSAGE: *Adults:* Opioid Overdose: Initial: 0.4-2mg IV every 2-3 minutes up to 10mg. IM/SQ if IV route not available. Post-op Opioid Depression: 0.1-0.2mg IV every 2-3 minutes to desired response. May repeat in 1-2 hr intervals. Supplemental IM doses last longer. Narcan Challenge Test: IV: 0.1-0.2mg, observe 30 secs for signs of withdrawal, then 0.6mg, observe for 20 minutes. SQ: 0.8mg, observe for 20 minutes. ***Pediatrics:*** Opioid Overdose: Initial: 0.01mg/kg IV. Inadequate Response: repeat 0.01mg/kg once. IM/SQ in divided doses if IV route not available. Post-op Opioid Depression: 0.005-0.01mg IV every 2-3 minutes to desired response. May repeat in 1-2 hr intervals. Supplemental IM doses last longer. Neonates: Opioid-induced Depression: 0.01mg/kg IV/IM/SQ, may repeat every 2-3 minutes until desired response.
WARNINGS/PRECAUTIONS: Caution in patients including newborns of mothers known or suspected of opioid physical dependence. May precipitate acute withdrawal syndrome. Have other resuscitative measures available. Caution with cardiac, renal, or hepatic disease. Monitor patients satisfactorily responding due to extended opioid duration of action. Abrupt postoperative opioid depression reversal may result in serious adverse effects leading to death.
PREGNANCY: Category B, caution in nursing.
INTERACTIONS: Caution using drugs with potential adverse cardiac effects. Reversal of buprenorphine-induced respiratory depression may be incomplete.
ADVERSE REACTIONS: Hypotension, hypertension, ventricular tachycardia and fibrillation, dyspnea, pulmonary edema, cardiac arrest, nausea, vomiting, sweating, seizures, body aches, fever, nervousness.

GLANDERS TREATMENT

CEFTAZIDIME

Fortaz *(GlaxoSmithKline)*, Ceptaz *(GlaxoSmithKline)*, Tazicef *(Hospira)*
Tazidime *(Lilly)*
HOW SUPPLIED: Fortaz: Inj: 500mg, 1g, 1g/50mL, 2g, 2g/50mL, 6g.
Ceptaz: Inj: 10g. Tazicef: Inj: 1g, 2g, 6g. Tazidime: Inj: 1g, 2g, 6g.
THERAPEUTIC CLASS: Cephalosporin (3rd generation)
INDICATION: Treatment of Glanders caused by *Burkholderia mallei.*[†]
DOSAGE: *Adults:* Usual: 1-2g IM/IV q8-12h.[†]
Pediatrics: 1 month-12 yrs: 30-50mg/kg IV q8h. Max: 6g/day. Neonates (0-4 weeks): 30mg/kg IV q12h.[†]
WARNINGS/PRECAUTIONS: Monitor renal function; potential for nephrotoxicity. Prolonged use may result in overgrowth of nonsusceptible organisms. Possible cross-sensitivity between penicillins, cephalosporins, and other beta-lactam antibiotics. Pseudomembranous colitis reported. Elevated levels with renal insufficiency can lead to seizures, encephalopathy, coma, asterixis and neuromuscular excitability. Possible decrease in PT; caution with renal or hepatic impairment, poor nutritional state; monitor PT and give vitamin K if needed. Caution with colitis, other GI diseases, and the elderly. Distal necrosis can occur after inadvertent intra-arterial administration. Continue therapy for 2 days after the signs and symptoms of infection have disappeared, but in complicated infections longer therapy may be required. False positive for urine glucose with Benedict's solution, Fehling's solution, and Clinitest® tablets.
DRUG INTERACTIONS: Nephrotoxicity reported with cephalosporins or potent diuretics (eg, furosemide). Avoid with chloramphenicol; may decrease effect of beta-lactam antibiotics. Possible decrease in PT; caution with a protracted course of antimicrobial therapy; monitor PT and give vitamin K if needed.
ADVERSE REACTIONS: Phlebitis and inflammation at injection site, pruritus, rash, fever, diarrhea.

DOXYCYCLINE

Doryx *(Warner Chilcott)*, Monodox *(Watson)*, Vibramycin *(Pfizer)*
HOW SUPPLIED: Doryx: Cap, Delayed-Release: (doxycycline hyclate) 75mg, 100mg. Monodox: Cap: (doxycycline monohydrate) 50mg, 100mg.

Vibramycin: Cap: (doxycycline hyclate) 50mg, 100mg; Inj: (vial) 100mg, 200mg; Syrup: (doxycycline calcium) 50mg/5mL [473mL]; Sus: (doxycycline monohydrate) 25mg/5mL [60mL]; Tab: (Vibra-Tabs) 100mg
THERAPEUTIC CLASS: Tetracycline derivative
INDICATION: Treatment of Glanders caused by *Burkholderia mallei.*[†]
DOSAGE: *Adults:* Usual: 100mg q12h on day 1, then 100mg qd or 50mg q12h. Severe Infection: 100mg q12h.[†]
Pediatrics: >8 yrs: ≤100 lbs: 1mg/lb bid on day 1, then 1mg/lb qd or 0.5mg/lb bid. Severe Infections: Maint: 2mg/lb. >100 lbs: Usual: 100mg q12h on day 1, then 100mg qd or 50mg q12h. Severe Infection: 100mg q12h.[†]
CONTRAINDICATIONS: Hypersensitivity to any of the tetracyclines.
WARNINGS/PRECAUTIONS: May cause fetal harm during pregnancy. Use during tooth development (last half of pregnancy, infancy, <8 yrs) may cause permanent discoloration of the teeth or enamel hypoplasia. Photosensitivity, increased BUN, superinfection may occur. Monitor hematopoietic, renal, and hepatic values periodically with long term therapy. Bulging fontanels in infants and benign intracranial HTN in adults reported. May decrease bone growth in premature infants.
PREGNANCY: Category D, not for use in nursing.
INTERACTIONS: May require downward adjustments of anticoagulant dosage. May interfere with bactericidal action of penicillin; avoid concurrent use when possible. Avoid antacids containing aluminum, calcium, or magnesium, sodium bicarbonate, and iron-containing preparations.
ADVERSE REACTIONS: Anorexia, nausea, vomiting, diarrhea, dysphagia, enterocolitis, rash, exfoliative dermatitis, renal toxicity, hypersensitivity reactions, blood dyscrasias.

IMIPENEM/CILASTATIN

Primaxin I.M. *(Merck)*, Primaxin I.V. *(Merck)*
HOW SUPPLIED: Primaxin I.V.: Inj: (Imipenem-Cilastatin) 250mg-250mg, 500mg-500mg. Primaxin I.M.: Inj: (Imipenem-Cilastatin) 500mg-500mg
THERAPEUTIC CLASS: Thienamycin/dehydropeptidase I inhibitor
INDICATION: Treatment of Glanders caused by *Burkholderia mallei.*[†]
DOSAGE: *Adults:* ≥70kg and CrCl >70mL/min: Dose based on imipenem component. Mild Infection: 250mg q6h. Moderate Infection: 500mg q6-8h or 1g q8h. Severe, Life Threatening Infection: 500mg-1g q6h or 1g q8h. Max dose: 50mg/kg/day or 4g/day, whichever is lower. Renal Impairment and/or <70kg: Refer to prescribing information. CrCl 6-20mL/min: 125-250mg q12h. CrCl ≤5mL/min: Administer hemodialysis within 48 hrs of dose.[†]
Pediatrics: ≥3 months: Dose based on imipenem component. 15-25mg/kg q6h. Max: 2g/day if susceptible or 4g/day if moderately susceptible.[†]
WARNINGS/PRECAUTIONS: Serious, fatal hypersensitivity reactions reported. Increased incidence of reactions with previous hypersensitivity to cephalosporins, penicillins, other beta-lactams and other allergens. Pseudomembranous colitis reported. Prolonged use may result in overgrowth of non-susceptible organisms. CNS adverse events (eg, myoclonic activity, confusion, seizures) reported most commonly with CNS disorders and renal dysfunction.
PREGNANCY: Category C, caution in nursing.
DRUG INTERACTIONS: Seizures reported with ganciclovir; avoid concomitant use. Avoid probenecid. Do not mix or physically add to other antibiotics. May give concomitantly with other antibiotics.
ADVERSE REACTIONS: Phlebitis/thrombophlebitis, nausea, diarrhea, vomiting, rash, fever, hypotension, seizures, dizziness, pruritus, urticaria, somnolence.

PIPERACILLIN

Pipracil *(Wyeth)*
HOW SUPPLIED: Inj: 2g, 3g, 4g
THERAPEUTIC CLASS: Broad-spectrum penicillin
INDICATION: Treatment of Glanders caused by *Burkholderia mallei.*[†]
DOSAGE: *Adults:* Usual: 3-4g IM/IV q4-6h. Max: 24g/day; IM: 2g/site. Renal Impairment: Serious Infection: CrCl 20-40mL/min: 4g q8h. CrCl <20mL/min: 4g q12h. Hemodialysis: Give 1g additional dose after each dialysis. Max: 2g q8h.[†]
Pediatrics: ≥12 yrs: Usual: 3-4g IM/IV q4-6h. Max: 24g/day; IM: 2g/site. Serious Infections: 200-300mg/kg/day IV divided q4-6h. Serious Infection: CrCl 20-40mL/min: 4g q8h. CrCl <20mL/min: 4g q12h. Hemodialysis: Give 1g additional dose after each dialysis. Max: 2g q8h.[†]
CONTRAINDICATIONS: Hypersensitivity to cephalosporins.
WARNINGS/PRECAUTIONS: Serious hypersensitivity reactions reported; increased risk with sensitivity to multiple allergens. Cross sensitivity to cephalosporins. Monitor renal, hepatic and hematopoietic functions with prolonged use. Discontinue if bleeding manifestations occur; increased risk with renal failure. Prolonged use may cause superinfections. May experience neuromuscular excitability or convulsions with higher than recommended doses. Contains 1.85mEg/g sodium; caution with salt restriction. Monitor electrolytes periodically with low potassium levels.

[†] Not FDA-approved for this indication.

May mask symptoms of syphilis. Increased incidence of rash and fever in cystic fibrosis. ADD-Vantage vial is not for IM use. Continue treatment for at least 48-72 hrs after patient becomes asymptomatic.
PREGNANCY: Category B, caution in nursing.
INTERACTIONS: Do not mix with aminoglycoside in a syringe or infusion bottle; may cause inactivation of aminoglycoside. May prolong neuromuscular blockade of non-depolarizing muscle relaxants (eg, vecuronium). Increased risk of hypokalemia with cytotoxic therapy or diuretics.
ADVERSE REACTIONS: Thrombophlebitis, erythema and pain at injection site, diarrhea, headache, dizziness, anaphylaxis, rash, superinfections.

MELIOIDOSIS TREATMENT

CEFTAZIDIME
Fortaz *(GlaxoSmithKline)*, Ceptaz *(GlaxoSmithKline)*, Tazicef *(Hospira)* Tazidime *(Lilly)*
HOW SUPPLIED: Fortaz: Inj: 500mg, 1g, 1g/50mL, 2g, 2g/50mL, 6g. Ceptaz: Inj: 10g. Tazicef: Inj: 1g, 2g, 6g. Tazidime: Inj: 1g, 2g, 6g.
THERAPEUTIC CLASS: Cephalosporin (3rd generation)
INDICATION: Treatment of Melioidosis caused by *Burkholderia pseudomallei.*[†]
DOSAGE: *Adults:* Usual: 1-2g IM/IV q8-12h.[†]
Pediatrics: 1 month-12 yrs: 30-50mg/kg IV q8h. Max: 6g/day. Neonates (0-4 weeks): 30mg/kg IV q12h.[†]
WARNINGS/PRECAUTIONS: Monitor renal function; potential for nephrotoxicity. Prolonged use may result in overgrowth of nonsusceptible organisms. Possible cross-sensitivity between penicillins, cephalosporins, and other beta-lactam antibiotics. Pseudomembranous colitis reported. Elevated levels with renal insufficiency can lead to seizures, encephalopathy, coma, asterixis and neuromuscular excitability. Possible decrease in PT; caution with renal or hepatic impairment, poor nutritional state; monitor PT and give vitamin K if needed. Caution with colitis, other GI diseases, and the elderly. Distal necrosis can occur after inadvertent intra-arterial administration. Continue therapy for 2 days after the signs and symptoms of infection have disappeared, but in complicated infections longer therapy may be required. False positive for urine glucose with Benedict's solution, Fehling's solution, and Clinitest® tablets.
DRUG INTERACTIONS: Nephrotoxicity reported with cephalosporins or potent diuretics (eg, furosemide). Avoid with chloramphenicol; may decrease effect of beta-lactam antibiotics. Possible decrease in PT; caution with a protracted course of antimicrobial therapy; monitor PT and give vitamin K if needed.
ADVERSE REACTIONS: Phlebitis and inflammation at injection site, pruritus, rash, fever, diarrhea.

DOXYCYCLINE
Doryx *(Warner Chilcott)*, Monodox *(Watson)*, Vibramycin *(Pfizer)*
HOW SUPPLIED: Doryx: Cap, Delayed-Release: (doxycycline hyclate) 75mg, 100mg. Monodox: Cap: (doxycycline monohydrate) 50mg, 100mg. Vibramycin: Cap: (doxycycline hyclate) 50mg, 100mg; Inj: (vial) 100mg, 200mg; Syrup: (doxycycline calcium) 50mg/5mL [473mL]; Sus: (doxycycline monohydrate) 25mg/5mL [60mL]; Tab: (Vibra-Tabs) 100mg.
THERAPEUTIC CLASS: Tetracycline derivative
INDICATION: Treatment of Melioidosis caused by *Burkholderia pseudomallei.*[†]
DOSAGE: *Adults:* Usual: 100mg q12h on day 1, then 100mg qd or 50mg q12h. Severe Infection: 100mg q12h.[†]
Pediatrics: >8 yrs: ≤100 lbs: 1mg/lb bid on day 1, then 1mg/lb qd or 0.5mg/lb bid. Severe Infections: Maint: 2mg/lb. >100lbs: Usual: 100mg q12h on day 1, then 100mg qd or 50mg q12h. Severe Infection: 100mg q12h.[†]
CONTRAINDICATIONS: Hypersensitivity to any of the tetracyclines.
WARNINGS/PRECAUTIONS: May cause fetal harm during pregnancy. Use during tooth development (last half of pregnancy, infancy, <8 yrs) may cause permanent discoloration of the teeth or enamel hypoplasia. Photosensitivity, increased BUN, superinfection may occur. Monitor hematopoietic, renal, and hepatic values periodically with long term therapy. Bulging fontanels in infants and benign intracranial HTN in adults reported. May decrease bone growth in premature infants.
PREGNANCY: Category D, not for use in nursing.
INTERACTIONS: May require downward adjustments of anticoagulant dosage. May interfere with bactericidal action of penicillin; avoid concurrent use when possible. Avoid antacids containing aluminum, calcium, or magnesium, sodium bicarbonate, and iron-containing preparations.
ADVERSE REACTIONS: Anorexia, nausea, vomiting, diarrhea, dysphagia, enterocolitis, rash, exfoliative dermatitis, renal toxicity, hypersensitivity reactions, blood dyscrasias.

TRIMETHOPRIM-SULFAMETHOXAZOLE
Bactrim *(Women First)*, Septra *(King)*
HOW SUPPLIED: Bactrim: (Sulfamethoxazole [SMX]-Trimethoprim [TMP]) Tab: 400mg-80mg*; Tab, DS: 800mg-160mg* *scored. Septra:

(Sulfamethoxazole [SMX]-Trimethoprim [TMP]) Inj: (Septra) 80mg-16mg/mL; Sus: (Sulfatrim Pediatric, Septra) 200mg-40mg/5mL [100mL, 473mL]; Tab: (Septra) 400mg-80mg*; Tab, DS: (Septra) 800mg-160mg* *scored
THERAPEUTIC CLASS: Sulfonamide/tetrahydrofolic acid inhibitor
INDICATION: Treatment of Melioidosis caused by *Burkholderia pseudomallei.*[†]
DOSAGE: *Adults:* 800mg SMX-160mg TMP q12h. CrCl: 15-30mL/min: 50% usual dose. CrCl: <15mL/min: Not recommended.[†]
CONTRAINDICATIONS: Megaloblastic anemia due to folate deficiency, pregnancy, nursing, infants <2 months, marked hepatic damage, severe renal insufficiency if cannot monitor renal status.
WARNINGS/PRECAUTIONS: Fatal hypersensitivity reactions (eg, Stevens-Johnson syndrome, toxic epidermal necrolysis, fulminant hepatic necrosis, agranulocytosis, aplastic anemia) may occur. Pseudomembranous colitis, cough, SOB, and pulmonary infiltrates reported. Avoid with group A beta-hemolytic streptococcal infections. Caution with hepatic/renal impairment, elderly, folate deficiency (eg, chronic alcoholics, anticonvulsants, malabsorption, malnutrition), bronchial asthma, and other allergies. In G6PD deficiency, hemolysis may occur. Increased incidence of adverse events with AIDS. Ensure adequate fluid intake and urinary output. Caution with porphyria, thyroid dysfunction.
PREGNANCY: Category C, contraindicated in nursing.
INTERACTIONS: Diuretics (especially thiazides) may increase risk of thrombocytopenia with purpura in elderly patients. Caution with warfarin, may prolong PT. Increased effects of phenytoin, oral hypoglycemics. Increased plasma levels of methotrexate, digoxin (especially in elderly). Marked but reversible nephrotoxicity reported with cyclosporine. May develop megaloblastic anemia with pyrimethamine >25mg/week. Increased levels with indomethacin. May decrease effects of TCAs. Single case of toxic delirium with amantadine.
ADVERSE REACTIONS: Nausea, vomiting, anorexia, rash, urticaria.

NERVE GAS TREATMENT

ATROPINE
Atropine Sulfate *(Various)*
HOW SUPPLIED: Inj: 0.05mg/mL, 0.1mg/mL, 0.4mg/mL, 0.5mg/mL, 1mg/mL
THERAPEUTIC CLASS: Anticholinergic
INDICATION: Indicated as an antisialagogue for preanesthetic medication to prevent or reduce secretions of the respiratory tract, to restore cardiac rate and arterial pressure during anesthesia when vagal stimulation produced by intra-abdominal surgical traction causes a sudden decrease in pulse rate and cardiac action, to lessen degree of AV heart block when increased vagal tone is a major factor in the conduction defect (possibly due to digitalis), to overcome severe bradycardia and syncope due to hyperactive carotid sinus reflex, as an antidote (with external cardiac massage) for cardiovascular collapse from the injudicious use of choline ester (cholinergic) drug, in treatment of anticholinesterase poisoning from organophosphorus insecticides, and as an antidote for the "rapid" type of mushroom poisoning due to presence of the alkaloid muscarine, in certain species of fungus such as *Amanita muscaria.*
DOSAGE: *Adults:* Usual: 0.5mg IM/IV/SC. Range: 0.4-0.6mg. If used as an antisialogogue, inject IM prior to anesthesia induction. Bradyarrhythmias: 0.4-1mg every 1-2 hrs prn. Max: 2mg/dose. May be used as an antidote for cardiovascular collapse resulting from injudicious administration of choline ester. When cardiac arrest has occurred Anticholinesterase Poisoning From Insecticide Poisoning: 2-3mg IV. Repeat until signs of atropine intoxication appear. Mushroom Poisoning: Administer sufficient doses to control parasympathomimetic signs before coma and cardiovascular collase supervene.
Pediatrics: Doses range from 0.6mg in >12 yrs and 0.1mg in newborns. Inject SC 30 minutes before surgery. Bradyarrhythmias: 0.01-0.03mg/kg IV.
CONTRAINDICATIONS: Glaucoma, pyloric stenosis, or prostatic hypertrophy except in doses used for preanesthetic medication.
WARNINGS/PRECAUTIONS: Avoid overdose in IV administration. Increased susceptibility to toxic effects in children. Caution in patients >40 yrs. Conventional doses may precipitate glaucoma in susceptible patients, convert partial organic pyloric stenosis into complete obstruction, lead to complete urinary retention in patients with prostatic hypertrophy or cause inspissation of bronchial secretions and formation of dangerous viscid plugs in patients with chronic lung disease.
PREGNANCY: Category C, safety in nursing not known.
ADVERSE REACTIONS: Dryness of the mouth, blurred vision, photophobia, tachycardia, anhidrosis.

[†] Not FDA-approved for this indication.

PLAGUE *(YERSINIA PESTIS)* TREATMENT

CHLORAMPHENICOL
Chloramphenicol *(Various)*

> Aplastic anemia, hypoplastic anemia, thrombocytopenia, and granulocytopenia may occur. Also reported is aplastic anemia terminating in leukemia. Blood dyscrasias occurred after both short-term and prolonged therapy. Do not use when less potentially dangerous drugs are effective. Not to be used for trivial infections, prophylaxis of bacterial infections, or to treat colds, flu, or throat infections. Perform adequate blood studies during treatment.

HOW SUPPLIED: Cap: 250mg; Inj: 100mg/mL
THERAPEUTIC CLASS: Bacteriostatic antibiotic
INDICATION: Alternative treatment for pneumonic plague.[†]
DOSAGE: *Adults:* Treatment: 25mg/kg q6h for 10 days. Postexposure Prophylaxis: 25mg/kg qid for 7 days.[†]
CONTRAINDICATIONS: Hypersensitivity to chloramphenicol; pregnancy, especially near term and during labor. Avoid with other drugs that may depress bone marrow.
WARNINGS/PRECAUTIONS: Caution in patients with intermittent porphyria; G6PD deficiency; premature and full-term infants.
PREGNANCY: Category D, not for use in nursing.
INTERACTIONS: Decreased liver breakdown and increased effect of anticoagulants, barbiturates, tacrolimus, phenytoin, and oral antidiabetic agents with concomitant use. Acetaminophen increases serum levels of chloramphenicol; rifampin decreases chloramphenicol effect.
ADVERSE REACTIONS: Nausea, vomiting, diarrhea, headache, glossitis, stomatitis.

CIPROFLOXACIN
Cipro *(Schering/Bayer)*
HOW SUPPLIED: Inj: (vial) 200mg/20mL, 400mg/40mL, (flexible container) 200mg/100mL, 400mg/200mL; Sus: 250mg/5mL, 500mg/5mL [100mL]; Tab: 250mg, 500mg, 750mg
THERAPEUTIC CLASS: Fluoroquinolone
INDICATION: Alternative treatment/prophylaxis for plague.[†]
DOSAGE: *Adults:* Treatment: 400mg IV bid for 10 days. Prophylaxis: 500mg po bid for 7 days.[†]
Pediatrics: Prophylaxis: 20mg/kg po bid for 7 days.[†]
CONTRAINDICATIONS: History of hypersensitivity to ciprofloxacin or any member of the quinolone class of antimicrobial agents.
WARNINGS/PRECAUTIONS: Convulsions, increased intracranial pressure and toxic psychosis reported. Caution with CNS disorders or if predisposed to seizures. Severe, fatal hypersensitivity reactions may occur. Pseudomembranous colitis, achilles and other tendon ruptures reported. Discontinue at first sign of rash or if pain, inflammation, or ruptured tendon occurs. Maintain hydration; avoid alkaline urine. Avoid excessive sunlight and UV light. Do not give via feeding tube. Monitor renal, hepatic, and hematopoietic function with prolonged use. Dose adjustment with renal dysfunction.
PREGNANCY: Category C, not for use in nursing.
Interactions: Increases theophylline and caffeine levels and prolongs effects. Fatal reactions have occurred with theophylline. Magnesium or aluminum containing antacids, sucralfate, Videx® (didanosine) chewable/buffered tablets or pediatric powder, and products containing calcium, iron, or zinc decrease serum and urine levels; space doses at least 2 hrs before or 6 hrs after administration. Altered serum levels of phenytoin. Severe hypoglycemia with glyburide (rare). Potentiated by probenecid. Transient serum creatinine elevations with cyclosporine. Enhances oral anticoagulant effects. Monitor PT. Caution with drugs that lower seizure threshold.
ADVERSE REACTIONS: Nausea, dizziness, headache, CNS disturbances, vomiting, diarrhea, rash, abdominal pain/discomfort.

DOXYCYCLINE
Doryx *(Warner Chilcott)*, Monodox *(Watson)*, Vibramycin *(Pfizer)*
HOW SUPPLIED: Doryx: Cap, Delayed-Release: (doxycycline hyclate) 75mg, 100mg. Monodox: Cap: (doxycycline monohydrate) 50mg, 100mg. Vibramycin: Cap: (doxycycline hyclate) 50mg, 100mg; Inj: (vial) 100mg, 200mg; Syrup: (doxycycline calcium) 50mg/5mL [473mL]; Sus: (doxycycline monohydrate) 25mg/5mL [60mL]; Tab: (Vibra-Tabs) 100mg
THERAPEUTIC CLASS: Tetracycline derivative
INDICATION: Treatment of plague due to *Yersinia pestis*.
DOSAGE: *Adults:* Treatment: Usual: 100mg q12h on 1st day, followed by 100mg qd. Severe Infections: 100mg q12h. Prophylaxis: 100mg bid for 7 days.

[†] Not FDA-approved for this indication.

Pediatrics: >8 yrs: >100lbs: 100mg q12h on 1st day, followed by 100mg qd. Severe Infections: 100mg q12h. ≤100lbs: 2mg/lb given bid on day 1, followed by 1mg/lb given qd-bid thereafter. Severe Infections: Up to 2mg/lb. Prophylaxis: >8 yrs: >100lbs: 100mg bid for 7 days. <100lbs: 2.2mg/kg PO bid for 7 days.
CONTRAINDICATIONS: Hypersensitivity to any of the tetracyclines.
WARNINGS/PRECAUTIONS: May cause fetal harm during pregnancy. Use during tooth development (last half of pregnancy, infancy, <8 yrs) may cause permanent discoloration of the teeth or enamel hypoplasia. Photosensitivity, increased BUN, superinfection may occur. Monitor hematopoietic, renal and hepatic values periodically with long term therapy. Bulging fontanels in infants and benign intracranial HTN in adults reported. May decrease bone growth in premature infants.
PREGNANCY: Category D, not for use in nursing.
INTERACTIONS: May require downward adjustments of anticoagulant dosage. May interfere with bactericidal action of penicillin; avoid concurrent use when possible. Avoid antacids containing aluminum, calcium, or magnesium, sodium bicarbonate, and iron-containing preparations.
ADVERSE REACTIONS: Anorexia, nausea, vomiting, diarrhea, dysphagia, enterocolitis, rash, exfoliative dermatitis, renal toxicity, hypersensitivity reactions, blood dyscrasias.

GENTAMICIN SULFATE
Gentamicin sulfate *(Various)*

> Potential nephrotoxicity, neurotoxicity, ototoxicity. Risk of toxicity is greater with impaired renal function, high dosage, or prolonged therapy. Monitor serum concentrations closely. Avoid prolonged peak levels >12mcg/mL and trough levels >2mcg/mL. Monitor renal and eight cranial nerve function, urine, BUN, serum creatinine, and CrCl. Obtain serial audiograms. Advanced age and dehydration increase risk of toxicity. Adjust dose or discontinue use with evidence of ototoxicity or nephrotoxicity. May cause fetal harm during pregnancy. Avoid concurrent and/or sequential systemic or topical use of other potentially neurotoxic and/or nephrotoxic drugs, such as cisplatin, cephaloridine, kanamycin, amikacin, neomycin, polymyxin B, colistin, paromomycin, streptomycin, tobramycin, vancomycin, and viomycin. Avoid concurrent use with potent diuretics, such as ethacrynic acid or furosemide.

HOW SUPPLIED: Inj: 10mg/mL, 40mg/mL
THERAPEUTIC CLASS: Aminoglycoside
INDICATION: Treatment of plague due to *Yersinai pestis*.
DOSAGE: *Adults:* IM/IV: Serious Infections: 3mg/kg/day given q8h. Life-Threatening Infections: 5mg/kg/day tid-qid; reduce to 3mg/kg/day as soon as clinically indicated. Treat for 7-10 days; may need longer course in difficult and complicated infections. Renal Impairment: Reduced dose given q8h or usual dose given at prolonged intervals based on either CrCl or serum creatinine. Dialysis: 1-1.7mg/kg, depending on severity of infection, at end of each dialysis period. Obese Patients: Calculate dose based on estimated lean body mass.
Pediatrics: Children: 6-7.5mg/kg/day (2-2.5mg/kg given q8h). Infants and Neonates: 7.5mg/kg/day (2.5mg/kg given q8h). Premature and Full-Term Neonates ≤1 week: 5mg/kg/day (2.5mg/kg given q12h). Treat for 7-10 days; may need longer course in difficult and complicated infections. Renal Impairment: Reduced dose given q8h or usual dose given at prolonged intervals based on either CrCl or serum creatinine. Dialysis: 2mg/kg at end of each dialysis period. Obese Patients: Calculate dose based on estimated lean body mass.
CONTRAINDICATIONS: Hypersensitivity to aminoglycosides.
WARNINGS/PRECAUTIONS: Contains metabisulfite. Neuromuscular blockade, respiratory paralysis, ototoxicity, and nephrotoxicity may occur after local irrigation or topical application during surgical procedures. Caution with neuromuscular disorders (eg, myasthenia gravis, parkinsonism). Caution in elderly; monitor renal function. Keep patients well-hydrated during treatment. May cause fetal harm when administered to pregnant women.
PREGNANCY: Category D, safety not known in nursing.
INTERACTIONS: Increased nephrotoxicity with cephalosporins. Do not premix with other drugs; administer separately. Neuromuscular blockade and respiratory paralysis may occur in anesthetized patients or those receiving neuromuscular blockers (eg, succinylcholine, tubocurarine, decamethonium). See Black Box Warning.
ADVERSE REACTIONS: Nephrotoxicity, neurotoxicity, rash, fever, urticaria, nausea, vomiting, headache, lethargy, confusion, depression, decreased appetite, weight loss, BP changes, blood dyscrasias, elevated LFTs.

MINOCYCLINE
Dynacin *(Par)*, Minocin *(Lederle)*
HOW SUPPLIED: Dynacin: Cap: 50mg, 75mg, 100mg; Tab: 50mg, 75mg, 100mg. Minocin: Cap: 50mg, 100mg

THERAPEUTIC CLASS: Tetracycline derivative
INDICATION: Treatment of plague due to *Yersinai pestis*.
DOSAGE: *Adults:* Usual: 200mg initially, then 100mg q12h; alternative is 100-200mg initially, then 50mg qid.
Pediatrics: >8 yrs: 4mg/kg initially followed by 2mg/kg q12h. Take with plenty of fluids.
CONTRAINDICATIONS: Hypersensitivity to any of the tetracyclines.
WARNINGS/PRECAUTIONS: May cause fetal harm during pregnancy. Use during tooth development (last half of pregnancy, infancy, <8 yrs) may cause permanent discoloration of the teeth or enamel hypoplasia; avoid use during this period. Renal toxicity, hepatotoxicity, photosensitivity, increased BUN, superinfection, pseudotumor cerebri may occur; perform hematopoietic, renal, and hepatic monitoring. May impair mental/physical abilities. Use alternate form of contraception other than oral contraceptives. May decrease bone growth in premature infants.
PREGNANCY: Category D, not for use in nursing.
INTERACTIONS: May require downward adjustments of anticoagulant dosage. May interfere with bactericidal action of penicillin; avoid concurrent use when possible. May decrease efficacy of oral contraceptives. Impaired absorption with antacids containing aluminum, calcium, or magnesium and iron-containing products. Fatal renal toxicity with methoxyflurane has been reported.
ADVERSE REACTIONS: Anorexia, nausea, vomiting, diarrhea, dysphagia, enterocolitis, pancreatitis, increased LFTs, hepatitis, liver failure, renal toxicity, rash, exfoliative dermatitis, Stevens-Johnson syndrome, skin and mucous membrane pigmentation, blood dyscrasias, headache, tooth discoloration.

STREPTOMYCIN SULFATE
Streptomycin sulfate *(Various)*

Risk of severe neurotoxic reactions (eg, vestibular and cochlear disturbances) increased significantly with renal dysfunction or pre-renal azotemia. Optic nerve dysfunction, peripheral neuritis, arachnoiditis, and encephalopathy may occur. Monitor renal function; reduce dose with renal impairment and/or nitrogen retention. Do not exceed peak serum level of 20-25mcg/mL with kidney damage. Avoid other neurotoxic and/or nephrotoxic drugs (eg, neomycin, kanamycin, gentamicin, cephaloridine, paromomycin, viomycin, polymyxin B, colistin, tobramycin, cyclosporine). Respiratory paralysis can occur, especially if given soon after anesthesia or muscle relaxants. Reserve parenteral form when adequate lab and audiometric testing is available.

HOW SUPPLIED: Inj: 1g
THERAPEUTIC CLASS: Aminoglycoside
INDICATION: Treatment of moderate to severe infections such as plague.
DOSAGE: *Adults:* IM only. Plague: 1g bid for minimum of 10 days. Renal Impairment: Reduce dose. Moderate/Severe Infections: 1-2g/day in divided doses q6-12h. Max: 2g/day.
Pediatrics: Moderate/Severe Infections: 20-40mg/kg/day (8-20mg/lb/day) in divided doses q6-12h.
CONTRAINDICATIONS: Hypersensitivity to aminoglycosides.
WARNINGS/PRECAUTIONS: Vestibular and auditory dysfunction may occur. Contains sodium metabisulfite. Can cause fetal harm in pregnancy. Caution with dose selection in renal impairment. Alkalinize urine to minimize or prevent renal irritation with prolonged therapy. CNS depression (eg, stupor, flaccidity) reported in infants with higher than recommended doses. If syphilis is suspected when treating venereal infections, perform dark field exam before initiating treatment, and monthly serologic tests for at least 4 months. Overgrowth of nonsusceptible organisms may occur. Terminate therapy when toxic symptoms appear, when impending toxicity is feared, when organisms become resistant, or when full treatment effect has been obtained
PREGNANCY: Category D, not for use in nursing.
INTERACTIONS: See Black Box Warning. Increased ototoxicity with ethacrynic acid, furosemide, mannitol and possibly other diuretics.
ADVERSE REACTIONS: Vestibular ototoxicity (nausea, vomiting, vertigo), paresthesia of face, rash, fever, urticaria, angioneurotic edema, eosinophilia.

TETRACYCLINE
Sumycin *(Par)*
HOW SUPPLIED: Sus: 125mg/5mL [473mL]; Tab: 250mg, 500mg
THERAPEUTIC CLASS: Streptomyces aureofaciens derivative
INDICATION: Treatment of plague due to *Yersinia pestis*.
DOSAGE: *Adults:* Mild-Moderate: 250mg qid or 500mg bid. Severe: 500mg qid. Renal Dysfunction: Reduce dose or extend dose interval.
Pediatrics: >8 yrs: Usual: 25-50mg/kg divided bid-qid. Renal Dysfunction: Reduce dose or extend dose interval.

† Not FDA-approved for this indication.

CONTRAINDICATIONS: Hypersensitivity to any of the tetracyclines.
WARNINGS/PRECAUTIONS: May cause fetal harm with pregnancy, permanent tooth discoloration during tooth development (last half of pregnancy and children <8 yrs). May increase BUN. Photosensitivity, enamel hypoplasia reported. Superinfection with prolonged use. Suspension contains sodium metabisulfite. Bulging fontanels in infants and benign intracranial HTN in adults reported. Monitor renal/hepatic and hematopoietic function with long-term use. Caution with history of asthma, hay fever, urticaria, and allergy.
PREGNANCY: Category D, not for use in nursing.
INTERACTIONS: May decrease PT; adjust anticoagulants. May interfere with bactericidal agents (eg, penicillin). May decrease effects of oral contraceptives. Take 1 hr before or 2 hrs after dairy products. Aluminum-, calcium-, iron- and magnesium-containing products impair absorption. Fatal renal toxicity reported with concurrent methoxyflurane.
ADVERSE REACTIONS: GI effects, photosensitivity, increased BUN, hypersensitivity reactions, blood dyscrasias, dizziness, headache.

PSITTACOSIS *(CHLAMYDOPHILA PSITTACI)* TREATMENT

DOXYCYCLINE
Doryx *(Warner Chilcott)*, Monodox *(Watson)*, Vibramycin *(Pfizer)*
HOW SUPPLIED: Doryx: Cap, Delayed-Release: (doxycycline hyclate) 75mg, 100mg. Monodox: Cap: (doxycycline monohydrate) 50mg, 100mg. Vibramycin: Cap: (doxycycline hyclate) 50mg, 100mg; Inj: (vial) 100mg, 200mg; Syrup: (doxycycline calcium) 50mg/5mL [473mL]; Sus: (doxycycline monohydrate) 25mg/5mL [60mL]; Tab: (Vibra-Tabs) 100mg
THERAPEUTIC CLASS: Tetracycline derivative
INDICATION: Treatment of *Chlamydia psittaci*.
DOSAGE: *Adults:* Usual: 100mg q12h on day 1, then 100mg qd or 50mg q12h for 10-21 days. Severe Infection: 100mg q12h for 10-21 days.
Pediatrics: >8 yrs: ≤100 lbs: 1mg/lb bid on day 1, then 1mg/lb qd or 0.5mg/lb bid for 10-21 days. Severe Infections: Maint: 2mg/lb. >100lbs: Usual: 100mg q12h on day 1, then 100mg qd or 50mg q12h for 10-21 days. Severe Infection: 100mg q12h for 10-21 days.
CONTRAINDICATIONS: Hypersensitivity to any of the tetracyclines.
WARNINGS/PRECAUTIONS: May cause fetal harm during pregnancy. Use during tooth development (last half of pregnancy, infancy, <8 yrs) may cause permanent discoloration of the teeth or enamel hypoplasia. Photosensitivity, increased BUN, superinfection may occur. Monitor hematopoietic, renal, and hepatic values periodically with long term therapy. Bulging fontanels in infants and benign intracranial HTN in adults reported. May decrease bone growth in premature infants.
PREGNANCY: Category D, not for use in nursing.
INTERACTIONS: May require downward adjustments of anticoagulant dosage. May interfere with bactericidal action of penicillin; avoid concurrent use when possible. Avoid antacids containing aluminum, calcium, or magnesium, sodium bicarbonate, and iron-containing preparations.
ADVERSE REACTIONS: Anorexia, nausea, vomiting, diarrhea, dysphagia, enterocolitis, rash, exfoliative dermatitis, renal toxicity, hypersensitivity reactions, blood dyscrasias.

MINOCYCLINE
Dynacin *(Par)*, Minocin *(Lederle)*
HOW SUPPLIED: Dynacin: Cap: 50mg, 75mg, 100mg; Tab: 50mg, 75mg, 100mg. Minocin: Cap: 50mg, 100mg
THERAPEUTIC CLASS: Tetracycline derivative
INDICATION: Treatment of *Chlamydia psittaci*.
DOSAGE: *Adults:* Usual: 200mg initially, then 100mg q12h for 10-21 days; alternative is 100-200mg initially, then 50mg qid for 10-21 days.
Pediatrics: >8 yrs: 4mg/kg initially followed by 2mg/kg q12h for 10-21 days. Take with plenty of fluids.
CONTRAINDICATIONS: Hypersensitivity to any of the tetracyclines.
WARNINGS/PRECAUTIONS: May cause fetal harm during pregnancy. Use during tooth development (last half of pregnancy, infancy, <8 yrs) may cause permanent discoloration of the teeth or enamel hypoplasia; avoid use during this period. Renal toxicity, hepatotoxicity, photosensitivity, increased BUN, superinfection, pseudotumor cerebri may occur; perform hematopoietic, renal, and hepatic monitoring. May impair mental/physical abilities. Use alternate form of contraception other than oral contraceptives. May decrease bone growth in premature infants.
PREGNANCY: Category D, not for use in nursing.
INTERACTIONS: May require downward adjustments of anticoagulant dosage. May interfere with bactericidal action of penicillin; avoid concurrent use when possible. May decrease efficacy of oral contraceptives. Impaired absorption with antacids containing aluminum, calcium, or magnesium and iron-containing products. Fatal renal toxicity with methoxyflurane has been reported.

ADVERSE REACTIONS: Anorexia, nausea, vomiting, diarrhea, dysphagia, enterocolitis, pancreatitis, increased LFTs, hepatitis, liver failure, renal toxicity, rash, exfoliative dermatitis, Stevens-Johnson syndrome, skin and mucous membrane pigmentation, blood dyscrasias, headache, tooth discoloration.

TETRACYCLINE
Sumycin *(Par)*

HOW SUPPLIED: Sus: 125mg/5mL [473mL]; Tab: 250mg, 500mg
THERAPEUTIC CLASS: Streptomyces aureofaciens derivative
INDICATION: Treatment of psittacosis due to *Chlamydia psittaci.*
DOSAGE: *Adults:* 500mg qid for 10-21 days.
Pediatrics: >8 yrs: Usual: 25-50mg/kg divided bid-qid for 10-21 days.
CONTRAINDICATIONS: Hypersensitivity to any of the tetracyclines.
WARNINGS/PRECAUTIONS: May cause fetal harm with pregnancy, permanent tooth discoloration during tooth development (last half of pregnancy and children <8 yrs). May increase BUN. Photosensitivity, enamel hypoplasia reported. Superinfection with prolonged use. Suspension contains sodium metabisulfite. Bulging fontanels in infants and benign intracranial HTN in adults reported. Monitor renal/hepatic and hematopoietic function with long-term use. Caution with history of asthma, hay fever, urticaria, and allergy.
PREGNANCY: Category D, not for use in nursing.
INTERACTIONS: May decrease PT; adjust anticoagulants. May interfere with bactericidal agents (eg, penicillin). May decrease effects of oral contraceptives. Take 1 hr before or 2 hrs after dairy products. Aluminum-, calcium-, iron- and magnesium-containing products impair absorption. Fatal renal toxicity reported with concurrent methoxyflurane.

Q FEVER *(COXIELLA BURNETII)* TREATMENT

CHLORAMPHENICOL
Chloramphenicol *(Various)*

> **Aplastic anemia, hypoplastic anemia, thrombocytopenia, and granulocytopenia may occur. Also reported is aplastic anemia terminating in leukemia. Blood dyscrasias occurred after both short-term and prolonged therapy. Do not use when less potentially dangerous drugs are effective. Not to be used for trivial infections, prophylaxis of bacterial infections, or to treat colds, flu, or throat infections. Perform adequate blood studies during treatment.**

HOW SUPPLIED: Cap: 250mg; Inj: 100mg/mL
THERAPEUTIC CLASS: Bacteriostatic antibiotic
INDICATION: Treatment of Q fever.
DOSAGE: *Adults:* 50-100mg/kg/day divided every 6 hours.
Pediatrics: 50-75mg/kg/day divided every 6 hours.
CONTRAINDICATIONS: Hypersensitivity to chloramphenicol; pregnancy, especially near term and during labor. Avoid with other drugs that may depress bone marrow.
WARNINGS/PRECAUTIONS: Caution in patients with intermittent porphyria; G6PD deficiency; premature and full-term infants.
PREGNANCY: Category D, not for use in nursing.
INTERACTIONS: Decreased liver breakdown and increased effect of anticoagulants, barbiturates, tacrolimus, phenytoin, and oral antidiabetic agents with concomitant use. Acetaminophen increases serum levels of chloramphenicol; rifampin decreases chloramphenicol effect.
ADVERSE REACTIONS: Nausea, vomiting, diarrhea, headache, glossitis, stomatitis.

DOXYCYCLINE
Doryx *(Warner Chilcott)*, Monodox *(Watson)*, Vibramycin *(Pfizer)*

HOW SUPPLIED: Doryx: Cap, Delayed-Release: (doxycycline hyclate) 75mg, 100mg. Monodox: Cap: (doxycycline monohydrate) 50mg, 100mg. Vibramycin: Cap: (doxycycline hyclate) 50mg, 100mg; Inj: (vial) 100mg, 200mg; Syrup: (doxycycline calcium) 50mg/5mL [473mL]; Sus: (doxycycline monohydrate) 25mg/5mL [60mL]; Tab: (Vibra-Tabs) 100mg
THERAPEUTIC CLASS: Tetracycline derivative
INDICATION: Rocky Mountain spotted fever, typhus fever, and typhus group, Q fever, rickettsialpox, and tick fevers caused by Rickettsiae.
DOSAGE: *Adults:* 100mg bid for 2-3 weeks.
Pediatrics: >8 yrs: <100lbs: 1mg/lb bid day 1. Maint: 1mg/lb/day as single dose or divided bid. Severe Infection: Maint: 2mg/lb/day. ≥100lbs: 100mg bid for 60 days. Initial: 200mg day 1. Maint: 100mg/day as single dose or 50mg q12h. Severe Infection: Maint: 100mg q12h.
CONTRAINDICATIONS: Hypersensitivity to any of the tetracyclines.
WARNINGS/PRECAUTIONS: May cause fetal harm during pregnancy. Use during tooth development (last half of pregnancy, infancy, <8 yrs) may

cause permanent discoloration of the teeth or enamel hypoplasia. Photosensitivity, increased BUN, superinfection may occur. Monitor hematopoietic, renal, and hepatic values periodically with long term therapy. Bulging fontanels in infants and benign intracranial HTN in adults reported. May decrease bone growth in premature infants.
PREGNANCY: Category D, not for use in nursing.
INTERACTIONS: May require downward adjustments of anticoagulant dosage. May interfere with bactericidal action of penicillin; avoid concurrent use when possible. Avoid antacids containing aluminum, calcium, or magnesium, sodium bicarbonate, and iron-containing preparations.
ADVERSE REACTIONS: Anorexia, nausea, vomiting, diarrhea, dysphagia, enterocolitis, rash, exfoliative dermatitis, renal toxicity, hypersensitivity reactions, blood dyscrasias.

MINOCYCLINE
Dynacin *(Par)*, Minocin *(Lederle)*

HOW SUPPLIED: Dynacin: Cap: 50mg, 75mg, 100mg; Tab: 50mg, 75mg, 100mg. Minocin: Cap: 50mg, 100mg
THERAPEUTIC CLASS: Tetracycline derivative
INDICATION: Rocky Mountain spotted fever, typhus fever, and typhus group, Q fever, rickettsialpox, and tick fevers caused by Rickettsiae.
DOSAGE: *Usual:* 200mg initially, then 100mg q12h; alternative is 100-200mg initially, then 50mg qid.
Pediatrics: >8 yrs: 4mg/kg initially followed by 2mg/kg q12h. Take with plenty of fluids.
CONTRAINDICATIONS: Hypersensitivity to any of the tetracyclines.
WARNINGS/PRECAUTIONS: May cause fetal harm during pregnancy. Use during tooth development (last half of pregnancy, infancy, <8 yrs) may cause permanent discoloration of the teeth or enamel hypoplasia; avoid use during this period. Renal toxicity, hepatotoxicity, photosensitivity, increased BUN, superinfection, pseudotumor cerebri may occur; perform hematopoietic, renal, and hepatic monitoring. May impair mental/physical abilities. Use alternate form of contraception other than oral contraceptives. May decrease bone growth in premature infants.
PREGNANCY: Category D, not for use in nursing.
INTERACTIONS: May require downward adjustments of anticoagulant dosage. May interfere with bactericidal action of penicillin; avoid concurrent use when possible. May decrease efficacy of oral contraceptives. Impaired absorption with antacids containing aluminum, calcium, or magnesium and iron-containing products. Fatal renal toxicity with methoxyflurane has been reported.
ADVERSE REACTIONS: Anorexia, nausea, vomiting, diarrhea, dysphagia, enterocolitis, pancreatitis, increased LFTs, hepatitis, liver failure, renal toxicity, rash, exfoliative dermatitis, Stevens-Johnson syndrome, skin and mucous membrane pigmentation, blood dyscrasias, headache, tooth discoloration.

TETRACYCLINE
Sumycin *(Par)*

HOW SUPPLIED: Sus: 125mg/5mL [473mL]; Tab: 250mg, 500mg
THERAPEUTIC CLASS: Streptomyces aureofaciens derivative
INDICATION: Treatment of Q Fever due to *Coxiella burnetii.*
DOSAGE: *Adults:* 500mg qid for 2-3 weeks.
Pediatrics: >8 yrs: Usual: 25mg/kg/day in divided doses for 2-3 weeks. Renal Dysfunction: Reduce dose or extend dose interval.
CONTRAINDICATIONS: Hypersensitivity to any of the tetracyclines.
WARNINGS/PRECAUTIONS: May cause fetal harm with pregnancy, permanent tooth discoloration during tooth development (last half of pregnancy and children <8 yrs). May increase BUN. Photosensitivity, enamel hypoplasia reported. Superinfection with prolonged use. Suspension contains sodium metabisulfite. Bulging fontanels in infants and benign intracranial HTN in adults reported. Monitor renal/hepatic and hematopoietic function with long-term use. Caution with history of asthma, hay fever, urticaria, and allergy.
PREGNANCY: Category D, not for use in nursing.
INTERACTIONS: May decrease PT; adjust anticoagulants. May interfere with bactericidal agents (eg, penicillin). May decrease effects of oral contraceptives. Take 1 hr before or 2 hrs after dairy products. Aluminum-, calcium-, iron- and magnesium-containing products impair absorption. Fatal renal toxicity reported with concurrent methoxyflurane.

RADIATION EXPOSURE TREATMENT

PENTETATE CALCIUM TRISODIUM
Pentetate Calcium Trisodium *(Akorn)*

HOW SUPPLIED: Inj: 200mg/mL
THERAPEUTIC CLASS: Chelating agent
INDICATION: Treatment of individuals with known or suspected internal contamination with plutonium, americium, or curium to increase the rate of elimination.

† Not FDA-approved for this indication.

DOSAGE: *Adults:* Initial: 1g IV. Maint: 1g IV qd. Most effective if given within first 24 hrs. Preferable to switch to pentetate zinc trisodium for maintenance therapy due to safety concerns.
Pediatrics: ≥12 yrs: 1g IV. Maint: 1g IV qd. ≤12 yrs: 14mg/kg IV. Maint: 14mg/kg IV qd. Max: 1g. Most effective if given within first 24 hrs. Preferable to switch to pentetate zinc trisodium for maintenance therapy due to safety concerns.
CONTRAINDICATIONS: None known.
WARNINGS/PRECAUTIONS: Depletion of endogenous trace metals. Caution in severe hemochromatosis, reports of death. Exacerbation of asthma when administered nebulized.
PREGNANCY: Category C, not for use in nursing.
ADVERSE REACTIONS: Headache, lightheadedness, chest pain, allergic reaction, dermatitis, metallic taste, nausea, diarrhea, injection site reactions.

PENTETATE ZINC TRISODIUM
Pentetate Zinc Trisodium *(Akorn)*
HOW SUPPLIED: Inj: 200mg/mL
THERAPEUTIC CLASS: Chelating agent
INDICATION: Treatment of individuals with known or suspected internal contamination with plutonium, americium, or curium to increase the rate of elimination.
DOSAGE: *Adults:* Initial: 1g IV. Maint: 1g IV qd. Most effective if given within first 24 hrs.
Pediatrics: ≥12 yrs: 1g IV. Maint: 1g IV qd. ≤12 yrs: 14mg/kg IV. Maint: 14mg/kg IV qd. Max: 1g. Most effective if given within first 24 hrs.
CONTRAINDICATIONS: None known.
WARNINGS/PRECAUTIONS: Depletion of endogenous trace metals. Caution in severe hemochromatosis, reports of death. Exacerbation of asthma when administered nebulized.
PREGNANCY: Category C, not for use in nursing.
ADVERSE REACTIONS: Headache, lightheadedness, chest pain, allergic reaction, dermatitis, metallic taste, nausea, diarrhea, injection site reactions.

POTASSIUM IODIDE
Potassium Iodide *(Various)*
HOW SUPPLIED: Sol: 1 g/mL; Syrup: 325 mg/5mL; Tab: 65mg, 30mg
THERAPEUTIC CLASS: Antithyroid agent
INDICATION: Treatment of irradiation hypothyroidism.
DOSAGE: *Adults:* 18-40 yrs: 130mg/day po when estimated exposure is 10 cGy or greater. >40 yrs: 130mg/day po when estimated exposure is 500 cGy or greater. Pregnant/Lactating: 130mg/day po when estimated exposure is 5 cGy. Therapy should be started prior to or as soon as possible after radioiodine exposure, preferably within 3-4 hr, and continued for 10 days after exposure has stopped.
Pediatrics: 3-18 yrs: 65mg/day po when estimated exposure is 5 cGy or greater. 1 month-3 yrs: 32mg/day po when estimated exposure is 5 cGy or greater. Birth-1 month: 16mg/day po when estimated exposure is 5 cGy or greater. Therapy should be started prior to or as soon as possible after radioiodine exposure, preferably within 3-4 hr, and continued for 10 days after exposure has stopped.
CONTRAINDICATIONS: Renal disorders, iodine-induced goiter.
WARNINGS/PRECAUTIONS: Caution in acute bronchitis, Addison's disease, dehydration, goiter, autoimmune thyroid disease, hyperthyroidism, tuberculosis, pregnancy, and lactation.
DRUG INTERACTIONS: Increased hypothyroid effect with lithium. Decreased anticoagulant effectiveness with warfarin
ADVERSE REACTIONS: Rash, GI irritation, paresthesia, goiter, hypothyroidism.

SALMONELLA TREATMENT

CEFTRIAXONE
Rocephin *(Roche)*
HOW SUPPLIED: Inj: 250mg, 500mg, 1g, 2g, 10g
THERAPEUTIC CLASS: Cephalosporin (3rd generation)
INDICATION: Treatment of *Salmonella* species.[†]
DOSAGE: *Adults:* Usual: 1-2g/day IV/IM given qd-bid. Max: 4g/day.[†]
Pediatrics: 50-75mg/kg/day IM/IV given q12h. Max: 2g/day.[†]
WARNINGS/PRECAUTIONS: Cross sensitivity to penicillins and other cephalosporins may occur. Pseudomembranous colitis reported. May result in overgrowth of nonsusceptible organisms. Altered PT, transient BUN and serum creatinine elevations may occur. Do not exceed 2g/day and monitor blood levels with both hepatic and renal dysfunction. Caution with history of GI disease. Discontinue if develop gallbladder disease. May alter PT; monitor with impaired vitamin K synthesis or low vitamin K stores. Avoid in hyperbilirubinemic neonates, especially prematures.
PREGNANCY: Category B, caution in nursing.

ADVERSE REACTIONS: Injection site reactions, eosinophilia, thrombocytosis, diarrhea, SGOT and SGPT elevations.

CIPROFLOXACIN
Cipro *(Schering/Bayer)*
HOW SUPPLIED: Inj: (vial) 200mg/20mL, 400mg/40mL, (flexible container) 200mg/100mL, 400mg/200mL; Sus: 250mg/5mL, 500mg/5mL [100mL]; Tab: 250mg, 500mg, 750mg
THERAPEUTIC CLASS: Fluoroquinolone
INDICATION: Treatment of *Salmonella typhi*.
DOSAGE: *Adults:* 500mg po q12h for 10 days.
CONTRAINDICATIONS: History of hypersensitivity to ciprofloxacin or any member of the quinolone class of antimicrobial agents.
WARNINGS/PRECAUTIONS: Convulsions, increased intracranial pressure and toxic psychosis reported. Caution with CNS disorders or if predisposed to seizures. Severe, fatal hypersensitivity reactions may occur. Pseudomembranous colitis, achilles and other tendon ruptures reported. Discontinue at first sign of rash or if pain, inflammation, or ruptured tendon occurs. Maintain hydration; avoid alkaline urine. Avoid excessive sunlight and UV light. Do not give via feeding tube. Monitor renal, hepatic, and hematopoietic function with prolonged use. Dose adjustment with renal dysfunction.
PREGNANCY: Category C, not for use in nursing.
INTERACTIONS: Increases theophylline and caffeine levels and prolongs effects. Fatal reactions have occurred with theophylline. Magnesium or aluminum containing antacids, sucralfate, Videx® (didanosine) chewable/buffered tablets or pediatric powder, and products containing calcium, iron, or zinc decrease serum and urine levels; space doses at least 2 hrs before or 6 hrs after administration. Altered serum levels of phenytoin. Severe hypoglycemia with glyburide (rare). Potentiated by probenecid. Transient serum creatinine elevations with cyclosporine. Enhances oral anticoagulant effects. Monitor PT. Caution with drugs that lower seizure threshold.
ADVERSE REACTIONS: Nausea, dizziness, headache, CNS disturbances, vomiting, diarrhea, rash, abdominal pain/discomfort.

TRIMETHOPRIM-SULFAMETHOXAZOLE
Bactrim *(Women First)*, Septra *(King)*, Sulfatrim Pediatric *(Alpharma)*
HOW SUPPLIED: Bactrim: (Sulfamethoxazole [SMX]-Trimethoprim [TMP]) Tab: 400mg-80mg*; Tab, DS: 800mg-160mg*. Septra: (Sulfamethoxazole [SMX]-Trimethoprim [TMP]) Inj: (Septra) 80mg-16mg/mL; Sus: (Sulfatrim Pediatric, Septra) 200mg-40mg/5mL [100mL, 473mL]; Tab: (Septra) 400mg-80mg*; Tab, DS: (Septra) 800mg-160mg* *scored
THERAPEUTIC CLASS: Sulfonamide/tetrahydrofolic acid inhibitor
INDICATION: Treatment of *Salmonella species*.[†]
DOSAGE: *Adults:* 800mg-160mg PO q12h for 5-7 days.[†]
CONTRAINDICATIONS: Megaloblastic anemia due to folate deficiency, pregnancy at term, nursing, infants <2 months old.
WARNINGS/PRECAUTIONS: Fatal hypersensitivity reactions (eg, Stevens-Johnson syndrome, toxic epidermal necrolysis, fulminant hepatic necrosis, agranulocytosis, aplastic anemia) may occur. Pseudomembranous colitis, cough, SOB, and pulmonary infiltrates reported. Avoid with group A beta-hemolytic streptococcal infections. Caution with hepatic/renal impairment, elderly, folate deficiency (eg, chronic alcoholics, anticonvulsants, malabsorption, malnutrition), bronchial asthma, and other allergies. In G6PD deficiency, hemolysis may occur. Increased incidence of adverse events in AIDS patients. Maintain adequate fluid intake.
PREGNANCY: Category C, contraindicated in nursing.
INTERACTIONS: Increase risk of thrombocytopenia with purpura with diuretics (especially thiazides) in the elderly. Caution with warfarin; may prolong PT. Increased effects of phenytoin, methotrexate.
ADVERSE REACTIONS: Anorexia, nausea, vomiting, rash, urticaria, cholestatic jaundice, agranulocytosis, anemia, hyperkalemia, renal failure, interstitial nephritis, hyponatremia, convulsions, arthralgia, myalgia, weakness.

SARIN TREATMENT

ATROPINE
Atropine Sulfate *(Various)*
HOW SUPPLIED: Inj: 0.05mg/mL, 0.1mg/mL, 0.4mg/mL, 0.5mg/mL, 1mg/mL
THERAPEUTIC CLASS: Anticholinergic
INDICATION: Indicated as an antisialagogue for preanesthetic medication to prevent or reduce secretions of the respiratory tract, to restore cardiac rate and arterial pressure during anesthesia when vagal stimulation produced by intra-abdominal surgical traction causes a sudden decrease in pulse rate and cardiac action, to lessen degree of AV heart block when increased vagal tone is a major factor in the conduction defect (possibly due to digitalis), to overcome severe bradycardia and syncope due to hyperactive carotid sinus reflex, as an antidote (with external cardiac massage) for cardiovascular collapse from the injudicious

use of choline ester (cholinergic) drug, in treatment of anticholinesterase poisoning from organophosphorus insecticides, and as an antidote for the "rapid" type of mushroom poisoning due to presence of the alkaloid muscarine, in certain species of fungus such as *Amanita muscaria*.

DOSAGE: *Adults:* Usual: 0.5mg IM/IV/SC. Range: 0.4-0.6mg. If used as an antisialogogue, inject IM prior to anesthesia induction. Bradyarrhythmias: 0.4-1mg every 1-2 hrs prn. Max: 2mg/dose. May be used as an antidote for cardiovascular collapse resulting from injudicious administration of choline ester. When cardiac arrest has occurred Anticholinesterase Poisoning From Insecticide Poisoning: 2-3mg IV. Repeat until signs of atropine intoxication appear. Mushroom Poisoning: Administer sufficient doses to control parasympathomimetic signs before coma and cardiovascular collase supervene. Sarin Poisoning: 6mg may be required initially.[†] *Pediatrics:* Doses range from 0.6mg in >12 yrs and 0.1mg in newborns. Inject SC 30 minutes before surgery. Bradyarrhythmias: 0.01-0.03mg/kg IV. Sarin Poisoning: 0.01-0.02 mg/kg IV or IM.[†]
CONTRAINDICATIONS: Glaucoma, pyloric stenosis, or prostatic hypertrophy except in doses used for preanesthetic medication.
WARNINGS/PRECAUTIONS: Avoid overdose in IV administration. Increased susceptibility to toxic effects in children. Caution in patients >40 yrs. Conventional doses may precipitate glaucoma in susceptible patients, convert partial organic pyloric stenosis into complete obstruction, lead to complete urinary retention in patients with prostatic hypertrophy or cause inspissation of bronchial secretions and formation of dangerous viscid plugs in patients with chronic lung disease.
PREGNANCY: Category C, safety in nursing not known.
ADVERSE REACTIONS: Dryness of the mouth, blurred vision, photophobia, tachycardia, anhidrosis.

PRALIDOXIME
Protopam *(Baxter)*
HOW SUPPLIED: Inj: 1g
THERAPEUTIC CLASS: Nerve gas antidote
INDICATION: Used together with atropine to treat poisoning caused by organophosphates and to treat anticholinesterase overdose.
DOSAGE: *Adults:* Anticholinesterase Overdose: Initial: 1-2g IV. Maint: 250mg IV every 5 minutes. Organophosphate Poisoning: Initial: 1-2g in 100mL NS infused over 15-30 minutes or 5% solution in SWFI over not less than 5 minutes. Repeat 1-2g in 1 hour if muscle weakness persists. *Pediatrics:* Organophosphate Poisoning (Mild). 1-2 g PO, may repeat in 3 hrs if necessary. Organophosphate Poisoning (Moderate to Severe): Intermittent: 25-50mg/kg IV; may repeat in 1-2 hrs, then at 10-12 hr intervals if necessary. Continuous: 25mg/kg IV single dose, then begin infusion at 10-20mg/kg/hr.[†]
WARNINGS/PRECAUTIONS: Caution in myasthenia gravis, may precipitate myasthenic crisis. Not effective in poisonings due to organophosphates without anticholinesterase activity or due to phosphorus/inorganic phosphates. Caution in renal impairment. Slow IV infusion prevents tachycardia, laryngospasm, and muscle rigidity.
PREGNANCY: Unkown.
ADVERSE REACTIONS: Blurred vision, double vision, difficulty in speaking, difficult or rapid breathing, dizziness, fast heartbeat, drowsiness, headache, nausea, muscle stiffness/weakness, injection site pain, difficulty in focusing of eyes.

SHIGELLA TREATMENT

CIPROFLOXACIN
Cipro *(Schering/Bayer)*
HOW SUPPLIED: Inj: (vial) 200mg/20mL, 400mg/40mL, (flexible container) 200mg/100mL, 400mg/200mL; Sus: 250mg/5mL, 500mg/5mL [100mL]; Tab: 250mg, 500mg, 750mg
THERAPEUTIC CLASS: Fluoroquinolone
INDICATION: Treatment of *Shigella boydii, Shigella dysenteriae, Shigella flexneri*, and *Shigella sonnei*.
DOSAGE: *Adults:* 500mg po q12h for 5 to 7 days.
CONTRAINDICATIONS: History of hypersensitivity to ciprofloxacin or any member of the quinolone class of antimicrobial agents.
WARNINGS/PRECAUTIONS: Convulsions, increased intracranial pressure and toxic psychosis reported. Caution with CNS disorders or if predisposed to seizures. Severe, fatal hypersensitivity reactions may occur. Pseudomembranous colitis, achilles and other tendon ruptures reported. Discontinue at first sign of rash or if pain, inflammation, or ruptured tendon occurs. Maintain hydration; avoid alkaline urine. Avoid excessive sunlight and UV light. Do not give via feeding tube. Monitor renal, hepatic, and hematopoietic function with prolonged use. Dose adjustment with renal dysfunction.
PREGNANCY: Category C, not for use in nursing.

INTERACTIONS: Increases theophylline and caffeine levels and prolongs effects. Fatal reactions have occurred with theophylline. Magnesium or aluminum containing antacids, sucralfate, Videx® (didanosine) chewable/buffered tablets or pediatric powder, and products containing calcium, iron, or zinc decrease serum and urine levels; space doses at least 2 hrs before or 6 hrs after administration. Altered serum levels of phenytoin. Severe hypoglycemia with glyburide (rare). Potentiated by probenecid. Transient serum creatinine elevations with cyclosporine. Enhances oral anticoagulant effects. Monitor PT. Caution with drugs that lower seizure threshold.
ADVERSE REACTIONS: Nausea, dizziness, headache, CNS disturbances, vomiting, diarrhea, rash, abdominal pain/discomfort.

DOXYCYCLINE
Doryx *(Warner Chilcott)*, Monodox *(Watson)*, Vibramycin *(Pfizer)*
HOW SUPPLIED: Doryx: Cap, Delayed-Release: (doxycycline hyclate) 75mg, 100mg. Monodox: Cap: (doxycycline monohydrate) 50mg, 100mg. Vibramycin: Cap: (doxycycline hyclate) 50mg, 100mg; Inj: (vial) 100mg, 200mg; Syrup: (doxycycline calcium) 50mg/5mL [473mL]; Sus: (doxycycline monohydrate) 25mg/5mL [60mL]; Tab: (Vibra-Tabs) 100mg
THERAPEUTIC CLASS: Tetracycline derivative
INDICATION: Treatment of *Shigella* species.
DOSAGE: *Adults:* Usual: 100mg q12h on day 1, then 100mg qd or 50mg q12h. Severe Infection: 100mg q12h.
Pediatrics: >8 yrs: ≤100lbs: 1mg/lb bid on day 1, then 1mg/lb qd or 0.5mg/lb bid. Severe Infections: Maint: 2mg/lb. >100lbs: Usual: 100mg q12h on day 1, then 100mg qd or 50mg q12h. Severe Infection: 100mg q12h.
CONTRAINDICATIONS: Hypersensitivity to any of the tetracyclines.
WARNINGS/PRECAUTIONS: May cause fetal harm during pregnancy. Use during tooth development (last half of pregnancy, infancy, <8 yrs) may cause permanent discoloration of the teeth and enamel hypoplasia. Photosensitivity, increased BUN, superinfection may occur. Monitor hematopoietic, renal and hepatic values periodically with long term therapy. Bulging fontanels in infants and benign intracranial HTN in adults reported. May decrease bone growth in premature infants.
PREGNANCY: Category D, not for use in nursing.
INTERACTIONS: May require downward adjustments of anticoagulant dosage. May interfere with bactericidal action of penicillin; avoid concurrent use when possible. Avoid antacids containing aluminum, calcium, or magnesium, sodium bicarbonate, and iron-containing preparations.
ADVERSE REACTIONS: Anorexia, nausea, vomiting, diarrhea, dysphagia, enterocolitis, rash, exfoliative dermatitis, renal toxicity, hypersensitivity reactions, blood dyscrasias.

TRIMETHOPRIM-SULFAMETHOXAZOLE
Bactrim *(Women First)*, Septra *(King)*, Sulfatrim Pediatric *(Alpharma)*
HOW SUPPLIED: Bactrim: (Sulfamethoxazole [SMX]-Trimethoprim [TMP]) Tab: 400mg-80mg*; Tab, DS: 800mg-160mg*. Septra: (Sulfamethoxazole [SMX]-Trimethoprim [TMP]) Inj: (Septra) 80mg-16mg/mL; Sus: (Sulfatrim Pediatric, Septra) 200mg-40mg/5mL [100mL, 473mL]; Tab: (Septra) 400mg-80mg*; Tab, DS: (Septra) 800mg-160mg* *scored
THERAPEUTIC CLASS: Sulfonamide/tetrahydrofolic acid inhibitor
INDICATION: Treatment of enteritis caused by susceptible strains of *Shigella flexneri* and *Shigella sonnei*.
DOSAGE: *Adults:* 800mg-160mg PO q12h for 5 days.
Pediatrics: 4mg/kg TMP and 20mg/kg SMX q12h for 5 days.
CONTRAINDICATIONS: Megaloblastic anemia due to folate deficiency, pregnancy at term, nursing, infants <2 months old.
WARNINGS/PRECAUTIONS: Fatal hypersensitivity reactions (eg, Stevens-Johnson syndrome, toxic epidermal necrolysis, fulminant hepatic necrosis, agranulocytosis, aplastic anemia) may occur. Pseudomembranous colitis, cough, SOB, and pulmonary infiltrates reported. Avoid with group A beta-hemolytic streptococcal infections. Caution with hepatic/renal impairment, elderly, folate deficiency (eg, chronic alcoholics, anticonvulsants, malabsorption, malnutrition), bronchial asthma, and other allergies. In G6PD deficiency, hemolysis may occur. Increased incidence of adverse events in AIDS patients. Maintain adequate fluid intake.
PREGNANCY: Category C, contraindicated in nursing.
INTERACTIONS: Increase risk of thrombocytopenia with purpura with diuretics (especially thiazides) in the elderly. Caution with warfarin; may prolong PT. Increased effects of phenytoin, methotrexate.
ADVERSE REACTIONS: Anorexia, nausea, vomiting, rash, urticaria, cholestatic jaundice, agranulocytosis, anemia, hyperkalemia, renal failure, interstitial nephritis, hyponatremia, convulsions, arthralgia, myalgia, weakness.

SMALLPOX TREATMENT

SMALLPOX VACCINE, DRIED
Dryvax *(Wyeth)*

HOW SUPPLIED: Inj: 100 million PFU
THERAPEUTIC CLASS: Vaccine
INDICATION: For active immunization against smallpox disease.
DOSAGE: *Adults/Pediatrics:* >12 months: Give IM into deltoid muscle or posterior aspect of arm over triceps muscle. Use 2 or 3 needle punctures for primary vaccination and 15 punctures for revaccination. May cover vaccination site with a porous bandage, until scab separates and underlying skin has healed. Inspect vaccination site 6-8 days later to interpret response.
CONTRAINDICATIONS: (Routine non-emergency use) Hypersensitivity to polymyxin B sulfate, dihydrostreptomycin sulfate, chlortetracycline HCl, and neomycin sulfate; infants <12 months of age; eczema, history of eczema, or other acute, chronic, or exfoliative skin conditions (including household contacts of such persons); systemic corticosteroid use at doses ≥2mg/kg or ≥20mg/day of prednisone for ≥2 weeks, or immunosuppressive use (eg, alkylating agents, antimetabolites), or radiation (including household contacts of such persons); congenital or acquired immune deficiencies (including household contacts of such persons); immunosuppressed individuals (including household contacts of such persons); pregnancy (including household contacts of such persons).
WARNINGS/PRECAUTIONS: Vial stopper contains dry natural rubber; caution with latex sensitivity. Patients susceptible to adverse effects of caccinia virus should avoid contact with persons with active vaccination lesions. Vaccinia virus may be cultured from site of primary vaccine from time of papule development until scab separates from skin lesion. Not recommended for elderly in non-emergency conditions.
PREGNANCY: Category C, not for use in nursing in non-emergency conditions.
INTERACTIONS: Avoid salves or ointments on vaccination site.
ADVERSE REACTIONS: Fever, rash, secondary pyogenic infections at vaccination site, inadvertent inoculation at other sites, regional lymphadenopathy, malaise.

TABUN TREATMENT

ATROPINE
Atropine Sulfate *(Various)*

HOW SUPPLIED: Inj: 0.05mg/mL, 0.1mg/mL, 0.4mg/mL, 0.5mg/mL, 1mg/mL
THERAPEUTIC CLASS: Anticholinergic
INDICATION: Indicated as an antisialagogue for preanesthetic medication to prevent or reduce secretions of the respiratory tract, to restore cardiac rate and arterial pressure during anesthesia when vagal stimulation produced by intra-abdominal surgical traction causes a sudden decrease in pulse rate and cardiac action, to lessen degree of AV heart block when increased vagal tone is a major factor in the conduction defect (possibly due to digitalis), to overcome severe bradycardia and syncope due to hyperactive carotid sinus reflex, as an antidote (with external cardiac massage) for cardiovascular collapse from the injudicious use of choline ester (cholinergic) drug, in treatment of anticholinesterase poisoning from organophosphorus insecticides, and as an antidote for the "rapid" type of mushroom poisoning due to presence of the alkaloid muscarine, in certain species of fungus such as *Amanita muscaria.*
DOSAGE: *Adults:* Usual: 0.5mg IM/IV/SC. Range: 0.4-0.6mg. If used as an antisialogogue, inject IM prior to anesthesia induction. Bradyarrhythmias: 0.4-1mg every 1-2 hrs prn. Max: 2mg/dose. May be used as an antidote for cardiovascular collapse resulting from injudicious administration of choline ester. When cardiac arrest has occurred Anticholinesterase Poisoning From Insecticide Poisoning: 2-3mg IV. Repeat until signs of atropine intoxication appear. Mushroom Poisoning: Administer sufficient doses to control parasympathomimetic signs before coma and cardiovascular collase supervene. Tabun Poisoning: 6mg may be required initially.†
Pediatrics: Doses range from 0.6mg in >12 yrs and 0.1mg in newborns. Inject SC 30 minutes before surgery. Bradyarrhythmias: 0.01-0.03mg/kg IV. Tabun Poisoning: 0.01-0.02 mg/kg IV or IM.†
CONTRAINDICATIONS: Glaucoma, pyloric stenosis, or prostatic hypertrophy except in doses used for preanesthetic medication.
WARNINGS/PRECAUTIONS: Avoid overdose in IV administration. Increased susceptibility to toxic effects in children. Caution in patients >40 yrs. Conventional doses may precipitate glaucoma in susceptible patients, convert partial organic pyloric stenosis into complete obstruction, lead to complete urinary retention in patients with prostatic hypertrophy or cause inspissation of bronchial secretions and formation of dangerous viscid plugs in patients with chronic lung disease.
PREGNANCY: Category C, safety in nursing not known.
ADVERSE REACTIONS: Dryness of the mouth, blurred vision, photophobia, tachycardia, anhidrosis.

PRALIDOXIME
Protopam *(Baxter)*

HOW SUPPLIED: Inj: 1g
THERAPEUTIC CLASS: Nerve gas antidote
INDICATION: Used together with atropine to treat poisoning caused by organophosphates and to treat anticholinesterase overdose.
DOSAGE: *Adults:* Anticholinesterase Overdose: Initial: 1-2g IV. Maint: 250mg IV every 5 minutes. Organophosphate Poisoning: Initial: 1-2g in 100mL NS infused over 15-30 minutes or 5% solution in SWFI over not less than 5 minutes. Repeat 1-2g in 1 hour if muscle weakness persists.
Pediatrics: Organophosphate Poisoning (Mild). 1-2 g PO, may repeat in 3 hrs if necessary. Organophosphate Poisoning (Moderate to Severe): Intermittent: 25-50mg/kg IV; may repeat in 1-2 hrs, then at 10-12 hr intervals if necessary. Continuous: 25mg/kg IV single dose, then begin infusion at 10-20mg/kg/hr.†
WARNINGS/PRECAUTIONS: Caution in myasthenia gravis, may precipitate myasthenic crisis. Not effective in poisonings due to organophosphates without anticholinesterase activity or due to phosphorus/inorganic phosphates. Caution in renal impairment. Slow IV infusion prevents tachycardia, laryngospasm, and muscle rigidity.
PREGNANCY: Unkown.
ADVERSE REACTIONS: Blurred vision, double vision, difficulty in speaking, difficult or rapid breathing, dizziness, fast heartbeat, drowsiness, headache, nausea, muscle stiffness/weakness, injection site pain, difficulty in focusing of eyes.

TULAREMIA TREATMENT

CHLORAMPHENICOL
Chloramphenicol *(Various)*

Aplastic anemia, hypoplastic anemia, thrombocytopenia, and granulocytopenia may occur. Also reported is aplastic anemia terminating in leukemia. Blood dyscrasias occurred after both short-term and prolonged therapy. Do not use when less potentially dangerous drugs are effective. Not to be used for trivial infections, prophylaxis of bacterial infections, or to treat colds, flu, or throat infections. Perform adequate blood studies during treatment.

HOW SUPPLIED: Cap: 250mg; Inj: 100mg/mL
THERAPEUTIC CLASS: Bacteriostatic antibiotic
INDICATION: Alternative treatment of tularemia.†
DOSAGE: *Adults:* 15mg/kg IV qid for 14 days.†
Pediatrics: 15mg/kg IV qid for 14 days.†
CONTRAINDICATIONS: Hypersensitivity to chloramphenicol; pregnancy, especially near term and during labor. Avoid with other drugs that may depress bone marrow.
WARNINGS/PRECAUTIONS: Caution in patients with intermittent porphyria; G6PD deficiency; premature and full-term infants.
PREGNANCY: Category D, not for use in nursing.
INTERACTIONS: Decreased liver breakdown and increased effect of anticoagulants, barbiturates, tacrolimus, phenytoin, and oral antidiabetic agents with concomitant use. Acetaminophen increases serum levels of chloramphenicol; rifampin decreases chloramphenicol effect.
ADVERSE REACTIONS: Nausea, vomiting, diarrhea, headache, glossitis, stomatitis.

CIPROFLOXACIN
Cipro *(Schering/Bayer)*

HOW SUPPLIED: Inj: (vial) 200mg/20mL, 400mg/40mL, (flexible container) 200mg/100mL, 400mg/200mL; Sus: 250mg/5mL, 500mg/5mL [100mL]; Tab: 250mg, 500mg, 750mg
THERAPEUTIC CLASS: Fluoroquinolone
INDICATION: Preferred treatment choice of both adults and children in mass casualty.† Preferred choice postexposure prophylaxis in mass casualty setting.†
DOSAGE: *Adults:* Treatment: 400mg IV bid for 10 days. Postexposure Prophylaxis: 500mg PO bid for 14 days; for pregnant women 100mg PO bid for 14 days.†
Pediatrics: Treatment: 15mg/kg IV bid for 10 days. Postexposure Prophylaxis: 15mg/kg PO bid for 14 days†. Administer at least 2 hrs before or 6 hrs after magnesium or aluminum containing antacids, sucralfate, Videx® (didanosine) chewable/buffered tablets or pediatric powder, or other products containing calcium, iron, or zinc.
CONTRAINDICATIONS: History of hypersensitivity to ciprofloxacin or any member of the quinolone class of antimicrobial agents.
WARNINGS/PRECAUTIONS: Convulsions, increased intracranial pressure and toxic psychosis reported. Caution with CNS disorders or if predisposed to

seizures. Severe, fatal hypersensitivity reactions may occur. Pseudomembranous colitis, achilles and other tendon ruptures reported. Discontinue at first sign of rash or if pain, inflammation, or ruptured tendon occurs. Maintain hydration; avoid alkaline urine. Avoid excessive sunlight and UV light. Do not give via feeding tube. Monitor renal, hepatic, and hematopoietic function with prolonged use. Dose adjustment with renal dysfunction.
PREGNANCY: Category C, not for use in nursing.
INTERACTIONS: Increases theophylline and caffeine levels and prolongs effects. Fatal reactions have occurred with theophylline. Magnesium or aluminum containing antacids, sucralfate, Videx® (didanosine) chewable/buffered tablets or pediatric powder, and products containing calcium, iron, or zinc decrease serum and urine levels; space doses at least 2 hrs before or 6 hrs after administration. Altered serum levels of phenytoin. Severe hypoglycemia with glyburide (rare). Potentiated by probenecid. Transient serum creatinine elevations with cyclosporine. Enhances oral anticoagulant effects. Monitor PT. Caution with drugs that lower seizure threshold.
ADVERSE REACTIONS: Nausea, dizziness, headache, CNS disturbances, vomiting, diarrhea, rash, abdominal pain/discomfort.

DOXYCYCLINE

Doryx *(Warner Chilcott)*, Monodox *(Watson)*, Vibramycin *(Pfizer)*
HOW SUPPLIED: Doryx: Cap, Delayed-Release: (doxycycline hyclate) 75mg, 100mg. Monodox: Cap: (doxycycline monohydrate) 50mg, 100mg. Vibramycin: Cap: (doxycycline hyclate) 50mg, 100mg; Inj: (vial) 100mg, 200mg; Syrup: (doxycycline calcium) 50mg/5mL [473mL]; Sus: (doxycycline monohydrate) 25mg/5mL [60mL]; Tab: (Vibra-Tabs) 100mg
THERAPEUTIC CLASS: Tetracycline derivative
INDICATION: Treatment of Tularemia due to *Francisella tularensis.*
DOSAGE: *Adults:* Treatment: 100mg IV bid for 14 to 21 days. Postexposure Prophylaxis: 100mg PO bid for 14 days.
Pediatrics: >45kg: 100mg IV bid for 14 to 21 days. <45kg: 2.2mg/kg IV bid for 14 to 21 days. Postexposure Prophylaxis: PO bid for 14 days. <45kg: 2.2mg/kg PO bid for 14 to 21 days.
CONTRAINDICATIONS: Hypersensitivity to any of the tetracyclines.
WARNINGS/PRECAUTIONS: May cause fetal harm during pregnancy. Use during tooth development (last half of pregnancy, infancy, <8 yrs) may cause permanent discoloration of the teeth or enamel hypoplasia. Photosensitivity, increased BUN, superinfection may occur. Monitor hematopoietic, renal and hepatic values periodically with long term therapy. Bulging fontanels in infants and benign intracranial HTN in adults reported. May decrease bone growth in premature infants.
PREGNANCY: Category D, not for use in nursing.
INTERACTIONS: May require downward adjustments of anticoagulant dosage. May interfere with bactericidal action of penicillin; avoid concurrent use when possible. Avoid antacids containing aluminum, calcium, or magnesium, sodium bicarbonate, and iron-containing preparations.
ADVERSE REACTIONS: Anorexia, nausea, vomiting, diarrhea, dysphagia, enterocolitis, rash, exfoliative dermatitis, renal toxicity, hypersensitivity reactions, blood dyscrasias.

GENTAMICIN SULFATE

Gentamicin sulfate *(Various)*

> Potential nephrotoxicity, neurotoxicity, ototoxicity. Risk of toxicity is greater with impaired renal function, high dosage, or prolonged therapy. Monitor serum concentrations closely. Avoid prolonged peak levels >12mcg/mL and trough levels >2mcg/mL. Monitor renal and eight cranial nerve function, urine, BUN, serum creatinine, and CrCl. Obtain serial audiograms. Advanced age and dehydration increase risk of toxicity. Adjust dose or discontinue use with evidence of ototoxicity or nephrotoxicity. May cause fetal harm during pregnancy. Avoid concurrent and/or sequential systemic or topical use of other potentially neurotoxic and/or nephrotoxic drugs, such as cisplatin, cephaloridine, kanamycin, amikacin, neomycin, polymyxin B, colistin, paromomycin, streptomycin, tobramycin, vancomycin, and viomycin. Avoid concurrent use with potent diuretics, such as ethacrynic acid or furosemide.

HOW SUPPLIED: Inj: 10mg/mL, 40mg/mL
THERAPEUTIC CLASS: Aminoglycoside
INDICATION: Treatment of Tularemia.[†]
DOSAGE: *Adults:* IM/IV: 5mg/kg qd for 10 days.[†]
Pediatrics: IM/IV: 2.5mg/kg tid for 10 days.[†]
CONTRAINDICATIONS: Hypersensitivity to aminoglycosides.
WARNINGS/PRECAUTIONS: Contains metabisulfite. Neuromuscular blockade, respiratory paralysis, ototoxicity, and nephrotoxicity may occur after local irrigation or topical application during surgical procedures. Caution with neuromuscular disorders (eg, myasthenia gravis, parkinsonism). Caution in elderly; monitor renal function. Keep patients well-hydrated during treat-

ment. May cause fetal harm when administered to pregnant women.
PREGNANCY: Category D, safety not known in nursing.
INTERACTIONS: Increased nephrotoxicity with cephalosporins. Do not premix with other drugs; administer separately. Neuromuscular blockade and respiratory paralysis may occur in anesthetized patients or those receiving neuromuscular blockers (eg, succinylcholine, tubocurarine, decamethonium). See Black Box Warning.
ADVERSE REACTIONS: Nephrotoxicity, neurotoxicity, rash, fever, urticaria, nausea, vomiting, headache, lethargy, confusion, depression, decreased appetite, weight loss, BP changes, blood dyscrasias, elevated LFTs.

STREPTOMYCIN SULFATE

Streptomycin sulfate *(Various)*

> Risk of severe neurotoxic reactions (eg, vestibular and cochlear disturbances) increased significantly with renal dysfunction or pre-renal azotemia. Optic nerve dysfunction, peripheral neuritis, arachnoiditis, and encephalopathy may occur. Monitor renal function; reduce dose with renal impairment and/or nitrogen retention. Do not exceed peak serum level of 20-25mcg/mL with kidney damage. Avoid other neurotoxic and/or nephrotoxic drugs (eg, neomycin, kanamycin, gentamicin, cephaloridine, paromomycin, viomycin, polymyxin B, colistin, tobramycin, cyclosporine). Respiratory paralysis can occur, especially if given soon after anesthesia or muscle relaxants. Reserve parenteral form when adequate lab and audiometric testing is available.

HOW SUPPLIED: Inj: 1g
THERAPEUTIC CLASS: Aminoglycoside
INDICATION: Treatment of moderate to severe infections such as tularemia.
DOSAGE: *Adults:* IM only. 1g IM bid for 10 days. Renal Impairment: Reduce dose.
Pediatrics: 15mg/kg IM bid. Max: 2g/day.
CONTRAINDICATIONS: Hypersensitivity to aminoglycosides.
WARNINGS/PRECAUTIONS: Vestibular and auditory dysfunction may occur. Contains sodium metabisulfite. Can cause fetal harm in pregnancy. Caution with dose selection in renal impairment. Alkalinize urine to minimize or prevent renal irritation with prolonged therapy. CNS depression (eg, stupor, flaccidity) reported in infants with higher than recommended doses. If syphilis is suspected when treating venereal infections, perform dark field exam before initiating treatment, and monthly serologic tests for at least 4 months. Overgrowth of nonsusceptible organisms may occur. Terminate therapy when toxic symptoms appear, when impending toxicity is feared, when organisms become resistant, or when full treatment effect has been obtained
PREGNANCY: Category D, not for use in nursing.
INTERACTIONS: See Black Box Warning. Increased ototoxicity with ethacrynic acid, furosemide, mannitol and possibly other diuretics.
ADVERSE REACTIONS: Vestibular ototoxicity (nausea, vomiting, vertigo), paresthesia of face, rash, fever, urticaria, angioneurotic edema, eosinophilia.

TYPHUS FEVER TREATMENT

CHLORAMPHENICOL

Chloramphenicol *(Various)*

> Aplastic anemia, hypoplastic anemia, thrombocytopenia, and granulocytopenia may occur. Also reported is aplastic anemia terminating in leukemia. Blood dyscrasias occurred after both short-term and prolonged therapy. Do not use when less potentially dangerous drugs are effective. Not to be used for trivial infections, prophylaxis of bacterial infections, or to treat colds, flu, or throat infections. Perform adequate blood studies during treatment.

HOW SUPPLIED: Cap: 250mg; Inj: 100mg/ml
THERAPEUTIC CLASS: Bacteriostatic antibiotic
INDICATION: Treatment of typhus fever.
DOSAGE: *Adults/Pediatrics:* 50mg/kg/day IV in 4 divided doses.
CONTRAINDICATIONS: Hypersensitivity to chloramphenicol; pregnancy, especially near term and during labor. Avoid with other drugs that may depress bone marrow.
WARNINGS/PRECAUTIONS: Caution in patients with intermittent porphyria; G6PD deficiency; premature and full-term infants.
PREGNANCY: Category D, not for use in nursing.
INTERACTIONS: Decreased liver breakdown and increased effect of anticoagulants, barbiturates, tacrolimus, phenytoin, and oral antidiabetic agents with concomitant use. Acetaminophen increases serum levels of chloramphenicol; rifampin decreases chloramphenicol effect.
ADVERSE REACTIONS: Nausea, vomiting, diarrhea, headache, glossitis, stomatitis.

DOXYCYCLINE

Doryx *(Warner Chilcott)*, Monodox *(Watson)*, Vibramycin *(Pfizer)*

HOW SUPPLIED: Doryx: Cap, Delayed-Release: (doxycycline hyclate) 75mg, 100mg. Monodox: Cap: (doxycycline monohydrate) 50mg, 100mg. Vibramycin: Cap: (doxycycline hyclate) 50mg, 100mg; Inj: (vial) 100mg, 200mg; Syrup: (doxycycline calcium) 50mg/5mL [473mL]; Sus: (doxycycline monohydrate) 25mg/5mL [60mL]; Tab: (Vibra-Tabs) 100mg
THERAPEUTIC CLASS: Tetracycline derivative
INDICATION: Rocky Mountain spotted fever, typhus fever, and typhus group, Q fever, rickettsialpox, and tick fevers caused by *Rickettsiae*.
DOSAGE: *Adults:* 100mg bid until 2-3 days after fever resolution
Pediatrics: >8 yrs: <100lbs: 1mg/lb bid day 1. Maint: 1mg/lb/day as single dose or divided bid. Severe Infection: Maint: 2mg/lb/day. ≥100lbs: 100mg bid for 60 days. Initial: 200mg day 1. Maint: 100mg/day as single dose or 50mg q12h. Severe Infection: Maint: 100mg q12h.
CONTRAINDICATIONS: Hypersensitivity to any of the tetracyclines.
WARNINGS/PRECAUTIONS: May cause fetal harm during pregnancy. Use during tooth development (last half of pregnancy, infancy, <8 yrs) may cause permanent discoloration of the teeth or enamel hypoplasia. Photosensitivity, increased BUN, superinfection may occur. Monitor hematopoietic, renal, and hepatic values periodically with long term therapy. Bulging fontanels in infants and benign intracranial HTN in adults reported. May decrease bone growth in premature infants.
PREGNANCY: Category D, not for use in nursing.
INTERACTIONS: May require downward adjustments of anticoagulant dosage. May interfere with bactericidal action of penicillin; avoid concurrent use when possible. Avoid antacids containing aluminum, calcium, or magnesium, sodium bicarbonate, and iron-containing preparations.
ADVERSE REACTIONS: Anorexia, nausea, vomiting, diarrhea, dysphagia, enterocolitis, rash, exfoliative dermatitis, renal toxicity, hypersensitivity reactions, blood dyscrasias.

MINOCYCLINE

Dynacin *(Par)*, Minocin *(Lederle)*

HOW SUPPLIED: Dynacin: Cap: 50mg, 75mg, 100mg; Tab: 50mg, 75mg, 100mg. Minocin: Cap: 50mg, 100mg
THERAPEUTIC CLASS: Tetracycline derivative
INDICATION: Rocky Mountain spotted fever, typhus fever, and typhus group, Q fever, rickettsialpox, and tick fevers caused by *Rickettsiae*.
DOSAGE: *Adults:* Usual: 200mg initially, then 100mg q12h; alternative is 100-200mg initially, then 50mg qid.
Pediatrics: >8 yrs: 4mg/kg initially followed by 2mg/kg q12h. Take with plenty of fluids.
CONTRAINDICATIONS: Hypersensitivity to any of the tetracyclines.
WARNINGS/PRECAUTIONS: May cause fetal harm during pregnancy. Use during tooth development (last half of pregnancy, infancy, <8 yrs) may cause permanent discoloration of the teeth or enamel hypoplasia; avoid use during this period. Renal toxicity, hepatotoxicity, photosensitivity, increased BUN, superinfection, pseudotumor cerebri may occur; perform hematopoietic, renal, and hepatic monitoring. May impair mental/physical abilities. Use alternate form of contraception other than oral contraceptives. May decrease bone growth in premature infants.
PREGNANCY: Category D, not for use in nursing.
INTERACTIONS: May require downward adjustments of anticoagulant dosage. May interfere with bactericidal action of penicillin; avoid concurrent use when possible. May decrease efficacy of oral contraceptives. Impaired absorption with antacids containing aluminum, calcium, or magnesium and iron-containing products. Fatal renal toxicity with methoxyflurane has been reported.
ADVERSE REACTIONS: Anorexia, nausea, vomiting, diarrhea, dysphagia, enterocolitis, pancreatitis, increased LFTs, hepatitis, liver failure, renal toxicity, rash, exfoliative dermatitis, Stevens-Johnson syndrome, skin and mucous membrane pigmentation, blood dyscrasias, headache, tooth discoloration.

VIRAL HEMORRHAGIC FEVER TREATMENT

RIBAVIRIN

Copegus *(Roche)*, Rebetol *(Schering)*

> Not for monotherapy treatment of chronic hepatitis C. Primary toxicity is hemolytic anemia. Avoid with significant or unstable cardiac disease. Contraindicated in pregnancy and male partners of pregnant women. Use 2 forms of contraception during therapy and for 6 months after discontinuation.

HOW SUPPLIED: Copegus: Tab: 200mg. Rebetol: Cap: 200mg; Sol: 40mg/mL [120mL]

† Not FDA-approved for this indication.

THERAPEUTIC CLASS: Nucleoside analogue
INDICATION: Reduction of mortality from Lassa fever (Adenavirus) in high-risk patients and presumably decreases morbidity in all patients with Lassa fever.† Clinically evident viral hemorrhagic fever of unknown etiology or secondary to Bunyarvirus (Rift Valley Fever).† Reduction of mortality and reduction of the incidence of oliguria and hemorrhage in hemorrhagic fever with renal syndrome caused by Hantaan Virus. †
DOSAGE: *Adults:* Lassa Fever/Rift Valley Fever: IV: Initial: 30mg/kg IV (Max: 2g). Followed by 16mg/kg IV (Max: 1g) every 6 hours for 4 days, followed by 8mg/kg IV (Max: 500mg) every 8 hours for 6 days. PO: Initial: 2g PO qd. Followed by 1.2g/day in 2 divided doses (≥75kg) or 1g/day PO in 2 divided doses (400mg qam and 600mg qpm; <75kg) for 10 days.† Hantaan Virus: IV: Initial: 33mg/kg IV. Followed by 16mg/kg IV every 6 hours for 4 days, followed by 8mg/kg IV (Max: 500mg) every 8 hours for 3 days.†
CONTRAINDICATIONS: Pregnancy, male partners of pregnant women, hemoglobinopathies (eg, thalassemia major, sickle cell anemia). Autoimmune hepatitis, and hepatic decompensation (Child-Pugh score greater than 6, Class B and C) in chirrotic CHC patients when used in combination with Pegasys.
WARNINGS/PRECAUTIONS: Discontinue with hepatic decompensation, confirmed pancreatitis, and hypersensitivity reaction. Severe depression, suicidal ideation, hemolytic anemia, bone marrow suppression, autoimmune and infectious disorders, pulmonary dysfunction, pancreatitis, and diabetes reported. Assess for underlying cardiac disease (obtain EKG); fatal and nonfatal MI reported with anemia. Caution with cardiac disease, discontinue if cardiovascular status deteriorates. Hemolytic anemia reported; monitor Hgb or Hct initially then at week 2 and 4 (or more if needed) of therapy. Suspend therapy if symptoms of pancreatitis arise. Avoid if CrCl <50mL/min. Obtain negative pregnancy test prior to initiation then monthly, and for 6 months post-therapy.
PREGNANCY: Category X, not for use in nursing.
INTERACTIONS: Avoid concomitant use with didanosine, stavudine and zidovudine.
ADVERSE REACTIONS: Fatigue/asthenia, pyrexia, rigors, nausea/vomiting, neutropenia, lymphopenia, anorexia, myalgia, arthralgia, headache, dizziness, irritability/anxiety/nervousness, insomnia, depression, dyspnea, alopecia, dermatitis.

YELLOW FEVER VACCINE

VF-Vax *(Aventis Pasteur)*

HOW SUPPLIED: Inj: 4.74 log^{10} PFU
THERAPEUTIC CLASS: Vaccine
INDICATION: Active immunization of persons 9 months of age and older in persons living or traveling to endemic areas or for international travel when required.
DOSAGE: *Adults/Pediatrics:* ≥9 months: Primary Vaccination: 0.5mL (4.74 log^{10} PFU). Booster: 0.5mL (4.74 log^{10} PFU) every 10 years. Desensitization: 0.05mL of 1:10 dilution, then 0.05mL of full strength, then 0.10mL of full strength, then 0.15mL of full strength, then 0.20mL of full strength SQ at 15-20 minute intervals.
CONTRAINDICATIONS: Hypersensitivity to eggs or egg products. Immunosuppressed patients due to illness (eg, HIV infection, leukemia, lymphoma, thymoma, generalized malignancy) or drug therapy (eg, corticosteriods, alkylating drugs, or antimetabolites) or radiation.
WARNINGS/PRECAUTIONS: Epinephrine (1:1000) should be immediately available. Vaccine-associated viscerotropic disease (rare) and vaccine-associated neurotropic disease (rare).
PREGNANCY: Category C, not for use in nursing.
INTERACTIONS: Prednisone and other corticosteroids may decrease immunogenicity and increase risk of adverse events.
ADVERSE REACTIONS: Systemic: Headache, myalgia, low-grade fevers. Local: Edema, hypersensitivity, pain, mass at injection site.

VX TREATMENT

ATROPINE

Atropine Sulfate *(Various)*

HOW SUPPLIED: Inj: 0.05mg/mL, 0.1mg/mL, 0.4mg/mL, 0.5mg/mL, 1mg/mL
THERAPEUTIC CLASS: Anticholinergic
INDICATION: Indicated as an antisialagogue for preanesthetic medication to prevent or reduce secretions of the respiratory tract, to restore cardiac rate and arterial pressure during anesthesia when vagal stimulation produced by intra-abdominal surgical traction causes a sudden decrease in pulse rate and cardiac action, to lessen degree of AV heart block when increased vagal tone is a major factor in the conduction defect (possibly due to digitalis), to overcome severe bradycardia and syncope due to hyperactive carotid sinus reflex, as an antidote (with external cardiac massage) for car-

diovascular collapse from the injudicious use of choline ester (cholinergic) drug, in treatment of anticholinesterase poisoning from organophosphorus insecticides, and as an antidote for the "rapid" type of mushroom poisoning due to presence of the alkaloid muscarine, in certain species of fungus such as *Amanita muscaria*.

DOSAGE: *Adults:* Usual: 0.5mg IM/IV/SC. Range: 0.4-0.6mg. If used as an antisialogogue, inject IM prior to anesthesia induction. Bradyarrhythmias: 0.4-1mg every 1-2 hrs prn. Max: 2mg/dose. May be used as an antidote for cardiovascular collapse resulting from injudicious administration of choline ester. When cardiac arrest has occurred Anticholinesterase Poisoning From Insecticide Poisoning: 2-3mg IV. Repeat until signs of atropine intoxication appear. Mushroom Poisoning: Administer sufficient doses to control parasympathomimetic signs before coma and cardiovascular collase supervene. VX Poisoning: 6mg may be required initially.[†]
Pediatrics: Doses range from 0.6mg in >12 yrs and 0.1mg in newborns. Inject SC 30 minutes before surgery. Bradyarrhythmias: 0.01-0.03mg/kg IV. VX Poisoning: 0.01-0.02 mg/kg IV or IM.[†]
CONTRAINDICATIONS: Glaucoma, pyloric stenosis, or prostatic hypertrophy except in doses used for preanesthetic medication.
WARNINGS/PRECAUTIONS: Avoid overdose in IV administration. Increased susceptibility to toxic effects in children. Caution in patients >40 yrs. Conventional doses may precipitate glaucoma in susceptible patients, convert partial organic pyloric stenosis into complete obstruction, lead to complete urinary retention in patients with prostatic hypertrophy or cause inspissation of bronchial secretions and formation of dangerous viscid plugs in patients with chronic lung disease.
PREGNANCY: Category C, safety in nursing not known.
ADVERSE REACTIONS: Dryness of the mouth, blurred vision, photophobia, tachycardia, anhidrosis.

PRALIDOXIME
Protopam *(Baxter)*
HOW SUPPLIED: Inj: 1g
THERAPEUTIC CLASS: Nerve gas antidote
INDICATION: Used together with atropine to treat poisoning caused by organophosphates and to treat anticholinesterase overdose.
DOSAGE: *Adults:* Anticholinesterase Overdose: Initial: 1-2g IV. Maint: 250mg IV every 5 minutes. Organophosphate Poisoning: Initial: 1-2g in 100mL NS infused over 15-30 minutes or 5% solution in SWFI over not less than 5 minutes. Repeat 1-2g in 1 hr if muscle weakness persists.
Pediatrics: Organophosphate Poisoning (Mild). 1-2 g PO, may repeat in 3 hrs if necessary. Organophosphate Poisoning (Moderate to Severe): Intermittent: 25-50mg/kg IV; may repeat in 1-2 hrs, then at 10-12 hr intervals if necessary. Continuous: 25mg/kg IV single dose, then begin infusion at 10-20mg/kg/hr.[†]
WARNINGS/PRECAUTIONS: Caution in myasthenia gravis, may precipitate myasthenic crisis. Not effective in poisonings due to organophosphates without anticholinesterase activity or due to phosphorus/inorganic phosphates. Caution in renal impairment. Slow IV infusion prevents tachycardia, laryngospasm, and muscle rigidity.
PREGNANCY: Unknown.
ADVERSE REACTIONS: Blurred vision, double vision, difficulty in speaking, difficult or rapid breathing, dizziness, fast heartbeat, drowsiness, headache, nausea, muscle stiffness/weakness, injection site pain, difficulty in focusing of eyes.

SUPPORTIVE CARE

ACETAMINOPHEN
Tylenol *(McNeil Consumer)*
HOW SUPPLIED: Drops: (Infants') 80mg/0.8mL; Sol: (Extra Strength) 500mg/15mL; Sus: (Children's) 160mg/5mL; Tab: (Regular Strength) 325mg, (Extra Strength) 500mg; Tab, Chewable: (Children's) 80mg, (Junior) 160mg
THERAPEUTIC CLASS: Analgesic
INDICATION: Temporary relief of minor aches and pains. Fever.
DOSAGE: *Adults:* (Regular Strength) 650mg q4-6h prn. Max: 3900mg/day. (Extra Strength) 1000mg q4-6h prn. Max: 4000mg/day.
Pediatrics: Max: 5 doses/day. 0-3 months (6-11 lbs): 40mg q4h prn. 4-11 months (12-17 lbs): 80mg q4h prn. 12-23 months (18-23 lbs): 120mg q4h prn. 2-3 yrs (24-35 lbs): 160mg q4h prn. 4-5 yrs (36-47 lbs): 240mg q4h prn. 6-8 yrs (48-59 lbs): 320mg q4h prn. 9-10 yrs (60-71 lbs): 400mg q4h prn. 11 yrs (72-95 lbs): 480mg q4h prn. 12 yrs: 640mg q4h prn. Older Children: Regular Strength: 6-11 yrs: 325mg q4-6h prn. Max: 1625mg/day. ≥12 yrs: 650mg q4-6h prn. Max: 3900mg/day. Extra Strength: ≥12 yrs: 1000mg q4-6h prn. Max: 4000mg/day.
WARNINGS/PRECAUTIONS: May cause hepatic damage.
PREGNANCY: Safety in pregnancy or nursing not known.
INTERACTIONS: Increased risk of hepatotoxicity with excessive alcohol use (≥3 drinks/day).

[†] Not FDA-approved for this indication.

ACTIVATED CHARCOAL
Actidose-Aqua *(Paddock)*, Char-Caps *(Key)*, Ez-Char *(Paddock)*
HOW SUPPLIED: Cap: 260mg; Powder: 25g/29.4g; Sus: 15g/72mL, 25g/120mL
THERAPEUTIC CLASS: Absorbent antidote
INDICATION: Indicated for use as an emergency antidote in the treatment of poisoning by most drugs and chemicals.
DOSAGE: *Adults/Pediatrics:* ≥13 yrs: Single-dose therapy: 25g to 100g as a slurry in water. Multiple-dose therapy: 50g to 100g as a slurry in water; then 12.5g every hour, 25g every two hours, 50g every four hours.
Pediatrics: 1-12 yrs: Single-dose therapy: 25g to 50g or 0.5g/kg to 1g/kg as a slurry in water. Multiple-dose therapy: 10g to 25g as a slurry in water; then 1g/kg to 2g/kg every 2-4 hours. ≤1 yr: 10g to 25g or 1g/kg as a slurry in water. Multiple-dose therapy: 10g to 25g as a slurry in water; then 1g/kg to 2g/kg every 2-4 hours.
CONTRAINDICATIONS: Absence of bowel sounds; risk of gastrointestinal obstruction, gastrointestinal perforation, recent surgery.
PREGNANCY: Unknown.
INTERACTIONS: Efficacy of other concurrently used oral medications may be decreased because of decreased absorption.
ADVERSE REACTIONS: Diarrhea, black stools, vomiting, constipation.

ALBUTEROL
Albuterol *(Various)*, Proventil *(Schering)*, Proventil HFA *(Schering)*, Ventolin *(GlaxoSmithKline)*, Ventolin HFA *(GlaxoSmithKline)*, Vospire ER *(Odyssey)*
HOW SUPPLIED: Aerosol: 0.09mg/inh [17g], (HFA) 0.09mg/inh [Proventil HFA: 6.7g; Ventolin HFA: 18g]; Sol (neb): 0.083% [3mL, 25″], 0.5% [20mL]; Syrup: 2mg/5mL; Tab: 2mg*, 4mg*; Tab, Extended Release (Vospire ER): 4mg, 8mg; (Proventil Repetabs): 4mg* *scored
THERAPEUTIC CLASS: Beta₂-agonist
INDICATION: (Aerosol) Prevention/treatment of bronchospasm with reversible obstructive airway disease and prevention of exercise-induced bronchospasm in patients ≥12 yrs and ≥4 yrs for HFA Aerosol. (Sol) Relief of bronchospasm with reversible obstructive airway disease and acute attacks of bronchospasm in patients ≥12 yrs. (Tab, Tab, Extended Release) Relief of bronchospasm with reversible obstructive airway disease in patients ≥6 yrs. (Syrup) Relief of bronchospasm in patients ≥2 yrs with reversible obstructive airway disease.
DOSAGE: *Adults:* Bronchospasm: (Aerosol, HFA Aerosol) 2 inh q4-6h or 1 inh q4h. (Repetabs/VoSpire ER) Initial: 4-8mg q12h. Max: 32mg/day. (Sol) 2.5mg tid-qid by nebulizer. (Syrup, Tabs) 2-4mg tid-qid. Max: 32mg/day (8mg qid). Elderly/Beta-Adrenergic Sensitivity: (Syrup, Tabs) Initial: 2mg tid-qid. Max: (Tabs) 8mg tid-qid. Exercise-Induced Bronchospasm: (Aerosol, HFA Aerosol) 2 inh 15 minutes (up to 30 minutes for HFA) before activity.
Pediatrics: Bronchospasm: >14 yrs: (Syrup) Initial: 2-4mg tid-qid. Max: 8mg qid. ≥12 yrs: (Aerosol, HFA Aerosol) 2 inh q4-6h or 1 inh q4h. (Sol) 2.5mg tid-qid by nebulizer. (Tabs) Initial: 2-4mg tid-qid. Max: 8mg qid. >12 yrs: (Repetabs/VoSpire ER) Initial: 4-8mg q12h. Max: 32mg/day. 6-14 yrs: (Syrup) Initial: 2mg tid-qid. Max: 24mg/day. 6-12 yrs: (Repetabs/VoSpire ER) Initial: 4mg q12h. Max: 24mg/day. (Tabs) Initial: 2mg tid-qid. Max: 24mg/day. 2-5 yrs: (Syrup) Initial: 0.1mg/kg tid (not to exceed 2mg tid). Titrate: May increase to 0.2mg/kg/day. Max: 4mg tid. ≥4 yrs: (HFA Aerosol) 2 inh q4-6h or 1 inh q4h. Exercise-Induced Bronchospasm: ≥12 yrs: (Aerosol) 2 inh 15 minutes before activity. ≥4 yrs: (HFA Aerosol) 2 inh 15-30 minutes before activity.
WARNINGS/PRECAUTIONS: Hypersensitivity reactions reported. Monitor for worsening asthma. Fatalities reported with excessive use. Caution with cardiovascular disorders, especially coronary insufficiency, arrhythmias and HTN. May need concomitant corticosteroids. Can produce paradoxical bronchospasm. Caution with DM, hyperthyroidism, seizures. May cause transient hypokalemia.
PREGNANCY: Category C, not for use in nursing.
INTERACTIONS: Avoid other sympathomimetic agents. Extreme caution with MAOIs and TCAs. Monitor digoxin. May worsen ECG changes and/or hypokalemia with nonpotassium-sparing diuretics. Antagonized by beta-blockers.
ADVERSE REACTIONS: Tachycardia, increased BP, tremor, nervousness, dizziness, nausea/vomiting, palpitations, paradoxical bronchospasm, heartburn, rhinitis, respiratory tract infection.

CALCIUM CHLORIDE
Calcium Chloride *(Various)*
HOW SUPPLIED: Inj: 100mg/mL
THERAPEUTIC CLASS: Calcium salt
INDICATION: Mild hypocalcemia due to neonatal tetany, tetany due to parathyroid deficiency or vitamin D deficiency, and alkalosis. Prophylaxis of hypocalcemia during exchange transfusions. Intestinal malabsorption. Treat effects of serious hyperkalemia as measured by ECG. Cardiac resuscitation after open heart surgery when epinephrine fails to improve weak

or ineffective myocardial contractions. Depression due to magnesium overdosage. Acute symptoms of lead colic. Rickets, osteomalacia. Reverse symptoms of verapamil overdosage.
DOSAGE: *Adults:* Hypocalcemia: 0.5-1g IV every 1-3 days, given at a rate not to exceed 13.6-27.3mg/min. Magnesium Intoxication: 0.5g IV. Cardiac Resuscitation: 0.5-1g IV or 0.2-0.8g injected into the ventricular cavity as a single dose.
Pediatrics: Hypocalcemia: 25mg/kg IV (0.2mL/kg up to 1-10mL/kg). Cardiac Resuscitation: 0.2mL/kg IV as single dose.
CONTRAINDICATIONS: Hypocalcemia of renal insufficiency. IM or SC use.
WARNINGS/PRECAUTIONS: Avoid in children due to possible tissue necrosis and sloughing.
PREGNANCY: Category C.
ADVERSE REACTIONS: Peripheral vasodilation, extravasation.

CALCIUM GLUCONATE
Calcium Gluconate *(Various)*
HOW SUPPLIED: Inj: 10%, 100mg/mL
THERAPEUTIC CLASS: Calcium salt
INDICATION: Mild hypocalcemia due to neonatal tetany, tetany due to parathyroid deficiency or vitamin D deficiency, and alkalosis. Prophylaxis of hypocalcemia during exchange transfusions. Intestinal malabsorption. Depression due to magnesium overdosage. Acute symptoms of lead colic. Rickets, osteomalacia. Reverse symptoms of verapamil overdosage. Decrease capillary permeability in allergic conditions, nonthrombocytopenic purpura, and exudative dermatoses. Pruritus due to certain drugs. Hyperkalemia to antagonize cardiac toxicity.
DOSAGE: *Adults:* Hypocalcemia: 2.3-9.3mEq (5-20mL of 10% solution) prn. Emergency Elevation of Serum Calcium: 7-14mEq (15-30.1mL). Hyperkalemia: 2.25-14mEq (4.8-30.1mL), if needed repeat after 1-2 minutes. Magnesium Intoxication: 4.5-9mEq (9.7-19.4mL). Exchange Transfusion: 1.35mEq (2.9mL) concurrent with each 100mL citrated blood.
Pediatrics: Hypocalcemia: 2.3mEq/kg/day (or 56mEq/m²/day) given well diluted and slowly in divided doses. Emergency Elevation of Serum Calcium: 1-7mEq (2.2-15mL). Hypocalcemic Tetany: 0.5-0.7mEq/kg (1.1-1.5mL/kg) tid-qid until tetany is controlled.
CONTRAINDICATIONS: IM, intramyocardial, or SC use due to severe tissue necrosis, sloughing, and abscess formation.

DEXAMETHASONE
Decadron *(Merck)*, Dexamethasone *(Various)*
HOW SUPPLIED: Inj: (Dexamethasone Sodium Phosphate) 4mg/mL, 10mg/mL; Sol: (Dexamethasone) 0.5mg/5mL, 1mg/mL; Tab: (Dexamethasone) 0.5mg*, 0.75mg*, 1mg*, 1.5mg*, 2mg*, 4mg*, 6mg* *scored
THERAPEUTIC CLASS: Glucocorticoid
INDICATION: Treatment of steroid responsive disorders.
DOSAGE: *Adults:* Individualize for disease and patient response. Withdraw gradually. (Tab) Initial: 0.75-9mg/day PO. Maint: Decrease in small amounts to lowest effective dose. Cushing's Syndrome Test: 1mg PO at 11pm; draw blood at 8am next morning. Or, 0.5mg PO q6h for 48 hrs; or 2mg (to distinguish if excess pituitary ACTH or other causes) PO q6h for 48 hrs; obtain 24 hr urine collections. (Inj) Initial: 0.5-9mg/day IV/IM. Cerebral Edema: Initial: 10mg IV, then 4mg IM q6h until edema subsides. Reduce dose after 2-4 days and gradually discontinue over 5-7 days. Palliative Management of Recurrent/Inoperable Brain Tumors: Maint: 2mg IV/PO bid-tid. Acute Allergic Disorders: 4-8mg IM on 1st day, then 1.5mg PO bid for 2 days, then 0.75mg PO bid for 1 day, then 0.75mg PO qd for 2 days. (Inj) Usual: 0.2-9mg. Maint: Decrease in small amounts to lowest effective dose. Intra-Articular/Intralesional/Soft Tissue Injection: Usual: 0.2-6mg once every 3-5 days to once every 2-3 weeks. See labeling for Shock Treatment. Take with meals and antacids to prevent peptic ulcer.
Pediatrics: Individualize for disease and patient response. Withdraw gradually. (Tab) Initial: 0.75-9mg/day PO. Maint: Decrease in small amounts to lowest effective dose. Cushing's Syndrome Test: 1mg PO at 11pm; draw blood at 8am next morning. Or, 0.5mg PO q6h for 48 hrs; or 2mg (to distinguish if excess pituitary ACTH or other causes) PO q6h for 48 hrs; obtain 24 hr urine collections. (Inj) Initial: 0.5-9mg/day IV/IM. Cerebral Edema: Initial: 10mg IV, then 4mg IM q6h until edema subsides. Reduce dose after 2-4 days and gradually discontinue over 5-7 days. Palliative Management of Recurrent/Inoperable Brain Tumors: Maint: 2mg IV/PO bid-tid. Acute Allergic Disorders: 4-8mg IM on 1st day, then 1.5mg PO bid for 2 days, then 0.75mg PO bid for 1 day, then 0.75mg PO qd for 2 days. (Inj) Usual: 0.2-9mg. Maint: Decrease in small amounts to lowest effective dose. Intra-Articular/Intralesional/Soft Tissue Injection: Usual: 0.2-6mg once every 3-5 days to once every 2-3 weeks. See labeling for Shock Treatment. Take with meals and antacids to prevent peptic ulcer.
CONTRAINDICATIONS: Systemic fungal infections.
WARNINGS/PRECAUTIONS: Increase dose before, during, and after stressful

situations. Avoid abrupt withdrawal. May mask signs of infection, activate latent amebiasis, elevate BP, cause salt/water retention, increase excretion of potassium and calcium. Prolonged use may produce cataracts, glaucoma, secondary ocular infections. Caution with recent MI, ocular herpes simplex, emotional instability, nonspecific ulcerative colitis, diverticulitis, peptic ulcer, renal insufficiency, HTN, osteoporosis, myasthenia gravis, threadworm infection, active tuberculosis. Enhanced effect with hypothyroidism, cirrhosis. Consider prophylactic therapy if exposed to measles or chickenpox. Risk of glaucoma, cataracts and eye infections. False negative dexamethasone suppression test with indomethacin.
PREGNANCY: Safety in pregnancy not known, not for use in nursing.
INTERACTIONS: Caution with ASA. Inducers of CYP3A4 (eg, phenytoin, phenobarbital, carbamazepine, rifampin) and ephedrine enhance clearance; increase steroid dose. Inhibitors of CYP3A4 (ketoconazole, macrolides) may increase plasma levels. Drugs that affect metabolism may interfere with dexamethasone suppression tests. Increased clearance of drugs metabolized by CYP3A4 (eg, indinavir, erythromycin). May increase or decrease phenytoin levels. Ketoconazole may inhibit adrenal corticosteroid synthesis and cause adrenal insufficiency during corticosteroid withdrawal. Antagonizes or potentiates coumarins. Hypokalemia with potassium-depleting diuretics. Live virus vaccines are contraindicated with immunosuppressive doses.
ADVERSE REACTIONS: Fluid/electrolyte disturbances, muscle weakness, osteoporosis, peptic ulcer, pancreatitis, ulcerative esophagitis, impaired wound healing, headache, psychic disturbances, growth suppression (children), glaucoma, hyperglycemia, weight gain, nausea, malaise.

DIAZEPAM
Valium *(Roche)*
HOW SUPPLIED: Tab: 2mg*, 5mg*, 10mg* *scored
THERAPEUTIC CLASS: Benzodiazepine
INDICATION: Management of anxiety disorders and short-term relief of anxiety symptoms. Symptomatic relief of acute alcohol withdrawal. Adjunct therapy in skeletal muscle spasm and convulsive disorders.
DOSAGE: *Adults:* Anxiety: 2-10mg bid-qid. Alcohol Withdrawal: 10mg tid-qid for 24 hours. Maint: 5mg tid-qid prn. Skeletal Muscle Spasm: 2-10mg tid-qid: Seizure Disorders: 2-10mg bid-qid. Elderly/Debilitated: Initial: 2-2.5mg qd-bid. Maint: Increase gradually as needed and tolerated.
Pediatrics: ≥6 months: 1-2.5mg tid-qid initially; increase gradually as needed and tolerated.
CONTRAINDICATIONS: Acute narrow angle glaucoma, untreated open angle glaucoma, patients <6 months (PO only).
WARNINGS/PRECAUTIONS: Monitor blood counts and LFTs in long-term use. Neutropenia and jaundice reported. Increase in grand mal seizures reported. Avoid abrupt withdrawal. Caution with kidney or hepatic dysfunction.
PREGNANCY: Not for use during pregnancy, safety in nursing not known.
INTERACTIONS: Phenothiazines, narcotics, barbiturates, MAOIs, and other antidepressants may potentiate effects. Delayed clearance with cimetidine. Avoid alcohol and other CNS-depressants. Risk of seizure with flumazenil.
ADVERSE REACTIONS: Drowsiness, fatigue, ataxia, paradoxical reactions, minor EEG changes.

DOPAMINE
Dopamine Hydrochloride *(Various)*
HOW SUPPLIED: Inj: 40mg/mL, 80mg/mL, 160mg/mL
THERAPEUTIC CLASS: Inotropic agent
INDICATION: For correction of hemodynamic imbalances present in shock due to MI, trauma, endotoxic septicemia, open-heart surgery, renal failure, and chronic cardiac decompensation.
DOSAGE: *Adults:* Initial: 2-5mcg/kg/min. Use 5mcg/kg/min in seriously ill. Increase in 5-10mcg/kg/min increments, up to 20-50mcg/kg/min.
CONTRAINDICATIONS: Pheochromocytoma, uncorrected tachyarrhythmias or ventricular fibrillation.
WARNINGS/PRECAUTIONS: Contains sulfites. Monitor BP, urine flow, cardiac output and pulmonary wedge pressure. Correct hypovolemia, hypoxia, hypercapnia, and acidosis prior to use. Reduce infusion rate with increase in diastolic BP/marked decrease in pulse pressure; increase rate if hypotension occurs. Discontinue if hypotension persists. Reduce dose if increased ectopic beats occurs. Caution with history of occlusive vascular disease (eg, atherosclerosis, arterial embolism, Raynaud's disease, cold injury, diabetic endarteritis, and Buerger's disease); monitor for changes in skin color or temperature. Administer phentolamine if extravasation is noted. Avoid abrupt withdrawal.
PREGNANCY: Category C, caution in nursing.
INTERACTIONS: Reduce dose to 1/10th of usual dose within 2 to 3 weeks of MAOI use. Potential additive effects on urine flow with diuretics. TCAs may potentiate pressor response. Antagonized by beta- and alpha-blockers, haloperidol. Extreme caution with cyclopropane or halogenated hydro-

carbon anesthetics. Possible severe HTN with some oxytocic drugs. Hypotension and bradycardia reported with phenytoin.
ADVERSE REACTIONS: Tachycardia, palpitation, ventricular arrhythmia (high doses), dyspnea, nausea, vomiting, headache, anxiety, bradycardia, hypotension, HTN, vasoconstriction.

HEPARIN
Heparin Sodium *(Wyeth)*
HOW SUPPLIED: Inj: 1000U/mL, 2500U/mL, 5000U/mL, 7500U/mL, 10,000U/mL
THERAPEUTIC CLASS: Glycosaminoglycan
INDICATION: Prophylaxis and treatment of venous thrombosis and its extension, PE in atrial fibrillation, and peripheral arterial embolism. Prevention of postoperative DVT and PE. Diagnosis and treatment of acute and chronic consumptive coagulopathies, for prevention of clotting in arterial and cardiac surgery.
DOSAGE: *Adults:* Based on 68kg: Initial: 5000U IV, then 10,000-20,000U SQ. Maint: 8000-10,000U q8h or 15,000-20,000U q12h. Intermittent IV Injection: Initial: 10,000U. Maint: 5000-10,000U q4-6h. Continuous IV Infusion: Initial: 5000U. Maint: 20,000-40,000U/24 hours. Adjust to coagulation test results. See labeling for details in specific disease states.
Pediatrics: Initial: 50U/kg IV drip. Maint: 100U/kg IV drip q4h or 20,000U/m²/24 hrs continuously.
CONTRAINDICATIONS: Severe thrombocytopenia, if cannot perform appropriate blood-coagulation tests (with full-dose heparin), uncontrollable active bleeding state (except in DIC).
WARNINGS/PRECAUTIONS: Not for IM use. Hemorrhage can occur at any site; caution with increased danger of hemorrhage (severe HTN, bacterial endocarditis, surgery, etc.). Monitor blood coagulation tests frequently. Thrombocytopenia reported; discontinue if platelets <100,000mm³ or if recurrent thrombosis develops. Contains benzyl alcohol. "White-clot syndrome" reported. Monitor platelets, Hct, and occult blood in the stool. Increased heparin resistance with fever, thrombosis, thrombophlebitis, infections with thrombosing tendencies, MI, cancer, and post-op. Higher bleeding incidence in women >60 yrs.
PREGNANCY: Category C, safe in nursing.
INTERACTIONS: Wait ≥5 hrs after last IV dose or 24 hrs after last SQ dose before measure PT for dicumarol or warfarin. Platelet inhibitors (eg, acetylsalicylic acid, dextran, phenylbutazone, ibuprofen, indomethacin, dipyridamole, hydroxychloroquine) may induce bleeding. Digitalis, tetracyclines, nicotine, or antihistamines may counteract anticoagulant action.
ADVERSE REACTIONS: Hemorrhage, local irritation, erythema, mild pain, hematoma, chills, fever, urticaria.

IBUPROFEN
Motrin *(Pharmacia)*
HOW SUPPLIED: Sus: 100mg/5mL [120mL, 480mL]; Tab: 400mg, 600mg, 800mg
THERAPEUTIC CLASS: NSAID
INDICATION: *Adults:* Mild to moderate pain. Dysmenorrhea. Rheumatoid arthritis (RA) Osteoarthritis (OA).
Pediatrics: Fever. Mild to moderate pain. Juvenile arthritis (JA).
DOSAGE: *Adults:* Pain: 400mg q4-6h prn. Dysmenorrhea: 400mg q4h prn. RA/OA: 300mg qid or 400mg, 600mg, or 800mg tid-qid. Max: 3200mg/day. Take with meals/milk. Renal Impairment: Reduce dose.
Pediatrics: Fever: 6 months-12 yrs: 5mg/kg for temp <102.5°F; 10mg/kg if temp ≥102.5°F q6-8h. Max: 40mg/kg/day. Pain: 6 months-12 yrs: 10mg/kg q6-8h. Max: 40mg/kg/day. JA: 30-40mg/kg/day divided into 3 or 4 doses. Milder disease may use 20mg/kg/day.
CONTRAINDICATIONS: Syndrome of nasal polyps, angioedema, and bronchospastic reactions to ASA or other NSAIDs.
WARNINGS/PRECAUTIONS: Risk of GI ulceration, bleeding, and perforation. Risk of anaphylactoid reactions. Caution with significantly impaired renal disease and intrinsic coagulation defects. Fluid retention/edema reported; caution with HTN or cardiac decompensation. Discontinue use if visual changes occur. May mask diagnostic signs of detecting infectious inflammatory painful conditions. Aseptic meningitis with fever and coma reported especially with SLE and related connective tissue diseases. Increased LFTs may occur; monitor for liver dysfunction. Decreases in Hgb/Hct reported.
PREGNANCY: Not recommended in pregnancy. Not for use in nursing.
INTERACTIONS: Use caution with anticoagulants. May enhance methotrexate toxicity. May decrease the natriuretic effects of furosemide or thiazides. Avoid use with aspirin. Decrease lithium clearance; monitor for toxicity.
ADVERSE REACTIONS: Nausea, epigastric pain, heartburn, dizziness, rash.

IPRATROPIUM/ALBUTEROL
Duoneb *(Dey)*
HOW SUPPLIED: Sol, Inhalation: (Albuterol-Ipratropium) 3mg-0.5mg/3mL [3mL, 30⁶ 60⁶].
THERAPEUTIC CLASS: Anticholinergic/beta₂-agonist
INDICATION: Treatment of bronchospasm in COPD in patients requiring more than one bronchodilator.
DOSAGE: *Adults:* 3mL qid via nebulizer. May give 2 additional doses/day.
CONTRAINDICATIONS: Hypersensitivity to atropine and its derivatives.
WARNINGS/PRECAUTIONS: Paradoxical bronchospasm and hypersensitivity reactions reported. Caution with cardiovascular disorders, convulsive disorders, hyperthyroidism, DM, narrow angle glaucoma, prostatic hypertrophy, and bladder-neck obstruction.
PREGNANCY: Category C, not for use in nursing.
INTERACTIONS: Additive interactions with anticholinergic agents. Increased risk of cardiovascular side effects with sympathomimetics. Use beta₁-selective blockers with hyperactive airways. Caution with or within 2 weeks of discontinuation of MAOIs or TCAs.
ADVERSE REACTIONS: Pain, chest pain, diarrhea, dyspepsia, nausea, leg cramps, bronchitis, lung disease, pharyngitis, pneumonia.

LORAZEPAM
Ativan *(Biovail)*
HOW SUPPLIED: Tab: 0.5mg, 1mg*, 2mg* *scored
THERAPEUTIC CLASS: Benzodiazepine
INDICATION: Management of anxiety.
DOSAGE: *Adults:* Initial: 2-3mg/day given bid-tid. Usual: 2-6mg/day in divided doses. Insomnia: 2-4mg qhs. Elderly/Debilitated: 1-2mg/day in divided doses.
Pediatrics: >12 yrs: Initial: 2-3mg/day given bid-tid. Usual: 2-6mg/day in divided doses. Insomnia: 2-4mg qhs.
CONTRAINDICATIONS: Acute narrow-angle glaucoma.
WARNINGS/PRECAUTIONS: Avoid with primary depression or psychosis. Withdrawal symptoms with abrupt discontinuation. Careful supervision if addiction-prone. Caution with elderly, and renal or hepatic dysfunction. Monitor for GI disease with prolonged therapy. Periodic blood counts and LFTs with long-term therapy.
PREGNANCY: Not for use in pregnancy or nursing.
INTERACTIONS: CNS-depressant effects with barbiturates, alcohol. Diminished tolerance to alcohol and other CNS depressants.
ADVERSE REACTIONS: Sedation, dizziness, weakness, unsteadiness, transient amnesia, memory impairment.

LORAZEPAM INJECTION
Ativan Injection *(Baxter)*
HOW SUPPLIED: Inj: 2mg/mL, 4mg/mL
THERAPEUTIC CLASS: Benzodiazepine
INDICATION: Treatment of status epilepticus and preanesthetic medication in adults.
DOSAGE: *Adults:* ≥18 yrs: Status Epilepticus: 4mg IV (given slowly at 2mg/min); may repeat 1 dose after 10-15 minutes if seizures recur or fail to cease. Preanesthetic Sedation: Usual: 0.05mg/kg IM; 2mg or 0.044mg/kg IV (whichever is smaller). Max: 4mg IM/IV.
CONTRAINDICATIONS: Acute narrow-angle glaucoma, sleep apnea syndrome, severe respiratory insufficiency. Not for intra-arterial injection.
WARNINGS/PRECAUTIONS: Monitor all parameters to maintain vital function. Risk of respiratory depression or airway obstruction in heavily sedated patients. May cause fetal damage during pregnancy. Increased risk of CNS and respiratory depression in elderly. Avoid with hepatic/renal failure. Caution with mild to moderate hepatic/renal disease. Avoid outpatient endoscopic procedures. Possible propylene glycol toxicity in renal impairment.
PREGNANCY: Category D, not for use in nursing.
INTERACTIONS: Additive CNS depression with other CNS depressants (eg, ethyl alcohol, phenothiazines, barbiturates, MAOIs). Increased sedation, hallucinations and irrational behavior with scopolamine. Decreased clearance with valproate, probenecid. Increased clearance with oral contraceptives. Severe adverse effects with clozapine and haloperidol reported.
ADVERSE REACTIONS: Respiratory depression/failure, hypotension, somnolence, headache, hypoventilation.

METHYLPREDNISOLONE
Medrol *(Pharmacia)*
HOW SUPPLIED: Tab: 2mg*, 4mg*, 8mg*, 16mg*, 32mg*; (Dose-Pak) 4mg* [21] *scored
THERAPEUTIC CLASS: Glucocorticoid
INDICATION: Steroid responsive disorders.
DOSAGE: *Adults:* Initial: 4-48mg/day depending on disease and response.

† Not FDA-approved for this indication.

Maint: Decrease dose by small amounts to lowest effective dose. MS: Initial: 160mg/day for 1 week. Maint: 64mg every other day for 1 month. Alternate Day Therapy: Twice the usual dose every other day for long-term therapy. *Pediatrics:* Initial: 4-48mg/day depending on disease and response. Maint: Decrease dose by small amounts to lowest effective dose. MS: Initial: 160mg/day for 1 week. Maint: 64mg every other day for 1 month. Alternate Day Therapy: Twice the usual dose every other day for long-term therapy.
CONTRAINDICATIONS: Systemic fungal infections.
WARNINGS/PRECAUTIONS: May need to increase dose before, during, and after stressful situations. May mask signs of infection or cause new infections. Prolonged use may produce glaucoma, optic nerve damage, secondary ocular infections. Increases BP, salt/water retention, potassium excretion. More severe/fatal course of infections reported with chickenpox, measles. Caution with Strongyloides, latent TB, hypothyroidism, cirrhosis, ocular herpes simplex, HTN, diverticulitis, fresh intestinal anastomoses, ulcerative colitis, osteoporosis, myasthenia gravis, renal insufficiency, peptic ulcer disease. Kaposi's sarcoma reported. Growth and development of children on prolonged therapy should be monitored. Monitor for psychic disturbances. Avoid abrupt withdrawal. The 24mg tabs contain tartrazine; caution with tartrazine sensitivity.
PREGNANCY: Safety in pregnancy and nursing not known.
INTERACTIONS: Reduced efficacy with hepatic enzyme inducers (eg, phenobarbital, phenytoin, and rifampin). Increases clearance of chronic high dose ASA. Caution with ASA in hypoprothrombinemia. Effects on oral anticoagulants are variable; monitor PT. Increased insulin and oral hypoglycemic requirements in DM. Avoid live vaccines with immunosuppressive doses. Possible decreased vaccine response with killed or inactivated vaccines with immunosuppressive doses. Mutual inhibition of metabolism with cyclosporine; convulsions reported. Potentiated by ketoconazole and troleandomycin.
ADVERSE REACTIONS: Fluid and electrolyte disturbances, HTN, osteoporosis, muscle weakness, cushingoid state, menstrual irregularities, nervousness, insomnia, impaired wound healing, DM, ulcerative esophagitis, excessive sweating, increases intracranial pressure, carbohydrate intolerance, glaucoma, cataracts, weight gain, nausea, malaise.

METOCLOPRAMIDE
Reglan *(Schwarz)*

HOW SUPPLIED: Inj: 5mg/mL; Syrup: 5mg/5mL; Tab: 5mg, 10mg* *scored
THERAPEUTIC CLASS: Dopamine antagonist/prokinetic
INDICATION: (PO) Symptomatic treatment of gastroesophageal reflux in patients who fail to respond to conventional therapy. (Inj, PO) Symptomatic relief of diabetic gastroparesis. (Inj) Prevention of post-op or chemo-induced nausea/vomiting. Diagnostic aid during radiological examination and facilitates intubation of small intestine.
DOSAGE: *Adults:* GERD: PO: 10-15mg qid 30 minutes ac and hs. Elderly: 5mg qid. Max: 12 weeks of therapy. Intermittent Symptoms: Up to 20mg single dose prior to provoking situation. Gastroparesis: 10mg PO 30 minutes ac and hs for 2-8 weeks. Severe Gastroparesis: May give same doses IV/IM for up to 10 days if needed. Antiemetic: (Postoperative) 10-20mg IM near end of surgery. (Chemotherapy-Induced) 1-2mg/kg 30 minutes before chemotherapy then q2h for two doses, then q3h for three doses. Give 2mg/kg for highly emetogenic drugs for initial 2 doses. Small Bowel Intubation/Radiological Exam: 10mg IV single dose. CrCl <40mL/min: 50% of normal dose.
Pediatrics: Small Bowel Intubation: 6-14 yrs: 2.5-5mg IV single dose. <6 yrs: 0.1mg/kg IV single dose. CrCl <40mL/min: 50% of normal dose.
CONTRAINDICATIONS: Where GI mobility stimulation is dangerous (eg, perforation, obstruction, hemorrhage), pheochromocytoma, seizure disorder, concomitant drugs that cause EPS effects.
WARNINGS/PRECAUTIONS: Caution with HTN, Parkinson's disease, depression. EPS, tardive dyskinesia, Parkinsonian-like symptoms, neuroleptic malignant syndrome reported. Administer IV injection slowly. Risk of developing fluid retention and volume overload especially with cirrhosis or CHF; discontinue if these occur. May increase pressure of suture lines.
PREGNANCY: Category B, caution with nursing.
INTERACTIONS: May decrease gastric absorption of drugs (eg, digoxin) and increase intestinal absorption of drugs (eg, APAP, tetracycline, levodopa, ethanol, and cyclosporine). Additive sedation with alcohol, hypnotics, narcotics, or tranquilizers. Caution with MAOIs. Antagonized by anticholinergics, narcotics. Insulin dose or timing of dose may need adjustment to prevent hypoglycemia. Contraindicated with drugs that cause EPS effects.
ADVERSE REACTIONS: Restlessness, drowsiness, fatigue, EPS effects (acute dystonic reactions), galactorrhea, hyperprolactinemia, hypotension, arrhythmia, diarrhea, dizziness, urinary frequency.

PROCHLORPERAZINE
Compazine *(GlaxoSmithKline)*

HOW SUPPLIED: Inj: (as edisylate) 5mg/mL; Sup: (as edisylate) 2.5mg; Tab: (as maleate) 5mg, 10mg
THERAPEUTIC CLASS: Phenothiazine derivative

† Not FDA-approved for this indication.

INDICATION: Control of severe nausea and vomiting. Management of psychotic disorders (eg, schizophrenia). Short-term treatment of generalized non-psychotic anxiety.
DOSAGE: *Adults:* Nausea/Vomiting: (Tab) Usual: 5-10mg tid-qid. Max: 40mg/day. (IM) 5-10mg IM q3-4h prn. Max: 40mg/day. (IV) 2.5-10mg IV (not bolus). Max: 10mg single dose and 40mg/day. Nausea/Vomiting with Surgery: 5-10mg IM 1-2 hrs or 5-10mg IV 15-30 minutes before anesthesia, or during or after surgery; repeat once if needed. Non-Psychotic Anxiety: (Tab) 5mg tid-qid; Psychosis: Mild/Outpatient: 5-10mg PO tid-qid. Moderate-Severe/Hospitalized: Initial: 10mg PO tid-qid. May increase in small increments every 2-3 days. Severe: (PO) 100-150mg/day. (IM) 10-20mg, may repeat q2-4 hrs if needed. Switch to oral after obtain control or if needed, 10-20mg IM q4-6h. Elderly: use lower dosing range and titrate more gradually.
Pediatrics: Nausea/Vomiting: >2 yrs and >20lbs: (PO/PR) 20-29 lbs: Usual: 2.5mg qd-bid. Max: 7.5mg/day. 30-39 lbs: 2.5mg bid-tid. Max: 10mg/day. 40-85 lbs: 2.5mg tid or 5mg bid. Max: 15mg/day. (IM) 0.06mg/lb, usually single dose for control. Psychosis: (PO/PR) 2-12 yrs: Initial: 2.5mg bid-tid, up to 10mg/day on 1st day. Max: 2-5 yrs: 20mg/day. 6-12 yrs: 25mg/day. (IM) <12 yrs: 0.06mg/lb single dose. Switch to oral after obtain control.
CONTRAINDICATIONS: Comatose states, concomitant large dose CNS depressants (alcohol, barbiturates, narcotics), pediatric surgery, pediatrics <2 yrs or <20 lbs.
WARNINGS/PRECAUTIONS: Secondary extrapyramidal symptoms can occur. Tardive dyskinesia, NMS may develop. Caution with activities requiring alertness. May mask symptoms of overdose of other drugs. May obscure diagnosis of intestinal obstruction, brain tumor, and Reye's syndrome. May interfere with thermoregulation. Caution with glaucoma, cardiac disorders. Caution in children with dehydration or acute illness. Discontinue 48 hrs before myelography and may resume after 24 hrs post-procedure.
PREGNANCY: Safety in pregnancy is not known; caution in nursing.
INTERACTIONS: Decreases oral anticoagulant effects. Potentiates alpha-adrenergic blockade. Thiazide diuretics potentiate orthostatic hypotension. Increased levels of both drugs with propranolol. Anticonvulsants may need adjustment. Risk of encephalopathic syndrome with lithium. Antagonizes antihypertensive effects of guanethidine and related compounds.
ADVERSE REACTIONS: Drowsiness, dizziness, amenorrhea, blurred vision, skin reactions, hypotension, NMS, cholestatic jaundice.

PREDNISONE
Prednisone *(Various)*

HOW SUPPLIED: Sol: 5mg/mL, 5mg/5mL; Tab: 1mg, 2.5mg*, 5mg*, 10mg*, 20mg*, 50mg* *scored
THERAPEUTIC CLASS: Glucocorticoid
INDICATION: Steroid responsive disorders.
DOSAGE: *Adults:* Initial: 5-60mg/day depending on disease and response. Maint: Decrease dose by small amounts to lowest effective dose.
Pediatrics: Initial: 5-60mg/day depending on disease and response. Maint: Decrease dose by small amounts to lowest effective dose.
CONTRAINDICATIONS: Systemic fungal infections.
WARNINGS/PRECAUTIONS: May need to increase dose before, during, and after stressful situations. May mask signs of infection or cause new infections. Prolonged use may produce glaucoma, optic nerve damage, secondary ocular infections. Increases BP, salt/water retention, potassium excretion. More severe/fatal course of infections reported with chickenpox, measles. Caution with latent TB, hypothyroidism, cirrhosis, ocular herpes simplex, HTN, diverticulitis, fresh intestinal anastomoses, ulcerative colitis, osteoporosis, myasthenia gravis, renal insufficiency, peptic ulcer disease. Growth and development of children on prolonged therapy should be monitored. Monitor for psychic disturbances. Avoid abrupt withdrawal.
PREGNANCY: Safety in pregnancy and nursing not known.
INTERACTIONS: Increases clearance of high dose ASA; caution in hypoprothrombinemia. Increased insulin and oral hypoglycemic requirements in DM. Avoid smallpox vaccine, and live vaccines with immunosuppressive doses. Possible decreased vaccine response with killed or inactivated vaccines with immunosuppressive doses. Increased clearance with hepatic enzyme inducers. Decreased metabolism with troleandomycin, ketoconazole. Variable effect on oral anticoagulants.
ADVERSE REACTIONS: Fluid and electrolyte disturbances, HTN, osteoporosis, muscle weakness, cushingoid state, menstrual irregularities, nervousness, insomnia, impaired wound healing, DM, ulcerative esophagitis, excessive sweating, increases intracranial pressure, carbohydrate intolerance, glaucoma, cataracts, weight gain, nausea, malaise.

SILVER SULFADIAZINE
Silvadene *(King)*

HOW SUPPLIED: Cre: 1% [20g, 50g, 85g, 400g, 1000g]
THERAPEUTIC CLASS: Sulfonamide antimicrobial
INDICATION: Adjunct for prevention and treatment of wound sepsis in patients with 2nd- and 3rd-degree burns.

DOSAGE: *Adults:* Apply under sterile conditions qd-bid to thickness of approximately 1/16 inch. Reapply if removed by patient activity. Continue until wound is healed.
CONTRAINDICATIONS: Late pregnancy, premature infants, newborns during 1st 2 months of life.
WARNINGS/PRECAUTIONS: Potential cross-sensitivity with other sulfonamides. Hemolysis may occur in G6PD deficient patients. Drug accumulation with hepatic and renal dysfunction. Monitor renal function and serum sulfa levels with extensive burns.
PREGNANCY: Category B, contraindicated in late pregnancy, and not for use in nursing.
INTERACTIONS: May inactivate topical proteolytic enzymes. Leukopenia increased with cimetidine.
ADVERSE REACTIONS: Transient leukopenia, skin necrosis, erythema multiforme, skin discoloration, burning sensation, rash, interstitial nephritis, fungal superinfection, systemic sulfonamide reactions.

SODIUM BICARBONATE

Sodium Bicarbonate *(Various)*

HOW SUPPLIED: Inj: 4%, 4.2%, 5%, 7.5%, 8.4%; Powder; Tab: 325mg, 520mg, 650mg
THERAPEUTIC CLASS: Alkalinizing agent/Electrolyte
INDICATION: Treatment of hyperacidity; severe diarrhea. Alkalization of the urine to treat drug toxicity. Treatment of acute mild to moderate metabolic acidosis due to shock, severe dehydration, anoxia, uncontrolled diabetes, renal disease, cardiac arrest, extracorporeal circulation of blood, severe primary lactic acidosis. Prophylaxis of renal calculi in gout. Prevention of renal calculi and nephrotoxicity during sulfonamide therapy. Neutralizing additive solution to decrease chemical phlebitis and client discomfort due to vein irritation at or near the site of infusion of IV acid solutions.
DOSAGE: *Adults:* Urinary Alkalinizer: Oral Powder: 1 tsp in a glass of water q4h. Tablets: Initial: 0.325-2g up to qid. Max: ≤60 yrs: 15g; >60yrs: 8g. Cardiac Arrest: 200-300mEq IV given rapidly as 7.5-8.4% solution. Severe Metabolic Acidosis: 90-180 mEq/L at a rate of 1-1.5 L during the first hour. Less Severe Metabolic Acidosis: 2-5mEq/kg given over a 4- to 8-hr period. Antacid: Oral Powder: ½ tsp in a glass of water q2h. Tablets: 0.325-2g qd-qid.
Pediatrics: Urinary Alkalinizer: 23-230mg/kg/day. Antacid: Tablets: 6-12 yrs: 520mg, may be repeated every 30 minutes.
CONTRAINDICATIONS: Chloride loss due to vomiting or from continuous GI suction. With diuretics known to produce a hypochloremic alkalosis. Metabolic and respiratory alkalosis. Hypocalcemia in which alkalosis may cause tetany. HTN, convulsions, CHF, and other situations where administration of sodium can be dangerous. As systemic alkalizer when used as a neutralizing additive solution. As an antidote for strong mineral acids because carbon dioxide is formed, which may cause discomfort and perforation.
WARNINGS/PRECAUTIONS: Caution in renal impairment, toxemia of pregnancy, oliguria or anuria, edema, CHF, liver cirrhosis, low-salt diets.
PREGNANCY: Category C, caution in nursing.
INTERACTIONS: Sodium bicarbonate can increase renal tubular reabsorption of many drugs leading to an increased effect (eg, amphetamines, tricyclic antidepressants, ephedrine, pseudoephedrine, quinidine). Alkalinization of the urine can cause an increased rate of excretion of many drugs including, benzodiazepines, chlorpropamide, iron, ketoconazole, methenamine compounds, methotrexate, nitrofurantoin, tetracyclines.
ADVERSE REACTIONS: Hypernatremia, alkalosis, hypercalcemia, nausea, vomiting, thrist.

SODIUM CHLORIDE IRRIGATION

Sodium Chloride Irrigation *(Various)*

HOW SUPPLIED: Sol: 1000mL, 3000mL, 5000mL
THERAPEUTIC CLASS: Irrigation solution
INDICATION: For use as an arthroscopic irrigation fluid with endoscopic instruments during arthroscopic procedures requiring distention and irrigation of the knee, shoulder, elbow, or other bone joints.
DOSAGE: *Adults:* Irrigate as needed. May warm in overpouch to near body temperature in water bath or oven heated to not more than 45°C.
WARNINGS/PRECAUTIONS: Not for injection. Caution in CHF, severe renal insufficiency, and conditions where edema and sodium retention exists. Use opened containers promptly to reduce potential for bacterial contamination. Discard unused portion.
PREGNANCY: Safety in pregnancy and nursing is not known.
INTERACTIONS: Caution with corticosteroids or corticotropin; some of the fluid may be absorbed systemically.

TRIMETHOBENZAMIDE

Tigan *(King)*

HOW SUPPLIED: Cap: 300mg; Inj: 100mg/mL; Sup: (Benzocaine-Trimethobenzamide) 2%-200mg (Sup, Pediatric), 2%-100mg
THERAPEUTIC CLASS: Emetic response modifier
INDICATION: Treatment of postoperative nausea and vomiting and for nausea associated with gastroenteritis.
DOSAGE: *Adults:* (Cap) 300mg tid-qid. (Inj) 200mg IM tid-qid. (Sup) 200mg tid-qid.
Pediatrics: (Sup; Sup, Pediatric) 30-90 lbs: 100-200mg tid-qid. <30 lbs: 100mg tid-qid.
CONTRAINDICATIONS: Injection in children, suppositories in premature or newborn Infants, suppositories if hypersensitive to similar local anesthetics.
WARNINGS/PRECAUTIONS: Caution in children; may cause EPS, which may be confused with CNS signs of undiagnosed primary disease (eg, Reye's syndrome) and may unfavorably alter the course of Reye's syndrome due to hepatotoxic potential. Caution with acute febrile illness, encephalitides, gastroenteritis, dehydration, electrolyte imbalance, and in elderly; CNS reactions reported. May produce drowsiness.
PREGNANCY: Safety in pregnancy and nursing not known.
INTERACTIONS: Caution with CNS agents (eg, phenothiazines, barbiturates, belladonna derivatives) in acute febrile illness, encephalitides, gastroenteritis, dehydration, and electrolyte imbalance. Adverse drug interactions reported with alcohol.
ADVERSE REACTIONS: Hypersensitivity reactions, parkinson-like symptoms, hypotension (inj), blood dyscrasias, blurred vision, coma, convulsions, mood depression, diarrhea, disorientation, dizziness, drowsiness, headache, jaundice, muscle cramps, opisthotonos.

† Not FDA-approved for this indication.